Physiotherapy Pain A...

T0103252

Topical Issues in Pain 4

Placebo and nocebo
Pain management
Muscles and pain

Editor
Louis Gifford FCSP BSc MAppSc

Foreword
Liz Macleod BSc(HONS) MCSP SRP

authorHOUSE®

AuthorHouse™ UK Ltd.
1663 Liberty Drive
Bloomington, IN 47403 USA
www.authorhouse.co.uk
Phone: 0800.197.4150

This book was first published by CNS Press in 2002

Published by AuthorHouse 08/30/2013

ISBN: 978-1-4918-7677-0 (sc)
ISBN: 978-1-4918-7678-7 (hc)
ISBN: 978-1-4918-7679-4 (e)

Foreword

In October 1998 a group of Scottish Physiotherapy Pain Association members hosted, by popular demand, a successful study day titled, 'Whiplash: science and management'. This coincided with the launch of the first book in the Topical Issues in Pain series appropriately named *Whiplash—science and management. Fear-avoidance beliefs and behaviour.* In his review of this first title Pat Wall stated, 'It is not an exaggeration to say that this book marks a milestone not only for an understanding of pain but also for the maturation of Physiotherapy.' He concludes,

> I look forward to this series and to the activities of the Physiotherapy Pain Association because they promise to revolutionise the morale, dignity and way of thinking of physiotherapists and thereby to affect everyone concerned with pain.

I too have looked forward to this series, and four years on I am eager to see how both Topical Issues in Pain 3 and 4 will be received. Four books in four years; this is quite an achievement and I believe that the Editor, Louis Gifford, should be congratulated. First, for the original idea of committing to print the excellent material presented at Physiotherapy Pain Association study days, and secondly, for delivering the goods.

Four books in four years. So what has happened to physiotherapy and 'pain' in the last four years? Notably: the growth of pain management programmes, the acknowledgement of biopsychosocial factors in pain treatment and management, the integration of 'Yellow flags and Red flags' in both the acute and chronic pain patient assessments, acknowledgement of patient and therapist fears in fear-avoidance beliefs and behaviours, and the demands of proving clinical effectiveness. I also believe that there has been a general increase in knowledge and awareness of the mechanisms and biology of pain and its impact on clinical pain management and pain relief.

If he were alive today, I think Pat Wall would be pleased with the progress that has been made.

Topical Issues in Pain 1 and 2 are key texts that have contributed to these changes and have helped the beneficial shift in the practice of many individual clinicians. These books are fast becoming standard texts for outpatient and student physiotherapists. Recently, and supported in full by The Private Practitioners Education Fund, every Physiotherapy School in the UK was provided with copies of the two volumes for their student libraries. It is hoped that the recently published third volume as well as this one will also be made available for students in a similar way.

Also, in the last four years, the PPA membership has increased and become far more proactive. For example, early in 2000 PPA North was established and has been organising and running courses and study days on pain management and measurement and the pain patient. PPA North members have also had representation on the Scottish Cross Party Group on Chronic Pain and were involved in February of this year when the Scottish Parliament held a members' debate on 'The plight of the chronic pain patient.' The complexity of chronic pain was acknowledged and appropriately trained physiotherapists were considered to be the key professionals equipped to deal with chronic pain. As a result of the debate The Cross Party for Chronic Pain will continue to press for improvements in pain services. PPA North has also embarked on a project to develop a 'practical pain management module' at Masters degree level. Hopefully this will begin taking students this year.

The PPA has quickly become a significant and respected special interest group. There is no doubt that the material contained in the Topical Issues in Pain volumes is a major reason for this. This volume, in particular, adds to the debate and controversies surrounding the problems that arise from pain. All clinicians should be obliged to understand and appreciate the nature and impact of the placebo, the importance of pain management in the context of both acute and chronic pain states, as well as some of the more controversial aspects and findings relating to muscle and musculoskeletal pain syndromes. This volume has them all—read on!

It is with great pride that I write this Foreword and would like to thank the Editor and all the authors for enabling the physiotherapy profession to embrace, and lead the field in, the many changes in practice that arise from the challenge of pain.

Liz Macleod
PPA North Chairperson
July 2002

Preface

I am so pleased with this book because it contains some of the most important pieces of the pain jigsaw—the placebo-nocebo puzzle; issues of function, communication, and change in managing pain; and a much needed and challenging sideways glance at some of the issues involved in relation to 'muscle' and 'musculoskeletal' pain states. I am sure that all who read this book will change how they think and will be impressed by the unique way the information is presented. There are a great many pages where I found myself saying, 'That's amazing, that's so interesting!'

The more I think about the difficulties and misunderstandings of those treating and managing pain, the more I think that *the* starting point for understanding pain should be with the placebo-nocebo phenomenon. In particular, the unique perspectives, interpretations and synthesis of the placebo-nocebo phenomenon and literature presented in Part 1 are those that are required for this understanding. I believe that if you can grasp this phenomenon in a broad and open-minded way, you grasp just about all the fundamental issues that cause so much trouble for such huge numbers of patients with pain. Understand placebo-nocebo and you immediately step into a more comfortable relationship with pain and the people it contains, restricts, and disables. Understanding the placebo and nocebo properly *must* change the way you think and work with your patients.

The authors of this section of the book are widely dispersed, and the information they provide is cutting edge! Huge thanks to Pat Roche over in Queensland, Nigel Lawes based in London, Mitch Noon down here in Cornwall, Richard Shortall in New Mexico, and Caroline Hafner in Wales.

To further set the scene I would like to make a few specific comments about two individual chapters and then the remaining two sections.

- At the back of any book like this there are usually one or two lonely chapters. While Ann Papageorgiou's chapter is 'at the back' it should not be considered as lonely or demoted! It demystifies epidemiology. It reviews the South Manchester Back Pain studies involving large numbers of patients and tries to seek answers to important questions relating to the occurrence and risk of back pain and chronicity. The study also asks similar questions about chronic widespread pains and the results are discussed here. The findings presented so clearly in this unique chapter add yet more weight to the validity and necessity of working within the framework of the biopsychosocial model.

• Good single patient case studies are useful sources of clinical information. Chapter 12, by Lorraine Moores, presents a single case study involving a fibromyalgia sufferer. This chapter is included for two reasons. The first is that it provides a useful clinical overview of how a difficult clinical problem can be managed, and of how fibromyalgia is complex and multifactorial. It has great clinical value. The second reason is that it stems from a highly praised MSc dissertation and provides a great model for the detail of research and the writing style required. Those readers embarking on an undergraduate or MSc research project should find this a very helpful chapter.

The two remaining chapters in the 'Muscles and Pain' section are by two world experts in pain-related research and the communication of their research to clinicians—Dr Paul Watson, who has the well earned honour of being the first Consultant Physiotherapist to be appointed; and Dr Trish Dolan, a well known researcher into the underlying causes of low back pain and impairment. Both chapters have considerable clinical impact and provide much food for thought.

Part II adds three more pieces of work to the 'pain management' chapters and sections of the Topical Issues in Pain series. Pain management is still a huge and challenging area that requires fundamental skills. We need to be careful, because there are a great many clinicians who profess to be skilled in this area when in reality they are far from it. I also believe that there are a great many clinicians, teachers, and bureaucrats in our profession who haven't a clue about what pain management is, what cognitive-behavioural therapy involves, or the broader implications of what the biopsychosocial model means for us all. I make no apologies for writing bluntly; challenge and change are uncomfortable, but a growing body of recent research is devaluing the basic tenets of our traditional treatment models and methods and so is forcing us to look elsewhere and to think from different perspectives. Chapters and work such as the three presented in Part II should help not only those who are new to the concepts promoted here but also those already working in the area. A big thank you to Heather Muncey and Babs Harper.

I have included Pat Wall's Introduction to the 4th edition of *Textbook of Pain* as the Introductory Essay to this Volume. It's brilliant, it's relevant to all the sections here, and I think you will all enjoy it! Much of Pat's life was devoted to grappling with the blinkered thinking on pain by his medical colleagues. Even though he was so respected and so eloquent with his messages, I know he struggled.

In a humble way it would be so good if this small book could take hold and spread its messages far and wide. This and previous volumes in the series are testament to the forward thinking clinicians who have listened to their patients, pondered the literature with them in mind and become involved in research so as to come up with something better.

I would like to thank and congratulate not only the authors of the work here, but also the team of key players who devote their time and patience to the continued success of the Physiotherapy Pain Association and all its work.

Louis Gifford
July 2002

Contributors

Patricia Dolan BSc PhD
Department of Anatomy
University of Bristol
Southwell Street
Bristol U.K

Louis Gifford MAppSc BSc FCSP
Chartered Physiotherapist
Kestrel
Swanpool
Falmouth
Cornwall TR11 5BD UK

Caroline Hafner MSc MCSP
Senior physiotherapist in pain management
Input Pain Management Centre
Bronllys Hospital
Bronllys
Brecon
Powys LD3 0LU UK

Babs Harper Grad Dip Phys HT MCSP
5 Heathfield Close
Keynsham
Bristol BS18 2HJ UK

Nigel Lawes MBBS
Senior Lecturer
Department of Anatomy & Developmental Biology
St George's Hospital Medical School
Cranmer Terrace,
London, SW17 0RE UK

Lorraine L Moores MSc MCSP
Clinical Specialist Physiotherapist in Pain Management
Manchester and Salford Pain Centre
Hope Hospital
Stott Lane
Salford M6 8HD UK

Heather Muncey BA Dip Grad Phys MCSP SRP MACP
Superintendent Physiotherapist in Pain Management Centre
Frenchay Hospital
Frenchay Park Road
Bristol BS16 1LE UK

Mitch Noon BA(Hons) MSc Psych D C Psychol
Consultant Clinical Psychologist and Head of Acute Trust
Psychology Services at Treliske Hospital
C/O Pain Management Unit
Treliske Hospital
Cornwall TR1 3JR UK

Ann C Papageorgiou SRN BA(Hons) MSc
Studies Co-ordinator, Arthritis Research Campaign
Epidemiology Unit
School of Epidemiology and Health Sciences
Stopford Building
University of Manchester
Oxford Road, Manchester M13 9PT UK

Patricia A Roche PhD MSc Psych BSc(Hons) MCSP
Lecturer, Physiotherapy
School of Health and Rehabilitation Sciences
University of Queensland
Brisbane
Queensland Australia

Richard Shortall BA BSc MSc MCSP
Physical therapist in private practice orthopedics
New Mexico USA

Paul Watson PhD MSc BSc(Hons) MCSP
Consultant AHP and Senior Lecturer in Pain Management and Rehabilitation
Department of Anaesthesia, Pain Management and Critical Care
University of Leicester
Leicester General Hospital
Leicester LE5 4PW UK

Contents

Introductory essay

Introduction to the fourth edition of *Textbook of Pain*

This chapter is reproduced with kind permission of the publishers, Churchill Livingstone, Edinburgh.

PATRICK D. WALL

Editor's comment

To make sense of the first paragraph and the last section of this chapter, readers need to remember that this first appeared as the introductory chapter to the 4th edition of *Textbook of Pain,* and it is to the chapters of that text that Pat Wall is referring.

The chapters in this book express the independent views of the selected authors. Everyone writing on pain has in mind a plan of how pain mechanisms operate. There are many different plans and some are complementary rather than contradictory. The editors have made no attempt to unify these concepts because we would rather leave the reader with the opportunity to select between the various widely held views. There are those who still believe pain can be adequately described as the result of activity in a dedicated pathway originating in peripheral nociceptors. Others propose a more complex approach which takes into account the plasticity of all the conduction pathways and the nature of pattern detection by parallel processing and the active participation of the brain in perception. The traditional scheme starts with a stimulus and follows the consequences through to a sensory-emotional response. In this introduction I propose a way to bring all the chapters together by a search beginning with the perception of pain.

Attention

No conscious awareness of anything is possible until it has captured our attention. Our sense organs in the eyes, ears, nose and body are in continuous action, day and night, awake or asleep. The central nervous system is receiving steady reports of all the events these sense organs are capable of detecting. Obviously, it would be a disaster of excess if we were continuously aware of the entire mass of arriving information. We completely ignore most of the information most of the time. And yet any fraction of this inflow is capable of riveting attention. For this to happen, there has to be a selective attention mechanism which must have a set of rules. Those rules are not arbitrary. Every species displays their rules which incorporate a selection of those events that are important to survival and well being. Some rules seem to be built in. Large, sudden novel events have precedence in their attention grabbing ability. And, I would propose, that the arrival in the nervous system of messages signaling tissue damage is another of these built in high priority events.

There is a learned component of our selective attention mechanism. The bored radar operator sits staring at the screen which is a snow storm of random blinking dots. Let one of these dots begin to move in a consistent line and attention locks onto that dot to the exclusion of all the others. Let the classical migraine sufferer detect a small twinkling area in the visual field and his attention is riveted on this trivial event because he has learned that the aura on his oncoming migraine attack begins with just such a scintillating area.

In social animals, subtle triggers of attention can be shared. In West Africa, two species of monkeys feed together in flocks but eat different fruits. Their main enemy is the monkey eagle and one species is quicker to spot arriving eagles so that both species benefit from the alarm of one. In Australia, a grouse selects her ground nest close to a tree containing a hawk nest because the hawks superior height and eyesight detects distant predators long before the earth bound grouse. And so it is with humans, where attention is infectious.

The attention mechanism must be continuously scanning the available information in the incoming messages and assigning a priority to the biological importance of the message. There are examples of 'thoughtless' decision as in, the switch of attention in the car driver in conversation with a passenger while engaged in 'unconscious' skilled driving until some fool cuts in front of her, whereupon attention promptly switches from conversation to avoidance. This brings out the second rule of selective attention which is that only one target at a time is permitted. Obviously it is possible to switch attention back and forth quite rapidly. However, at any one instant, only one collection of information is available for conscious sensory analysis. This one object can itself be pre-set. An example is the detection of the mention of your name in the random buzz of cocktail party conversation. It is possible to scan a long list of names and detect the one you seek with no recall of any of the other names.

It is not intuitively obvious that attention can only be directed to one subject at any one time. It would seem a rather ridiculous limitation in a mental process which clearly has freedom to rove over vast areas. Shoes and ships and sealing-wax, cabbages and kings. An explanation for this strict limit on attention could be that sensory events are analysed in terms of the action which might be appropriate to the event. If the aim of attention relates to appropriate action, then it follows that a fundamental requirement of nature is that only one action at a time is permitted. It is not possible to move forwards and backwards simultaneously. You must 'make up your mind'. The explanation for the singleness of momentary attention would then derive from the purpose of attention which is to assemble and highlight those aspects of the sensory input that would be relevant to carrying out one act.

Of course, rival sensory events may compete for attention. The myth of the ass who starves to death when placed equidistant between two bales of hay is indeed a myth which would never happen. There may be many events occurring simultaneously each demanding attention. They are rank ordered into a hierarchy in terms of biological importance. The practical consequence of this ordering is the apparent paradox of the painless injury. Each of these victims was involved in a situation where some action, other than attending to their wound, had top priority. Getting out of a burning aircraft is more urgent than attending to a broken leg. The attention does not oscillate between the two demands. One is assigned complete domination until safety is achieved. Only then is the alternate assigned the top position, attention shifts and pain occurs. The workman in the course of a skilled task and the tackled footballer about to score a goal carry on to complete the task with engrossed attention in spite the conflicting demands of their coincidental injury. Only when the conditions of the top priority fade, there is a reassessment of the next most urgent priority. In conditions of complete 'emergency analgesia', pain emerges as the dominant fact when the emergency is over. The priority ranking of importance of what deserves attention is partly built in and partly learned from personal experience and partly a component of culture.

From the first positron emission tomographic (PET) images of people in pain, intense activity was detected in the anterior cingulate. It is even apparent in patients with very chronic pain associated with a single nerve neuropathy and, even more surprising, it is only present on the right side irrespective of which side the pain is on. However, this general area is also active in many other situations including directed visual or auditory attention, precise eye and hand movements, and even during complex speech. The suggestion that this zone is involved in attention mechanisms fits with the results of surgical destruction of the area as a treatment of obsessional melancholic depression which I take to be a disorder of attention.

Therapy based on a moulding of attention is effective. It is called distraction. When a toddler trips, smacks into the pavement and howls, what does a parent do? Pick it up, dance about, coo, oo and ah, kiss it better. These are distractions. Because you can only attend to one thing at a time, it follows that you can only have one pain at a time. This fact led to many excellent folk remedies; hot poultices, horse linaments and mustard plasters. They are called counter-stimulants. When pain really sets in, attention is utterly monopolised and nothing else exists in the world but the pain. Many therapies attempt to intrude on this fixation. The distraction that is effective may be simple but it will depend on established priorities. A game of cards, letting the cat out or the sight of a hated neighbour can provide a brief interlude in pain. Some victims discover this for themselves and prolong their brief holidays from pain by inventing distractions while others get professional help in occupational therapy. In another distraction therapy given the pretentious title of cognitive therapy, the victim learns to day dream where they play out an internal fantasy. It may be that they are on a warm sunny beach or at a football match or in their favourite bar. Some people can become very skilled at these distractions and give themselves longer and longer respites from their miserable pain.

Alerting, orientation and exploration

As attention shifts to pain, alertness appears. There is something wrong. Alarm bells. Action stations. Muscles tense and the body stiffens to a ram rod. Unknown to the victim, these overt changes are part of a massive reorganisation of many parts of the body. The heart and vascular system get ready for action. The hormone system mobilises sugar and alerts the immune system. The gut becomes stationary. Sleep as an option is cancelled.

The eyes, head and neck turn to inspect where the pain seems located. The hands explore the area. Muscles are contracted to learn what makes the pain worse and what eases it and to seek a comfortable position and then hold it. The end result is a body fixed in an overall pain posture. Muscles are in steady contraction and, as time goes by, some muscles grow while joints and tendons deteriorate because this frozen posture itself sets off local changes. The vascular and endocrine systems hold their emergency state if pain is prolonged and these systems are not evolved to cope with this prolonged stress state. The quiet gut demonstrates its inactivity as constipation. Perhaps worst of all, sleep is impossible and chronic pain patients become completely exhausted. Even intermittent sleep deprivation drives the strongest of us into pretty peculiar ways of thinking as any doctor on night duty knows and as any parent with a new baby knows. Chronic pain patients get to their wits end as their grim experience is prolonged.

Clearly this state of affairs needs therapeutic attack. The key word is relaxation and much ingenuity has been used. The problem is to override a natural defence mechanism which has a protective role in brief emergencies but which becomes maladaptive when prolonged. Drugs to inhibit the overactive muscles are commonly prescribed but they are sedative and intellectually flattening. After a while, patients refuse them or become zombies. Physiotherapists have many ways of relaxing muscles and of re-establishing movement in frozen zones. First they have to overcome the patients natural fear that movement which produces pain does not necessarily increase the injury and that lack of movement which seemed at first to prevent pain eventually plays a role in prolonging the pain. Yoga and the Alexander technique are examples of posture training. Relaxation is not easy and training methods are needed. One successful version, 'bio-feedback' training, provides the patient with an electronic indicator of the amount of contraction in a muscle and allows the patient to judge second by second his success in relaxation. The patient has to learn how to relax and how to prolong the effect into real life outside the training sessions. Sleep follows relaxation but it may need additional help until the patient can sleep on his own.

The sensation of pain itself

We are used to discussing sensation as the consequence of stimulation in a series of boxes, firstly injury generates an announcement of its presence in sensory nerves; secondly the attention mechanism selects the incoming message as worthy of entry; thirdly the brain generates the sensation of pain. Now the question is 'how does the brain interpret the input?' The classical theory is that the brain analyses the sensory input to determine what has happened and presents the answer as a pure sensation. I propose an alternate theory that the brain analyses the input in terms of what action would be appropriate.

Let us explore the alternate theory as it has practical consequences for pain. If the classical theory were true, the first action of the brain is to identify the nature of the events which generated the sensory input. This should produce the first sensation of injury as pure pain. The next stage of the classical theory is that different parts of the brain perceive the pure sensation and generate an assessment of affect, that is to say 'is the pure pain miserable, dangerous, frightening and so on?' My first reaction, on introspection, is that I have never felt a pure pain. Pain for me arrives as a complete package. A particular pain is at the same time painful and miserable and disturbing and so on. I have never heard a patient speak of pain isolated from its companion affect. Because classical theory assigns different parts of the brain to the task of the primary sensory analysis and others for the task of adding affect, one would expect some disease to separate pain from misery. No such disease is known. During neurosurgical operations, very small areas of brain can be stimulated and some cause pain. There has never been a report of pain evoked which was not accompanied by fear or misery or other strong affects. Finally there are parts of brain, the primary sensory cortex, which has been classically assigned the role of primary sensory analysis and yet, in the imaging studies, these areas are often reported as silent while the subject reports pain. Even for the sympathetic pain on hearing of the death of a friend, the sensation is inseparable from the sadness and loneliness.

Therefore let us explore the alternative which is that the brain analyses its sensory input in terms of the possible action which would be appropriate to the event which triggered the whole process. There is in this absolutely no suggestion that any action need actually take place. Trained subjects and stoics may receive a clearly painful stimulus with no overt movement even though they can later report the nature of the pain they felt. There are elaborate and extensive areas of our brain concerned with motor planning as distinct from motor movement itself. It is precisely these areas that are most obviously active when the brain is imaged in subjects who are in pain but who are quite stationary with no movement. Chapter 8 by Ingvar [*Textbook of Pain 4th edn*] describes the areas found to be active while the subjects feel pain. The first area of surprise to be reported was the anterior cingulate which becomes active in any act of attention and this is exactly what is expected given the evidence that attention is a prerequisite of pain. The other areas consistently reported as active by many investigators are the premotor cortex, the frontal lobes, basal ganglia and cerebellum. All of the last hundred years of neurology have assigned these areas a role in the preparation for skilled planned movement.

Because I am proposing a quite new hypothesis here, one should explore widely to see if there are facts which support the possibility that sensory analysis is carried on in terms of motor action which would be appropriate to the input. Of the many imaging studies carried out on normal subjects or on patients in pain, some have shown no activation of the primary sensory cortex and even in those showing such activation, the area extends rostrally into the motor area in spite of the fact that no overt motor movement is detected. The marked activation of the cerebellum is a great surprise because classical opinion assigned no sensory role to the cerebellum. However, more recent work has clearly shown that the cerebellum plays a role in the analysis of sensory input in the course of establishing conditioned responses. Similarly the basal ganglia, putamen and globus pallidus were classically only given a function in overt movement and yet show marked activation in subjects in pain who show no signs of movement. However, muscle ache is a common prodromal sign of Parkinsonism and responds to L-DOPA which is reported to reduce neuropathic pain.

Sometimes the detection of a sensory input is demonstrated by motor movement. Mimicry is an example. The earliest sign that a baby is detecting complex visual stimuli is its mimicry of facial expression; opening the mouth, smiling etc. Cells in monkey cortex in the inferior precental area have been detected which respond when the animal carries out a complex hand movement such as grasping but astonishingly these same cells also become active when the animal observes someone else making the same movement even though the animal makes no such movement. The acquisition of bird song has been studied in great detail in the Zebra Finch and necessarily involves the motor system during the learning phase. Even in human speech, Chomsky and Halle described a form of recognition which they termed analysis by synthesis. Here the correct detection of a sound pattern is confirmed by imitation. In these examples, the brain is showing and proving that it has detected a sensory input and checks the correctness of its analysis by producing an imitative movement. Now we ask if the movement is necessary. The nature of the stimulus must also be represented in the premotor system which preceded the movement of mimicry.

Evidence for this is seen in the firing of single cells in the posterior parietal areas when the animal is presented with visual targets on which it will fixate. In a classical sensory system the target would first be located in a visual space after which the motor system would decide what would be the appropriate movement. What is found in fact is that the cells respond from the beginning in terms of the appropriate movement. Another example is observed in the best studied auditory cortex which is that of bats. The animal locates its prey by analysing return echoes. If this was a classical sensory system, the brain would analyse the echoes in order to locate the target's position when the sound bounced off the target. In fact the cortex also analyses the speed and vectors of target and the outcome is the collision course on where the target will be when the bat gets there. This is analogous to the display in modern aeroplanes on auto-pilot which show not primarily the position of the plane but the course to the chosen destination and at the same time the courses to all the alternate airports in range. The sensory information from the inertial navigation equipment is displayed in terms of appropriate action.

The most dramatic example in man is the unilateral neglect syndrome seen in patients with inferior parietal lobe destruction. If the lesion is on the right side, no visual or auditory or somatic stimuli on the left side are detected or identified. If such patients are asked to draw a clock face, they number correctly the hours 12-6 but fail completely on the left side. On classical theory, these patients have a hole smashed in their sensory map. Recently a new dimension of this large sensory deficit has been observed by a number of groups and has been imaged by PET scanning. If the vestibular system is stimulated by cooling one external ear canal, the patient has a nystagmus and experiences spinning in one direction. While this is going on, the neglect of the left sensory input disappears completely. There are three conclusions, (1) the sensory analysis mechanism had not been destroyed by the lesion, (2) sensory analysis is only possible in a predetermined frame of motor response and (3) one of the factors determining the location of that sensory frame is the vestibular system. The vestibular system determines the posture of appropriate motor action and evidently of sensory analysis. I propose that these are one and the same mechanism.

What would be the consequences of following the hypothesis that sensory events are analysed in terms of the appropriate potential motor responses? It would provide a more satisfactory explanation of the paradoxes produced by the classical hypothesis and the beginning of understanding of the facts just described. What are the appropriate motor responses to the arrival of injury signals? They attempt to (1) remove the stimulus; (2) adopt a posture to limit further injury and optimise recovery and (3) seek safety and relief and cure. The youngest most inexperienced animal may attempt a series of these response triggered by built-in mechanisms. As the animal grows in experience, the reactions will become more subtle, elaborate and sophisticated. If the sequence is frustrated at any stage, the sensation-posture remains fixed.

Humans develop and elaborate the three stage response from the moment of birth. Until about ten years ago, pain in the new born was neglected and even denied by professionals for two reasons. The first was that the human brain was seen as a hierarchy of levels; the spinal cord, the brain stem and the cortex. This view had been introduced by Hughlings Jackson in the nineteenth century. Each level was believed to dominate and control the level below. The hierarchy of levels was believed to be an evolutionary development and to be repeated in the development of each individual. The ability to feel pain, misery and suffering was assigned as a property unique to the cortex. All reactions to injury in the absence of cortex were called simple reflexes and thought to be mechanical and free of sensation or emotion. This view led Descartes to deny mind to lower creatures and was perpetuated in post-Darwinian neurology which assigned sensation and emotion to recently evolved structures such as the forebrain and cortex. It is true that we have a poorly developed cortex at birth. It takes two years for the major motor outflow from the cortex to establish control over the spinal cord. The second line of reasoning by professionals was that, because babies could not feel pain, there was no point in giving them potentially dangerous analgesic drugs.

Fortunately, thinking has changed and pain in babies and children has become a major focus of attention. The chapters in this book by Fitzgerald and by Berde demonstrate the progress *[see Textbook of Pain 4th edn, chs 9 & 42]*. Turning away from endless inconsequential philosophy on whether a baby feels pain, they and others turned to practical objective measures. The first question was whether a baby who must be operated on soon after birth prospers better if treated with a full battery of analgesics which would be given an adult. The answer was a powerful yes and the result has been a marked change in neonatal anaesthesia and in survival. The second question was to ask if the injuries commonly suffered by babies, especially premature ones, produce a long-term shift of behaviour. Again the answer is yes. Fitzgerald showed that even the act of taking a blood sample without anaesthesia changed the motor behaviour of premature babies. This has focused new studies on long-term effects. Most surprising is a Swedish study confirmed in Canada where a large group of boys who had been circumcised soon after birth were compared with similar boys who were not circumcised. These children were observed six months later when they received their standard immunisation injections. The circumcised boys struggled, shouted and cried far more than the others. Subtle controls showed that it was indeed the circumcision which had engendered the abnormal reaction to subsequent minor injury. In the child and the adult, there is a continuous development of the way in which the victim moves through the three stages of reaction. Experience teaches skills. Society adds its methods of help and its prohibitions. Expectation becomes tuned.

Finally, we need to re-examine the alternative either that pain signals presence of a stimulus or that it signals the stage reached in a sequence of possible actions. Obviously the placebo phenomenon represents a profound challenge to these alternatives. The placebo by definition is not active and therefore cannot change the signal produced by the stimulus. It can hardly be categorised as a distraction of attention. Someone who has received placebo treatment for pain does not actively switch attention to some alternate target. On the contrary, they await passively the onset of the beneficial effect of the placebo while continuing the active monitoring of the level of pain. If, however, the sensation of pain is associated with a series of potential actions; remove the stimulus, change posture, seek safety and relief, eventually the appropriate action is to apply therapy. If the person's experience has taught them that a particular action is followed by relief, then they respond if they believe the action has occurred. In this scheme of thinking, the placebo is not a stimulus but an appropriate action. As such the placebo terminates and cancels the sense of pain by fulfilling the expectation that appropriate action has taken.

When pain persists

The disease develops

In chapters in this book [*Textbook of Pain 4th edn*], repeated examples are given where damage to tissue is followed by inflammation. The quality of the pain and what to do about it changes. In post-operative pain, the initial acts of tissue damage were carried out under anaesthesia and the patient wakes up to sense only the later stages where the body attempts repair. In slow onset diseases such as arthritis, pain escalates as the disease process extends. Pain may grow in sudden jumps as in some cancer pains where the tumour has expanded into new territory and blocks the normal flow of blood or the intestines or urine or nerve impulses. Intermittent pains can grow with each episode. Someone of my age walking up hill may be struck by a chest pain. Stop walking and the pain goes. This is angina of effort where the heart is announcing that it can no longer pump enough blood around in response to the energy demand of walking up hill. As time goes by, the arteries continue to clog and their maximum blood flow drops. As this proceeds, the steepness of the hill which can be climbed drops, the amount of exercise which pain permits drops and rest periods prolong. Eventually, if untreated, the angina forbids even standing up. These are the expected reasons why pain may persist or escalate which it may be possible to attack at source. However, there are a series of quite different changes that accompany pain which we must now examine because they play an important role in pain intensity.

Fear and anxiety

Anyone who senses an unexpected new pain and does not feel fear is not normal. There is a natural fear of the unknown in all of us and this is coupled with a fear of the consequent future. As part of the innate urge to explore, there is an immediate urge to know what is going on. We fear the cause and its meaning. When a patient goes to the doctor with bad pain and tenderness in the abdomen, the doctor may diagnose appendicitis or cancer or an ulcer or constipation and so on. The patient may laugh with relief if the diagnosis is appendicitis because she has learnt to believe that this is cured with a minor operation. This is a socially educated 20th century response since two hundred years ago it might have been the worst of all the diagnoses because many patients with this disorder were in rapid decline and dead within days. Quite obviously the amount of fear and the target of the fear will depend crucially on the person and their experience and their situation. A middle-aged man from a family where all the men died of heart attacks in their 50s and 60s has good reason to blanche with terror at the first twinge of chest pain. There are those with reason to fear cancer who develop an obsessed phobia and become crippled by their inability to accept medical assurance that they do not have cancer. The fear may become the disease.

Fear of consequences can be even more widespread and wild and personally eccentric and therefore hidden to the witnesses. 'Who is going to marry me now' said an Israeli woman officer with the amputated leg. 'What a fool they will think of me to have let this happen' said a machine shop foreman with an accidentally amputated foot. Fears do not often relate to death but very frequently to the manner of the death. Fears relate to jobs, to sports, to sex and all manner of personal needs. There is a type of macho tough-guy who has 'never had a days illness in his life' who falls apart at the seams with his first experience of pain and fear which breaks into his accustomed absolute self-control. There is every reason for each person to identify fears of cause or of consequence.

Fear generates anxiety and anxiety focuses the attention. The more attention is locked, the worse the pain. Therefore there is a marked correlation between pain and anxiety. The anxiety may focus on the pain or it may be of the free floating variety with a feeling of general disquiet that something is wrong that cannot be identified. The anxiety of pain is generated by the unknown and grows worse as the pain persists and short-term expectations of relief fail to be fulfilled.

Therefore a major aim of therapy should be to identify, understand and treat the anxiety. This may need to start immediately after an accident. A type of very distressed patient can be seen in any emergency room who is agitated by the scare of the rough and tumble of what they have just been through although pain is their complaint. Of course, the pain should be treated but they respond best if they also get care to help them calm down. Unfortunately, most chronic pain patients have settled into a rather steady state of fear and anxiety which becomes progressively harder and harder to shift. This by itself is justification for early treatment. A very good example is the effect on post-operative pain produced by a quite brief talk with the anaesthetist before the operation. The aim is to educate the patient with a step-by-step explanation of the stages to be expected. The expectation allows the patient to face the progressive stages of her recovery with familiarity and therefore with less tension and anxiety. This points to the value of education in decreasing anxiety by illuminating the unknown. Well designed programmes for the relief of chronic pain teach as much as the patient wishes to understand of her own pain problem. It is always surprising to me what a revelation such courses are to the patients who have been carrying a load of magical mumbo-jumbo myths which nourish their anxiety. A crucial example which hinders recovery guided by physiotherapy is the myth that no movement is permitted which increases pain because that movement would increase injury. This myth helps freeze the patient into narrower and narrower ranges of movement. Ignorance is never blessed. Any knowledge which brings the patient into a clearer appreciation of her condition thereby decreases anxiety. For that reason, this book is written. It is true that there is a well recognised type of patient who sits in front of the doctor and says in effect 'Cure me' with the unspoken coda that they are totally passive and expect curative action to be impressed on them by others. One's heart sinks especially when you recognise that you are the twentieth doctor who has been invited to cure this patient. As I have presented pain as an active process involved with the brains analysis of appropriate behaviour, I would prefer to see the patient as an active member of the patients own treatment team. Anxiety has been a traditional subject for psychiatrists and psychologists and it is most encouraging that they are beginning to apply their skills to the specific anxiety component of pain.

Failure and depression

If pain persists and treatment fails, it is not surprising that depression sets in. Some patients plod sadly on, convinced that somewhere in the world a therapist exists with the answer. For some, it is a variation of the same answer but administered by a therapist with the right stuff. More than ten repeated operations on the same painful back are well known in affluent countries. Surgeons are nothing if not high in confidence and not above hinting to the patient that they had been unlucky to encounter incompetent butchers before they reached the right one. Early in his career, the Canadian neurosurgeon Wilder Penfield learned that his sister had a brain tumour and said 'She must be operated on by the best neurosurgeon in the world. Me!' Sometimes these charismatic fireworks are associated with success and sometimes not. The higher the patient scales the ladder of more and more distinguished therapists, the harder the fall. Frustration and anger are added to depression. Depression is a progressive certainty in a miserable future. Attention scans every detail of the pain to confirm that no change for the better has occurred and that it is in fact even worse than suspected. Every small change becomes a catastrophe for some.

This grim picture of anxiety and depression, phobia and fatalism are so commonly seen in chronic pain patients that there are those who claim that these conditions become the primary cause of the pain rather than being secondary to the pain which caused the anxiety and depression in the first instance. Needless to say this view is popular among doctors committed to some therapy which has failed a particular patient. Such doctors believe they have given the appropriate therapy to the patient and if the patient fails to respond, it must be the fault of the patient. There are, of course, psychologists of the 'mind over matter' psychosomatic school who are happy to support doctors who claim that the apparent body fault must be produced by faulty thinking because the patient has failed to respond to therapy. One important school of behaviour therapy believes that one can condition the patient out of his pain by ignoring any sign or word associated with pain and by rewarding and encouraging any sign or word associated with non-painful activity. Needless to say, smart patients soon learn what the therapists want and shut up about their pains. They are considered successes.

I have not seen a scrap of convincing evidence that the mood and attitude create the pain. A recent new successful therapy provides clear evidence that the pain drives the attitude. A rare urological disease 'flank pain with haematuria' is characterised by intense pain, no known pathology and no known therapy. The patients are anxious, depressed, heavy users of narcotics and at their wits end. The treatment consists of flushing the affected kidney under anaesthesia with capsaicin, a specific nerve poison. The patients become pain free and at the same time their anxious depressed personalities return into the normal range. These are not anxious depressed personalities liable to create or exaggerate kidney pain. However, there is no doubt that the pain produced anxiety, fear, depression and obsession feeds back onto attention and posture and makes pain and living with pain harder to bear. Therefore every effort made to treat these helps the patient. Rehabilitation programmes focusing on education and movement and relief of fear, depression and anxiety do not cure pains but give the patients a freer life style which persists.

Coping

Some fortunate patients can learn to cope with their ongoing pain. Coping is not ignoring. In fact, it is the opposite. These people have learned to live with their pain in a realistic context. The pain persists but no longer demands emergency responses. Pain is not necessarily a catastrophe, signalling impending annihilation. Patients obviously need help to reach this conclusion. It is the beginning of a series of steps which gives a sense of understanding and of a type of control. Berde's chapter on Pain in Children [see Ch. 42 Textbook of Pain 4th edn], lists characteristics of young people in prolonged pain of neuropathic origin which is demolishing their lives. They tend to be depressed, anxious, in wheelchairs or on crutches, missing school, stressed, with a distorted body image, with eating disorders and in awful relations with their parents and siblings. This gruesome picture contrasts with children of the same age with a painful disorder with obvious disease, rheumatoid arthritis, who have the example of fellow sufferers and learn to cope. I recommend going to talk with a Second World War amputee who has been in severe pain for fifty years. Give him a chance to talk and he will describe precisely his pain now and the misery of the early days after his injury. Somehow with the help of his comrades he learned to ignore the fool doctors who dismissed his pain and to weave a life around the pain. He will also tell you that some of those comrades coped by killing themselves with bullets or booze. Coping is clearly a skill which may be learned with help. There is no chance of coping if attention is monopolised by fear, anxiety and depression. There is no chance of coping while passively awaiting death or the invention of a cure. Coping is an active process directed at everything other than the pain itself. It needs inspiration and inspired help to live with pain.

Finally

This book *[Textbook of Pain 4ᵗʰ edn]* is about the many challenges of the many pains.

Inevitably the authors and the readers have repeatedly turned to tackle the urgent practical question of how to control pains. Beyond that question, there are deeper ones and the practical question will not be answered satisfactorily until we understand more of the context in which pain resides. Pain is one facet of the sensory world in which we live. It is inherently ridiculous to consider pain as an isolated entity although many do exactly that. Our understanding brains steadily combine all available information from the outside world and from within our own bodies and from our personal histories and our genetic histories. The outcomes are decisions of the tactics and strategies which could be appropriate to respond to the situation. We use the word pain as shorthand for one of these groupings of relevant response tactics and strategies.

Placebo and nocebo

1

Placebo and patient care

PATRICIA A ROCHE

Introduction

The physiotherapy profession has faced a crisis of confidence in recent years. The reason for the dilemma may be able to be traced to just two words—*placebo effects*. In this era of evidence based medicine, in which we are required to demonstrate scientifically validated practice (see Volume 3, Topical Issues in Pain), we are simultaneously confronted with a growing list of scientific publications which show that physical therapies give no greater symptom relief than do placebo administrations of the same therapy (Feine & Lund 1997). Most of our therapies are insufficiently tested against placebo control (Koes et al 1995). Of those so tested, some show inferior benefits compared with placebo (Hashish et al 1988).

Health professionals have traditionally taken a negative view of the placebo phenomenon (Wall 1994). Many physical therapists discuss placebo effects in tones of puzzlement or, sometimes, derision. Some regard the entire topic of the placebo phenomenon as a threat to the validity of the profession. We are, nevertheless, in an era of increasingly sophisticated research evidence of the extent and potency of placebo response in health therapy (see Chapter 4). It is therefore timely that physical therapists consider the evidence surrounding the placebo phenomenon objectively and ask if, and how, it could contribute to the scientific basis for physical therapy. The alternative is to deny the validity of the phenomenon, and, perhaps, to hope that it will conveniently disappear. I doubt that there are many physiotherapists who would choose the latter path. Most experienced therapists have encountered the placebo phenomenon in the clinical setting. There are probably few of us who cannot recall at least one patient who has reported symptom relief from a machine which, it is realised belatedly, was not switched on! As a mature profession we can view the evidence for the legitimacy of placebo phenomenon with an open mind. The evidence is that placebo effects are mediated by psychological mechanisms of learned expectancy and, at least some of the time, by descending and opioid based mechanisms of analgesia (Roche 2002) (see also, Chapter 2).

There has been an increase in scientific interest in the placebo phenomenon in recent years. A Medline search on the number of papers including placebo as a key word reveals that placebo was mentioned less than 900 times in pharmaceutical drug trials between 1971 and 1975. This number rose to over 17 000 citations between 1991 and 1995 (Kuypers 1999). However—in a reflection of the dismissive attitude toward placebo as a topic worthy of serious scientific investigation—most placebo results are reported in almost cursory fashion. Only a minute fraction of the whole number has investigated the nature and mechanisms of the placebo phenomenon itself.

Pain is the symptom that is reported most commonly to respond to placebo therapy. Nowadays, there is an increasing focus among pain researchers on investigating the clinical effects and mechanisms of placebo analgesia. This chapter summarises essential points emerging from that research. Also in this chapter, I propose the placebo phenomenon as a means of improving our understanding of how *learning* affects the outcome of physical therapy and patient care. Readers of *Topical Issues in Pain, Volumes 1 and 2* (Gifford 1998, 2000) will know that 'learning' is also a foundation for biopsychosocial concepts of pain and pain therapy. I propose that placebo effects in health therapy are part of the evidence for the biopsychosocial model. From that basis, the chapter concludes with a view of the place of placebo in physiotherapy research and practice.

Placebo terms and definitions

There is considerable debate in scientific circles about the specific language, concepts and definitions surrounding placebo. Nevertheless, the following statements apply:

'Placebo' is thought to derive from the Latin verb *placebit* meaning 'it will please'. Wall (1994) argues that negative views toward placebo originate from its early use in the first line of vespers for the dead. Monks extorted money from relatives of the dead to sing these vespers. By the 16th century the word had become associated with the sense of 'untrustworthiness' and 'trickery'. The Concise English Dictionary defines placebo as 'a medicine having no therapeutic action'. Most people understand the word `placebo' as a term for false medicine and most would acknowledge that placebo is often 'given to humour the patient or as a control during an experiment to test the efficacy of a genuine medicine' (Hayward & Sparkes 1986).

The placebo analgesic **response** is the reduction in pain that occurs in an individual as a result of placebo administration. The placebo analgesic **effect** is the reduction of pain in a group of individuals given a placebo treatment (Fields & Price 1997). In addition, it has been suggested that the placebo phenomenon can best be understood by differentiating between the 'characteristic' and 'incidental' ingredients of a given therapy (Grunbaum 1986, cited in Richardson 1994). Characteristic ingredients are those medicinal ingredients, which are remedial for a particular disorder, for example, the anti-inflammatory component of non-steroidal anti-inflammatory drugs. Incidental ingredients have no specific remedial effect. One author stated:

> For a therapy to be a non-placebo, at least one of its characteristic ingredients should be remedial. Placebo effects are those which are produced by incidental ingredients, regardless of the presence of characteristic ingredients in the therapy (Richardson, 1994, p16.).

Iatroplacebogenic stimuli

Sources of placebo response related to interpersonal and environmental factors are 'iatroplacebogenic' (French 1997, Gracely 2000). Some researchers limit the meaning of 'iatroplacebogenesis' to the (conscious or unconscious) interpersonal effects of the clinician on treatment efficacy, for example a clinician's empathy or personal charisma (Shapiro 1971, Gracely 2000). I prefer to include the effects of environmental cues under the category 'iatroplacebogenic'. We have all learned, through personal experience or vicariously from another's person experience (or nowadays, from televised hospital dramas), to associate certain environmental cues with 'medical assistance' and 'cure'. The sight of pills, surgical gowns and theatre instruments, certain smells such as ether, and sounds such as an ambulance siren, are all part of a wealth of stimuli that many of us may associate with care, healing and pain relief.

Iatroplacebogenic cues produce positive placebo effects, such as the reduction of pain and other symptoms of illness. Health therapists also need to be aware of 'nocebo' effects. These are negative symptoms such as nausea and increased pain, which occur simply from the suggestion—and the belief—that they will occur (Max et al 1988, Hahn 1997). The potential for placebo and nocebo effects to contribute to positive and negative outcomes respectively, in physical therapy, is raised later in this chapter.

The legacy of negative attitudes toward placebo in clinical practice

First we can consider the legacy of negative views towards placebo. There has been a persistently reductionist view in medical thinking which sees the psyche as functioning separately from the soma. Genuine pain is associated with clinical evidence of pathology and/or tissue damage (biogenic model) but pain without such evidence is regarded as psychogenic (Gamsa 1994). One result is that placebo effects are often regarded in medical circles as 'a nuisance' or as 'an indication of medical charlatanism and quackery' (Richardson 1994, p 1 citing Wall 1992, 1994). The reductionist view also leads to negative views towards those patients who have the misfortune to have responded to a placebo therapy. Wall (1993, 1994) notes that such individuals are often viewed as having inadvertently revealed the falsity of their symptoms. Health practitioners, it appears, often believe that individuals who are persistent placebo responders are highly suggestible or have 'mistakenly confused true therapies with placebos'—ie. that placebo responders are in one way or another 'silly' (Wall, 1994). There is good survey evidence to show that the use of placebos in general medicine is common, but for all the wrong reasons. One study showed that 80% of 300 nurses and physicians anonymously admitted to recent placebo administration, most commonly for pain relief (Gray & Flynn 1981). Another cited the most common reasons for giving a placebo as punishing 'difficult' or 'undeserving' patients, and proving that the patients' symptoms were imaginary (Goodwin et al 1979).

Such attitudes have long-lasting and detrimental effects on health outcomes. For example, health practitioners do unconsciously relay their beliefs and attitudes to individual patients by means of body language and terms of description (Wall 1996, Harding 1998). It is highly likely that a strong link exists between health practitioners' negative attitudes toward placebo responders and the anxiety, even the affront, which patients show if it is suggested that their complaint may have a psychological component, or could benefit from psychological therapy. Even today, most of the population translates 'psychological' as 'imaginary' and 'without credibility'. There remains a legacy of denial towards the importance of psychological factors in pain and pain management in medical health practice and in our patients. One effect is that the job of incorporating an integrated biopsychosocial perspective into everyday clinical practice for pain is made considerably harder than it ought to be.

With this in mind, we can turn to examining some of the most commonly held misconceptions about the placebo phenomenon. Wall (1992, 1994, 1999)—who was a leading writer on this topic—considers these misconceptions as placebo 'myths', which have grown up in medical culture as mechanisms of professional self-defence. Just three of these myths (and the evidence to refute them) are considered next.

Errors and evidence in placebo analgesia

One-third of the population responds to placebo

The myth that placebo analgesia reliably accounts for at least 50% pain reduction in one-third (33%) of subjects is a misrepresentation of data from eleven studies conducted by Beecher (1955). Wall (1993) points out that the figure of 33% is dangerous as well as false because it labels 'a fraction of the population as mentally peculiar'. In fact, the percent of placebo responders varies from 0–100% of a study group depending on the circumstances of the study (Jospe 1978, Turner et al 1994, Wall 1994).

Despite earlier research, there is no good evidence for the assertions that placebo responders are neurotic, extroverted, introverted, lacking in sophistication—or simply over anxious to please! (White et al 1985). Placebo analgesia occurs in people with normal personalities, varied levels of education, and from all walks of life (Stam & Spanos 1987). It is a myth that placebos affect only imaginary illnesses. Placebo analgesia frequently occurs in people with real pathology and real clinical pain (for review, see Roche 2002). Patients with malignant and non-malignant diseases, and with acute as well as chronic pain frequently respond to placebo (Roche & Wright 1990, Roche et al 1993, Houde et al 1996). A review of placebo controlled studies of physical therapy for musculoskeletal pain (Feine & Lund 1997) indicates indistinguishable results from real and placebo treatments for epicondylitis (Binders et al 1985), osteoarthritis (Falconer et al 1992, Lewis et al 1994), rheumatoid arthritis (Heussler et al 1993), and chronic low back pain (Marchand et al 1993).

Placebos reduce anxiety

One hypothesis is that placebos reduce only the affective (unpleasant) component of pain, particularly anxiety. One study showed that placebo reduced anxiety in dental pain but left pain 'intensity' unaffected (Gracely et al 1978). Evidence is growing, however, which shows that placebos also reduce the sensory components of pain as well physiological, functional and behavioural symptoms of illness.

I, for one, am not at all convinced that placebos target only pain anxiety. In an investigation of active or placebo TENS for cancer pain, my colleagues and I observed that individual subjects experienced substantial and sustained pain relief from placebo TENS, on a daily basis, for up to 12 weeks (Roche et al 1993). McGill Pain Questionnaire (MPQ) subclass description prior to placebo TENS included several sensory subclasses, and the affective subclasses describing anxiety and the sense of punishment. Following placebo TENS, the MPQ profiles of the placebo responders no longer included sensory words, or punishment, but did include continued use of words describing anxiety.

There is growing number of well controlled, double-blind trials demonstrating significant physiological effects from placebo electrotherapy, in addition to analgesia. For example, a comparison of different intensities of ultrasound (including zero) clearly showed that placebo gave the greatest reduction in pain, *swelling and jaw tightness* following wisdom tooth extraction, compared with active ultrasound (Hashish et al 1988). Such evidence lays to rest the myth that placebos do not affect real physiological symptoms, such as tissue inflammation. The placebo effect was not due to the effect of tissue massage from the ultrasound head. The strongest effects occurred when the therapist and patient both believed that the ultrasound machine was on. This important study of ultrasound, and the additional evidence of the power of patient-therapist belief in effecting physiological change (Gracely 2000), should convince even the most sceptical amongst us that placebo research is important to physiotherapy research and practice.

23

Placebo-induced improvements in joint swelling, and improvements in walking distance and grip strength are quite commonly reported (Langley et al 1984, Moffett et al 1996). Perhaps the most dramatic example of placebo potency comes from a double-blind trial of real versus placebo surgery, conducted in the mid 1950s (Cobb et al 1959). The trial was conducted to review the value of surgical ligation of the mammary artery for symptoms of angina—a common and costly treatment for angina in those days. The effects of complete surgical ligation were compared with those of placebo surgery, in which the coronary arteries were exposed but no surgery was performed. The results showed significantly lower pain, less vasodilatory drug intake, and improved walking distance in the majority of subjects in *each* group. Some subjects in each group also showed improvement in the shape of their electrocardiogram. The results demonstrated the invalidity of the surgical treatment. They also led to the statement that 'surgery has the most potent placebo effect that can be exercised in medicine' (Finnieson 1969). It is a mystery why similarly controlled trials of surgery were not imposed in recent decades. That, however, has begun to change. The US Food and Drug Administration now requests controlled proof of efficacy for new surgical techniques (cited in Gracely 2000, p 1057). An article in *Time* magazine tells us that the National Institutes of Health in the US has been rejecting proposals for surgical innovations from researchers that do not employ double-blind placebo methodology (Thompson 1999).

Placebo effects are short-lived

Improvements from the placebo surgery in the study by Cobb and colleagues were maintained over six months (Cobb et al 1959). This was the first evidence to refute the myth that placebos have only fleeting benefits compared with the longer-term effects of real medicines. In fact, placebo effects can be very long-lasting. Although active TENS shows a greater cumulative effect overall, both placebo and active TENS relives back pain in some patients for up to 12 months (Marchand et al 1993). We obtained quite similar long-term results in our randomised clinical trial of TENS for pain in patients with spinal metastasis (Roche et al 1993). Self-reported diary scores of pain intensity, before and after twice-daily home applications of TENS for spinal pain, showed significant pain reduction from non-active TENS units in some patients. The placebo responders regularly recorded between 2 and 8 hours post-treatment pain relief. Three of these patients had significant daily reductions in pain for up to 6 weeks, and in two cases for 12 weeks. These data although somewhat limited in the number of subjects, tend to support the evidence that placebo analgesia can be enduring in some individuals.

It can be surprisingly simple to administer a placebo treatment. In the prostate cancer study, each subject was clearly informed that the study involved 'treatment' and 'no treatment' conditions. Subjects were informed that some of the TENS patterns being tested would not be felt by the skin. The placebo TENS units were doctored to prevent any electrical output.

However the external signals, such as the flashing light, were retained, so that the apparatus appeared to be working normally. Despite having been informed that they may be entered into a 'no treatment' condition, and despite experiencing no stimulus, placebo responders reported pain relief. Interestingly, and in line with other studies (Marchand et al 1993), some of our subjects reported a 'sensation' under the placebo electrodes.

Is clinical evidence enough?

It has been claimed that 20–30% of clinical improvement can be explained by placebo effects (Jospe 1978). Others argue that nearly all controlled studies of clinical analgesia fail to measure the placebo effect because they have not controlled for the 'natural history of the pain' (Price et al 1999). There is considerable variation in the normal temporal course of different clinical pains. For example postoperative pain initially rises slowly in intensity, headache pain follows the course of an inverted 'U', and rheumatoid arthritis pain, although variable on a day to day basis, is stable over time (Price 2000, Roche 1998). Clinical studies which do not include a non-treatment condition monitoring the natural course of the pain—as most do not—cannot justifiably claim to have demonstrated a placebo effect on pain (Price 2000).

Experimental models of pain and placebo research

Compared with clinical pain, researchers have relatively greater control over experimental pain models induced under laboratory conditions. Laboratory data has less inherent variability and greater validity compared to clinical pain (Price et al 1999). Induced ischaemic arm pain is a useful laboratory model of pain (Smith et al 1966) which is quite commonly used in placebo and pain research. The arm pain develops gradually over a period up to 25 minutes and is safe in healthy volunteers. It has some of the somatic and affective-emotional qualities of clinical pain (Roche et al 1984). The manufactured drug naloxone is another useful tool in laboratory pain research. As it is a direct antagonist of opioid activity, naloxone can be used to test whether analgesia is opioid-based. For instance, if a low or moderate dose of naloxone given after analgesia, reverses the analgesia and returns the pain to its pre-naloxone level, the analgesia is thought to be mediated via the 'descending' (opioid-based) system of pain relief associated with the mid-brain and periaqueductal grey regions of the brain (see Chapter 2).

Research in the 1970s and 1980s produced controversial evidence concerning the opiate basis to placebo analgesia. More conclusive answers resulting from more rigorous and imaginative research methodologies have been reported in recent years. To date, the evidence demonstrates that the placebo response, and placebo analgesia, is mediated by cognitive mechanisms such as expectancy, and is—at least in part—an opioid-based phenomenon.

Mechanisms explaining the placebo affect

Four principle mechanisms have been proposed to explain the placebo effect: classical conditioning (Wickramsekera 1980), response expectancy (Kirsch 1985), anxiety reduction (Sternbach 1968), and endorphin (i.e. opioid) release (Levine et al 1978). In the discussion that follows some of these mechanisms will be reviewed as well as some more contemporary perspectives.

Conditioning and learned expectancy

Classical conditioning is the elementary first step in the establishment of learned associations between a stimulus and a response. However, modern theorists prefer more of an informational role involving cognition and active mental reasoning in the occurrence of placebo analgesia, which is based on learned expectancy. Two teams of researchers in particular have indicated the role of conditioning and expectancy.

A series of experiments by Voudouris et al (1989, 1990) demonstrated the importance of classical conditioning in subjects' responses and ability to tolerate pain—and the speed with which the effect occurs. Increasing intensities of a painful electrical stimulus were first of all applied to the arm of a volunteer subject. Next the experimental groups were conditioned to *expect* lower levels of pain. Here, cream was applied to their arm which they were told was 'analgesic', but was in fact neutral. At the next trial, the strength of the pain stimulus was secretly lowered. Subjects in the groups with the sham 'analgesic cream' reported significantly less pain compared with the controls. At the next trial the pain stimuli were returned to their original level. Strong carry-over effect was shown. The sham 'analgesic cream' groups continued to report less pain and seemed not to register the return of the pain stimuli to original levels.

Montgomery and Kirsch (1997) believed that, in addition to an initial conditioning processes, placebo analgesia involved cognitive appraisal and learned experience which result in the establishment of habitual directions of response or 'response expectancy'. They replicated the research design used by Voudouris et al (1990), with the single difference that they informed some of the participants given the sham 'analgesic cream' (the informed group) that the stimulus was being lowered during the conditioning trials. Their results demonstrated significantly weaker placebo analgesia in the informed, compared to the uninformed, group. In this manner, the authors successfully showed that the conditioning procedure leading to a placebo response could be manipulated by the direction of response expectancy. In fact, conditioning did not occur when expectancy of pain relief was obstructed. The principle conclusion is that it is the nature and direction of expectancy, rather than simple conditioning processes, which mediate whether and to what extent placebo analgesic responses occur. These results support earlier studies which indicated that placebo respondents, and the positive or negative direction of their response, can be identified by simply asking subjects beforehand what is expected (White et al 1985).

Placebo analgesia and learning

The role of expectancy in mediating placebo analgesia should come as no surprise to those who acknowledge the role of cognitions in mediating physiological responses. In recent years, brain imaging techniques have shown that several areas of the mid-brain and cortex that are involved in arousal, attention, memory, expectation, motivation, conditioning and perception, are activated by nociceptive stimuli (Jones 1992, Treede et al 1999). These areas—intrinsically involved in *learning and emotion*—have either direct or indirect input into the mid-brain structures, which are involved in pain perception and descending mechanisms of analgesia. There is no doubt that associations exist between mechanisms of learning and emotion and the occurrence of placebo analgesia.

Placebo analgesia is sometimes opioid-based

A recent and remarkable series of experiments shows specifically that expectancy activates opioid-based placebo analgesia, but that not all placebo analgesia is opioid-based. First, an elaborate experimental design was constructed in which the effect of cognitive expectancy cues, drug conditioning, or a combination of both, was measured on subjects' tolerance of induced ischaemic pain (Amanzio & Benedetti 1999). There were 12 groups of subjects, each tested on five consecutive days. Some groups received hidden infusions of naloxone in order to test which responses were opioid-based. The principle results were that expectation cues, with and without morphine conditioning, produced analgesia that was completely blocked by naloxone. The results provided further evidence for the involvement of endogenous opioid mechanisms in expectancy-based placebo analgesia. However, conditioning with keterolac—a non-steroidal anti-inflammatory drug—also induced placebo analgesia, which was insensitive to naloxone. Placebo analgesia appears to be mediated by more than one descending system—opioid and non-opioid. Although only speculative, it is likely that the involvement of opioid-based mechanisms of analgesia may depend on whether cognitions of expectancy are involved.

The most recent experiment in this series examined the degree of variance in analgesic response following infusions of analgesic drugs for post-operative (clinical) or induced ischaemic (laboratory) pain. The manipulated conditions included hidden or open infusion of the drug, or simultaneous infusion of naloxone (Amanzio et al 2001). Analgesic effects were at their height under the 'open' condition—when the subject had a full view of the infusion. In contrast, the analgesic effects were consistently suppressed under hidden infusion. The findings showed that the non-specific placebo components of conditioning and expectancy determined individual variability in analgesic effectiveness to a large extent.

This study supports and expands previous work based on the hypothesis that psychological factors activate endogenous opiate mechanisms of analgesia (Benedetti et al 1999, Grevert et al 1983, Levine et al 1978), but the evidence is not yet entirely conclusive. For example, a recent study failed to find any relationship between expectancy and the release of beta-endorphin (Roelofs et al 2000). The researchers considered that their lack of results may have been due to the type of pain stimulus they employed—electrical stimulation of the sural nerve. It may be that the ischaemic arm stimulus, which has a longer duration and is more like clinical pain, is more reliably associated with endogenous activity.

For the moment, the cumulative results of placebo pain research do indicate that simple psychological manoeuvres, which reinforce the patient's belief that he/she has been given a pain-relieving procedure, are associated with activation of endogenous opiate systems. Importantly too, these same beliefs will amplify the effectiveness of real analgesia. Effective placebo manoeuvres can be as straightforward as giving the patient an open view of the analgesic procedure, or telling a patient that the 'agent to be injected is known to produce powerful reductions of pain in some people' (Price 2001).

Mimicry and specificity in placebo analgesia

Although quite easily engendered, placebo analgesic effects show complex patterns of behaviour such as mimicry. For example, placebo morphine shows similar analgesic duration and potency as a morphine infusion administered on previous days (Amanzio & Benedetti 1999). Expectancy also produces somatotopically specific placebo analgesia. Benedetti et al (1999) produced four areas of local inflammation simultaneously in the four limbs of healthy subjects. These researchers instructed the subjects that analgesic cream (in reality neutral cream) had been applied at just two of these sites. Placebo analgesia occurred in just these two sites. The results also excluded the possibility that placebo responses were mediated by anxiety. If central and global responses such as reduced anxiety had been involved, placebo analgesia would have occurred at all four sites.

Co-determination of placebo effects

Despite the important role of expectancy in placebo analgesia, most authors concede that several inter-related mechanisms are involved. Factors such as the patient's age, the type of pain, the specific pathology, the type of opioid-receptor activated, and pharmacodynamics, undoubtedly play additional roles in the *variance* of the placebo analgesic effect (Amanzio et al 2001). Inter-related mechanisms of conditioning, expectancy, anxiety and motivation probably co-determine the *magnitude* of the effect (for a review, see Price 2000).

There is little conclusive evidence to date for the role of motivation in placebo analgesia. Nevertheless, a moment's reflection of the lengths we—and our patients—will go to, to be rid of pain, demonstrates that the motivation and desire for pain relief can be overwhelming. Wall (1993) argues that the *need* for pain relief is not unlike the *need* to relieve hunger or thirst. He notes that attention is selective and that we generally attend to the event of highest biological importance. Pain—like extreme hunger or thirst—is often just such an event. When pain is perceived, we are highly motivated to perform sets of behaviours which, we believe, will result in—be consummated in—pain relief. These motivated behaviours range from common activities such as consulting a physician, to agreeing to be rendered unconscious and operated upon by a surgical team. In consulting a doctor or physical therapist, the behavioural milieu would normally include: accepting the expert's diagnosis (label) and prescribed instructions for rest, taking medications and resuming normal weight bearing and mobility, as appropriate. Thus motivated behaviours are a prelude to returning to normal activities and work responsibilities. They are based on the assumption that pain and tissue damage from the injury will quite quickly subside and that healing will occur.

Consummator actions

Wall (1999), in an inspiring chapter, proposes that such simple behaviours are the fundamental triggers of analgesia. He argues against viewing pain and analgesia in purely sensory terms. He proposes that pain be viewed as a state of need. As hunger or thirst need to be satiated, so pain must be alleviated if we are to reverse the emotional distress and biological threat implied by pain. He proposes that 'sensory input is analysed in terms of the *action* which might be appropriate to the event'. In this model, 'action' does not necessarily involve motor activity or movement. Appropriate action, for example, following recent injury, may be inaction and immobility. Nevertheless, a subconscious cognitive appraisal is implied, whereby the 'selection' of acts which are *appropriate* to tissue healing and pain relief— that is, acts which would normally consummate in the organism's recovery from injury—are themselves sufficient to trigger mechanisms of healing and analgesia. Placebo research shows that even the patient's (or clinician's) belief that such consummator acts have occurred is sufficient to trigger these mechanisms.

Central analysis, which favours such appropriate action, may then trigger the biophysiological events, which lead to healing and reduction, or removal, of pain. In a previous article, I refer to this mechanism in terms of 'setting a positive bias' towards recovery in the central nervous system (Roche 2002) (see also Chapter 6). The key issue underlining such concepts is that it requires an attentive, reasoning and constantly analysing system to select and appraise what is 'appropriate' action.

Iatroplacebogenesis: physician–patient factors

Even the mental decision to commit oneself to follow a prescribed physiotherapy exercise regime, or to engage in disease self-management courses, or to seek surgery, may be centrally 'analysed' as consummator cognitions and to effect some degree of positive bias. It is also likely that simply being a part of the therapist-patient interaction is analysed as 'consummator' in the emotional sense.

Putting one's trust in health professionals is axiomatic to the therapeutic relationship (see Chapter 3). Butler (1998, p 11) notes 'a deep–seated and universal belief in the willingness of physicians and health therapists to help'. Put simply, people believe that medical attention will relieve symptoms, particularly if the physician says it will (Richardson 1994). In addition, there is growing evidence to support health professionals' belief that the behaviour or personality of the practitioner influences treatment outcome.

The double-blind procedure in controlled clinical trials was introduced because of evidence of the Rosenthal effect—whereby the expectations of the researcher (or therapist) are conveyed to the experimental subject. Gracely (2000) discusses different examples of placebo effects from interpersonal effects between the patient and the clinician: for example, the typical initial high rates of efficacy with a new procedure or drug, and the equally typical decline in these success rates over time. Even though the actual efficacy of the new procedure has not changed, the falling rates of treatment success can only mean that the clinician's initial enthusiasm in the new procedure has declined as the new treatment fails to live up to expectations—and that that reduction in confidence is, directly or indirectly, communicated to the patient. In addition, huge differences exist in the success rates of identical active and placebo procedures in different hospitals, cities and countries, and from identical procedures conducted by different clinicians.

Iatroplacebogenesis: environmental factors

Therapeutic apparatus can also induce iatroplacebogenic effects. Langley et al (1984) used oscilloscope displays of a (placebo) TENS stimulus 'output' to create placebo analgesia in 50% of subjects. In an honours study into the effects of sham electrotherapy, we found that the simple application of non-functioning apparatus (placebo Inteferential or placebo TENS) extended pain threshold and endurance to induced ischaemic pain compared with controls (Roche & Tan 2000). Importantly, our results pointed to a generalised (and positive) learned response to medical apparatus in our subjects. No subjects had had prior experience of Inteferential or TENS, yet they responded positively to placebo electrotherapy, which they were told was therapeutic. The most plausible explanation is that carry-over effect occurred from previous successful treatments involving medical apparatus.

The analysing system

What is clear is that real biophysical changes, in this case placebo analgesia, are mediated, to a degree, by the individual's expectancies. Such expectancies are in turn, shaped and moulded by experience. Therefore the system which mediates placebo analgesia is a far cry from the passive, unadaptable system which has traditionally been held to mediate pain. The complexity of placebo effects and placebo analgesia reflects the unique plasticity of the system of pain perception and analgesia. Wall (1996) describes the system as 'unitary, integrated and constantly analysing', and, 'modified by experience'. Gifford (1998a) in describing pain in the biological context of stress biology, has described the same system as a 'mature organism' constantly scrutinising and sampling its internal and external environment, deriving meaning from it and testing its own knowledge, beliefs, past successful behaviours and the observed successful behaviours of others. I call it simply a system of 'learning'.

A learning system

Recent evidence from functional magnetic resonance imaging studies emphasises the learning basis of pain perception and analgesia. Widespread cortical and sub-cortical areas governing sensation, motivation and emotion are activated, even by a simple laboratory pain stimulus. These same areas are associated with diffuse, descending pathways of analgesia. The processes of learning are a major part of cortical processing, daily decision-making, and behaviour. Therefore any factor involved in experiencing pain or getting rid of pain, involves the cortical processes associated with learning. Placebo analgesia, being mediated by expectancies and expectancies being a learned construct, can therefore also be proposed as a direct neurophysiological result of learning.

It is interesting to point out at this stage that strong parallels exist between the mechanisms of placebo effects and successful physiotherapy outcome in that both depend on learning. Independent of the physiological effects on tissues of any of our specific treatment strategies, the overall success of each and every one of our therapies depends on the individual patient's ability to learn. Simply put, the bulk of physical therapy assessment and rehabilitation strategies aim to assist the patient to unlearn or modify dysfunctional movement patterns and behaviours, or to learn, or re-learn—and reinforce— adaptive movement patterns and behaviours. The goals of physical therapy are to engage and influence the same integrated, constantly analysing system of learning as is implicated in the perception and relief of pain and which is associated with placebo analgesia.

The meaning of placebo results

What implications do the results of placebo research have in health therapy? The first is that, contrary to popular opinion, placebo 'treatment' is not the same as 'no' treatment (Wall 1994) (also see Chapter 2). Incidental non-specific placebo factors activate the same descending mechanisms of analgesia, as do characteristic ingredients. The mimicry of placebo analgesia shows that even the nature of the analgesia triggered by incidental or characteristic ingredients can be similar. Perhaps most importantly, a placebo treatment which results in pain relief, develops or reinforces the same positive expectancies for further pain relief in later treatments, as does 'real' analgesic medicine.

Learned expectancies—which can also be referred to as anticipation, faith, trust or hope—are the product of the meaning we have derived from past experience. They represent an 'investment' of belief which each individual patient makes when accepting that the activities, or behaviours, advised by health practitioners will result in (be consummated in) recovery and freedom from pain. It is these cognate pathways which Gifford (1998a) describes as resulting from the 'scrutinising' analytical CNS, and which bring about changes in observable behaviour, autonomic, endocrine and immune activity, resulting in tissue healing and recovery. Such changes are retained for future learning and adaptation in tissue pathways of the brain and body (Gifford 1998a). Once reinforced, even a mere once or twice, these changes are to some degree, learned and are rarely completely extinguished even if rarely activated (Roche 2002). The next most logical inference is that the positive or negative direction of cognate 'action pathways' is set by the nature of the individual's learned experience in the clinical setting.

The significance of placebo research to physical therapy outcome

The results of the research cited earlier, for example by Voudouris (1989, 1990), demonstrate that the direction of a therapeutic response from non-specific factors is 'set' very quickly—within a few repetitions. A positive setting, once learned, can be mimicked at the next 'similar' occasion. The 'scrutinising' system will include previously successful cues from the clinical environment in its determination of the 'similar' setting. When a treatment for pain is successful, repeating the treatment—or even placing the patient in the same room as the previously successful treatment—should re-activate, and reinforce, a positive biophysical response to some extent. The research which shows that placebos taken immediately after an analgesic drug reproduce as much as 50% of the efficacy of the active drug, indicates the extent to which the repetition of a 'positive' setting may supplement medicinal treatment. The studies showing learned placebo responses can have a carry-over effect for six months or longer and reinforce the potency of these non-specific placebo responses in establishing a positive pattern of outcome. We do not know how much non-specific placebo responses contribute towards good physical therapy outcome. There is however, little doubt that 'success breeds success' and that the non-specific 'placebo' component of a treatment, or treatment setting, has a cumulative 'knock-on' effect on subsequent treatments.

To my mind, the importance of placebo in physiotherapy is not whether it does, or does not, pose a challenge to the validity of 'real' physical therapy techniques. Instead, it is that placebo effects demonstrate the major role played by plasticity and learning in pain perception, analgesia, and physical therapy outcome.

The placebo response is a part of the learned therapeutic response. Placebo effects, being positive, supplement the positive biophysical and psychophysical changes we bring about with specialised physiotherapy techniques. We should never forget that pain relief is a joy. It is freedom from what is, in all cases, a biological stress and a threat to well being. When pain is experienced, our hopes, actions and expectancies, as well as our mind and body well-being, are so powerfully programmed toward obtaining pain relief, that its opposite—enduring pain—is a significant, and often long-term, state of distress. An acknowledgment that placebo may have positive influences in physiotherapy and pain management does however mean that we must next consider the opposite situation—the occurrence and consequences of **nocebo** effects if our treatments fail to relieve pain.

Nocebo effects

The most common working definition of the nocebo phenomenon is the causation of sickness (or death) by expectations of sickness (or death) and by associated emotional states (Hahn 1997). Wall (1993) notes that phenomena such as 'voodoo death' or the 'giving-up-given-up' complex indicate that 'beliefs can sicken and kill.' Research in psychoneuroimmunology nowadays explores the link between beliefs and health.

Failed treatment is a primer for failed outcome

It is axiomatic, therefore, to propose that failed treatments for pain, by reversing expectancies of pain relief, and by engendering learned expectancies of treatment failure, produce negative biophysical responses— nocebo responses. In turn, nocebo responses reinforce failed treatments for pain. The repetition or persistence of this pattern contributes to the development of chronic pain.

Countless negative cognitions and beliefs are generated—in both the patient and the clinician—when expectancies of pain relief are frustrated and unfulfilled (Hildebrandt et al 1997, Loeser & Sullivan 1997). Doctors and patients implicitly challenge each other's credibility. A survey of doctors and patients suggests that clinicians tend to withdraw their belief in their patients' motivation to improve and in the credibility of the patients' symptoms, thus inadvertently reinforcing the patients' pain behaviour (Kenny unpublished data). Patients' loss of belief in their clinician's capability to relieve pain distresses the patient (Peyrot et al 1993, Okifuji et al 1999) and the doctor (Kenny unpublished data). In addition to the direct negative feedback which failed treatment has on a patient's expectancies, any non-specific negative cues (statements, beliefs or behaviours) from clinicians towards their patients, will create negative beliefs and negative biophysical consequences, i.e. nocebo effects.

Such nocebo effects can have serious consequences. Failed pain treatment can be the most frightening situation an individual ever has to confront. Furthermore, there is no reason to believe that nocebo effects are learned any the less quickly, or are less powerful, or long-lasting, than are the positive

33

responses of placebo interventions. Indeed, because of the importance of pain relief to the human psyche, nocebo responses are likely to be specifically associated with long-lasting negative emotions and beliefs. For example, enduring pain is associated with long-term feelings of anxiety, helplessness and despair, and with higher levels of pain (Roche 1995, 1998). Repeated failure of treatment for pain is associated with the patient's loss of self-esteem, heightened negative expectancies and persistent activity avoidance (Vlaeyen et al 1995, Crombez et al 1999, Watson & Kendall 2000), in short, with the development of chronic pain-related disability. Individuals' beliefs and their coping reactions are stronger predictors of pain-related disability in musculoskeletal disorders, such as low back pain, than are physical or biomedical factors (Waddel et al 1993, Vlaeyen & Linton 2000).

The main conclusion to be drawn from these factors is that the patient's cognitive appraisal (the extraction of meaning from a therapeutic interaction) and the subsequent establishment of positive or negative expectancies in the patient, is perhaps the most powerful of all learned inputs into the therapeutic setting. The importance of positive expectancy to physiotherapy is that, in order to maximise its supportive role in treatment outcome, we must establish the learned association with successful pain treatment—as *early* as possible. Placebo research provides an important reason to get our treatments right—first time. Its alternative is that we contribute inadvertently toward early learning and negative setting in the CNS and in so doing contribute to the creation of chronic pain (see also Chapter 6).

The biopsychosocial placebo

Peat (2000) notes that we can 'probably not' prove that positive (biophysical) changes in our patients can be attributed entirely to the parameters of the treatment. The results of placebo research support that view. There is now broad acknowledgment that non-specific effects account for a substantial proportion of the effectiveness of therapeutic interventions and 'should not be casually discounted' (NIH Consensus Statement Online, 1997).

The need to prove that X therapeutic manoeuvre results in Y biophysical change only becomes imperative if we adhere to the biomedical 'reductionist' approach to therapy. If we instead adopt the biopsychosocial paradigm as originally proposed by Engel (1977), we incorporate the 'analysing, scrutinising and learning' system (in brief, the biopsychosocial system) into our arena of assessment. Accepting the scientifically proven legitimacy of placebo—or, more precisely, of 'non-specific' phenomena—allows the physiotherapist to welcome placebo responses as additive and interactive with biophysical treatment. Since non-specific factors can, however, also be negative, we need a means of identifying nocebo, as well as placebo, influences. In short, the evidence regarding non-specific effects in health therapy supports the need for items of our evaluation which assess dimensions of the patient's beliefs and expectations from treatment.

A brief but useful method of biopsychosocial assessment in physiotherapy would complement evidence-based research. In the context of this article, 'evidence' has meant identifying which of our treatments has sufficient specific or 'characteristic' biophysical effects, over and above non-specific placebo effects, to be retained. However, 'evidence' should incorporate the quality of life and attitudinal scales. The results of placebo research invite us to integrate our treatment plans and management strategies with the wider psychosocial arena. How best do we plan to use the positive setting reflected by placebo responses? How do we integrate and reinforce the capacity for positive learning—without offering falsity, or our own naive over-enthusiastic expectancies? Perhaps one of the most urgent needs is to develop a capability for managing nocebo responses in patients in whom our own or previous practitioners' treatments have failed. It is surely, the most common complaint of 'failed' pain clinic patients, that their clinicians have not listened and that they have not been heard (Kenny unpublished data). Even if all of our treatment techniques do not relieve pain, physiotherapists should not abandon the patient to a solitary search for alternative treatment. We could utilise our understanding of the learning system to introduce a wider biopsychosocial basis to physiotherapy. This could include the capability to explore the patient's beliefs and expectations, and to explore which learning skills (for example, chronic disease education/self-management skills) and appropriate cognitive-behavioural input could better match expectancies to results and could improve coping and functional outcomes.

Conclusion

In conclusion, the outcome of placebo research to date provides an incontestable rationale for revision of traditional physiotherapy biomedical models of thinking. There is an urgent need to incorporate an approach, which includes the evidence, that non-specific factors influence all treatment interactions and can promote or impair successful treatment. That leaves the thorny question of demonstrating evidence-based practice. I believe that, far from being a threat to the evidence base for physiotherapy, the placebo phenomenon offers exciting opportunities for physical therapy researchers to work alongside the basic and social scientists towards a greater understanding of the science of therapeutics. The placebo-nocebo phenomenon is a mirror of the mechanisms of the active and analytical system in promoting or preventing analgesia and healing. It beckons us to become involved at the clinical and laboratory level with multidisciplinary and collaborative investigations into the healing system. It therefore offers areas of research that will provide multiple levels of evidence. The path will not be easy or short but it cannot be ignored. Placebo research, because it includes clinical and basic sciences, may provide the most solid evidence for physiotherapy efficacy. In the long run, the placebo phenomenon is friend to the therapist and the patient, not foe (Roche 2002).

REFERENCES

Amanzio M, Benedetti F 1999 Neuropharmacological dissection of placebo analgesia: Expectation-activated opioid systems versus conditioning-activated specific subsystems. The Journal of Neuroscience 19 (1):484–494

Amanzio A, Pollo A, Maggi G, Benedetti F 2001 Response variability to analgesics: a role of non-specific activation of endogenous opioids. Pain 90:205–215

Beecher H K 1955 The powerful placebo. Journal of the American Medical Association 159:1602–1606

Benedetti F, Arduinno C, Amanzio M 1999 Somatotopic activation of opioid systems by target-directed expectations of analgesia. Journal of Neuroscience 19(9):3639–3648

Binders A, Hodge G, Greenwood AM, Hazleman BL, Page TDP 1985 Is therapeutic ultrasound effective in treating soft tissue lesions? British Medical Journal 290:512–514

Butler D 1998 Integrating pain awareness into physiotherapy—wise action for the future. In: Gifford L (ed) Topical Issues in Pain 1, Whiplash—science and management. Fear-avoidance beliefs and behaviour. Physiotherapy Pain Association Yearbook. CNS Press, Falmouth 1–27

Cobb LA, Thomas GI, Dillard DM, Merendino KA, Bruce RA 1959 An evaluation of internal mammary artery ligation by a double-blind technique. New England Journal of Medicine 260:1115–1118

Crombez G, Vlaeyen JWS, Heuts PHTG, Lysens R 1999 Fear of pain is more disabling than pain itself: Evidence on the role of pain related fear in chronic back disability. Pain 80:329–340

Falconer J, Hayes KW, Chang RW 1992 Effect of ultrasound on mobility in osteoarthritis of the knee. A randomized clinical trial. Arthritis Care and Research 5:29–35

Feine JS, Lund JP 1997 An assessment of the efficacy of physical therapy and physical modalities for the control of chronic musculoskeletal pain. Pain 71:5–23

Fields HL, Price DD 1997 Toward a neurobiology of placebo analgesia. In: Harrington A (ed.) Placebo: Probing the Self-Healing Brain. Harvard University Press, Boston

Finneson BE 1969 Diagnosis and Management of Pain Syndromes. Saunders, Philadelphia

French S 1997 The powerful placebo. In: French S (ed) Physiotherapy: A psychosocial approach 2nd edn. Butterworth-Heinemann Ltd, Oxford 292–303

Gamsa, A 1994 The role of psychological factors in chronic pain II. A critical appraisal. Pain 57:17–31

Gifford LS (ed) 1998 Topical Issues in Pain 1. Whiplash—science and management. Fear-avoidance beliefs and behaviour. CNS Press, Falmouth

Gifford LS 1998a The mature organism model. In: Gifford LS (ed) Topical Issues in Pain 1. Whiplash—science and management. Fear-avoidance beliefs and behaviour. CNS Press, Falmouth 45–56

Gifford LS (ed) 2000 Topical Issues in Pain 2. Biopsychosocial assessment. Relationships and pain. CNS Press, Falmouth

Goodwin JS, Goodwin JM, Vogel JM 1979 Knowledge and use of placebo by house officers and nurses. Annals of Internal Medicine 91:106–110

Gracely RH 2000 Charisma and the art of healing, In: Devor M, Rowbotham MC, Wiesenfirld-Hallin Z (eds) Proceedings of the 9th World Congress on Pain: Progress in Pain Research and Management, Vol 16. IASP Press, Seattle 1045–1068

Gracely RH, McGrath P, Dubner R 1978 Validity and sensitivity of ratio scales. Manipulation of affect by diazepam. Pain 5:19–29

Gray G, Flynn P 1981 Survey of placebo use in a general hospital. General Hospital Psychiatry 3:199–203

Grevert P, Albert LH, Goldstein A 1983 Partial antagonism of placebo analgesia by naloxone. Pain 16:129–143

Hahn R A 1997 The nocebo phenomenon: concept, evidence, and implications for public health. Preventative Medicine 26:607–611

Harding V 1998 Minimising chronicity after whiplash injury. In: Gifford LS (ed) Topical Issues in Pain 1: Whiplash—science and management. Fear avoidance behaviour and beliefs CNS press, Falmouth 105–114

Hashish I, Feinman C, Harvey W 1988 Reduction of postoperative pain and swelling by ultrasound: a placebo effect. Pain 83:303–313

Hayward AL, Sparkes JJ 1986 The Concise English Dictionary. Omega Books, London 867

Heussler JK, Hinchey G, Margioot E, Quinn R, Butler P, Martin J, Sturgess AD 1993 A double-blind randomised trail of low power laser treatment in rheumatoid arthritis. Annals of Rheumatic Diseases 52:703–706

Hildebrandt J, Pfingsten M, Saur P, Jansen J 1997 Prediction of success from a multidisciplinary treatment program for chronic low back pain. Spine 22(9):990–1001

Houde RW, Beaver WT, Wallenstein SL, Rogers A 1966 A comparison of the analgesic effects of pentazine and morphine in patients with cancer. Clinical Pharmacology Therapeutics 7:740–751

Jones SL 1992 Descending control of nociception. In: Light AR (ed) The Initial Processing of Pain and its Descending Control: Spinal and trigeminal systems. Karger, New York

Jospe M 1978 The Placebo Effect in Healing. Lexington Books, Lexington MA 170

Kenny DT Pain making: doctor-patient relationship (submitted for publication)

Kirsch I 1985 Response expectancy as a determinant of experience and behaviour. American Psychologist 40:1202

Koes BW, Bouter LM, van der Heijden GJMG 1995 Methodological quality of randomized clinical trials on treatment efficacy in low back pain. Spine 20:228–235

Kuypers R 1999 Changing times: In: Placebo—Newsletter of the IASP Special Interest Group on Placebo, IASP Press, August

Langley GB, Sheppeard H, Johnson M, Wigley RD 1984 The analgesic effects of transcutaneous electrical nerve stimulation and placebo in chronic pain patients. Rheumatology International 2:1–5

Levine JD, Gordon NC, Fields HL 1978 The mechanisms of placebo analgesia. Lancet 2: 657

Lewis B, Lewis D, Cumming G 1994 The comparative analgesic effects of TENS and a non-steroidal anti-inflammatory drug for painful osteoarthritis. British Society of Rheumatology 33:455–460

Loeser JD, Sullivan M 1997 Doctors, diagnosis and disability: A disastrous diversion. Clinical Orthopaedics and Related Research 336:61–66

Marchand S, Charest J, Jinuxe Li, Chenard Jean-Rene, Lavignolle B, Laurencelle L 1993 Is TENS purely a placebo effect? A controlled study on chronic low back pain. Pain 54:99–106

Max MB, Schafer SC, Culnane M, Dubner R, Gracely RH 1988 Association of pain relief with drug side effects in postherpetic neuralgia: A single dose study of clonidine, codeine, ibuprofen and placebo. Clinical Pharmacology Therapy 43:363–371

Moffet JA, Richardson PH, Frost H, Osborn A 1996 A placebo controlled double blind trial to evaluate the effectiveness of pulsed short wave diathermy for osteoarthritic hip and knee pain. Pain 67:121–127

Montgomery GH, Kirsch I 1997 Classical conditioning and the placebo effect. Pain 72:107–113

NIH Consensus Statement Online 1997 Acupuncture. Nov 3–5 [24 June 1999] 15(5):1–34

Okifuji A, Turk DJ, Kalauokalani D 1999 Clinical outcome and economic evaluation of multidisciplinary pain centers. In: Block AR, Kremer AF, Fernandez E (eds) Handbook of Pain Syndromes. LEA Publishers, London

Peat G 2000 Interpreting the results of treatment. In: Gifford LS (ed) Biopsychosocial assessment and management. Relationships and pain. CNS Press, Falmouth 13–35

Peyrot M, Moody P, Wiese J 1993 Biogenic, psychogenic and sociogenic models of adjustment to chronic pain. An exploratory study. International Journal of Psychiatry in Medicine 23:63–80

Price DD 2000 Factors that determine the magnitude and presence of placebo anlagesia. In: Devor M, Rowbotham MC, Wiesenfeld-Hallin Z (eds) Proceedings of the 9th World Congress on Pain, Progress in Pain Research and Management, Volume 16. IASP Press, Seattle 1085–1095

Price DD 2001 Assessing placebo effects without placebo groups: an untapped possibility? Pain 90:201–203

Price DD, Milling LS, Kirsch I et al 1999 An analysis of factors that contribute to the magnitude of placebo analgesia. Pain 83(2):147–156

Richardson PH 1994 Placebo effects in pain management. Pain Reviews 1:15–32

Roche PA 1995 Anxiety, depression and the sense of helplessness: their relationship to pain from rheumatoid arthritis. In: Shacklock MO (ed) Moving in on Pain. Butterworth-Heineman Australia 90–97

Roche PA 1998 The course and prediction of pain in rheumatoid arthritis: a multivariate study over six years. PhD thesis, University of Queensland, Australia

Roche PA 2002 Placebo analgesia: friend not foe. In: Strong J, Unruth A, Wright A, Baxter GD (eds). Pain: a textbook for therapists. Chruchill Livingstone, Edinburgh 81–99

Roche PA, Gijsbers K, Belch JJF, Forbes CD 1984 Modification of induced ischaemic pain by transcutaneous electrical nerve stimulation. Pain 20:45–52

Roche PA, Wright A 1990 An investigation into the value of TENS for arthritis pain. Physiotherapy Theory and Practice 6:25–33

Roche PA, Heim H, Oei T, Ganendran A, Summers S 1993 Transcutaneous electrical nerve stimulation (TENS) for pain from metastatic carcinoma of the prostate: an interim report. Abstract 1126, 7th World Congress on Pain, Paris, France, IASP Press, Seattle 421

Roche PA, Tan H-Y, Stanton WR Modification of induced ischaemic pain by placebo electrotherapy, Physiotherapy Theory and Practice (in press)

Roelofs J, ter Riet G, Peters ML, Kessels GH, Reulen JPH, Menheere PPCA 2000 Expectations of analgesia do not affect spinal nociceptive R-III reflex activity: an experimental study into the mechanism of placebo-induced analgesia. Pain 89:75–80

Shapiro AK 1971 Placebo effects in medicine, psychotherapy and psychoanalysis. In: Nergina AE, Garfield SL (eds) Handbook of Psychotherapy and Behaviour Change: An empirical analysis. Wiley, New York

Smith GM, Egbert LD, Markowitz RA, Mosteller F, Beecher HK 1966 An experimental method sensitive to morphine in man. Journal of Pharmacology and Experimental Therapeutics 154:324–332

Stam HJ, Spanos NP 1987 Hypnotic analgesia, placebo analgesia and ischaemic pain: the effects of contextual variables. Journal of Abnormal Psychology 96:313–320

Sternbach RA 1968 Pain: a psychological analysis. Academic Press, New York

Thompson D 1999 Real knife, fake surgery. Time Magazine, February 22:52

Treede RD, Kenshalo DR, Gracely RH, Jones AKP 1999 The cortical representation of pain. Pain 79:105–111

Turner JA, Deyo RA, Loeser JD 1994 The importance of placebo effects in pain treatments and research. Journal of the American Medical Association 271(20):1609–1614

Vlaeyen JWS, Kole-Snijders AMJ, Boeren RGB, van Eck H 1995 Fear of movement (re) injury in chronic low back pain and its relations to behavioural performance. Pain 62:363–372

Vlaeyen JWS, Linton SJ 2000 Fear-avoidance and its consequences in chronic musculoskeletal pain: a state of the art. Pain 85:317–332

Voudouris NJ, Peck GL, Coleman G 1989 Conditioned response models of placebo phenomena: Further support. Pain 38:109–116

Voudouris NJ, Peck GL, Coleman G 1990 The role of conditioning and verbal expectancy in the placebo response. Pain 43:121–128

Waddell G, Somerville D, Henderson I, Newton M, Main C 1993 A fear-avoidance beliefs questionnaire (FABQ) and the role of fear-avoidance beliefs in chronic low-back pain and disability. Pain 1993 5:82–86

Wall PD 1992 The placebo effect: an unpopular topic. Pain 51:1–3

Wall PD 1993 Pain and the placebo response. In: Ciba Foundation Symposium: 174. 'Experimental and theoretical studies of consciousness.' Held at the Ciba Foundation, London, 7–9 July, 1992. 187–217

Wall PD 1994 The placebo and placebo response. In: Wall PD, Melzack RC (eds) Textbook of Pain. Churchill Livingstone, Edinburgh 1297–1307

Wall PD 1996 Comments After 30 years of the Gate Control Theory. Pain Forum 5:12–22

Wall PD 1999 The placebo and placebo response. In: Wall PD, Melzack RC (eds) Textbook of Pain, 4th edn. Churchill Livingstone, Edinburgh 1297–1307

Watson P, Kendall N 2000 Assessing psychosocial yellow flags. In: Gifford LS (ed) Topical Issues in Pain 2. Biopsychosocial assessment and management. Relationships and pain CNS Press, Falmouth 111–129

White L, Tursky B, Schwartz GE (eds) 1985 Placebo—theory, research and mechanisms. Guildford Press, New York 37–58

Wickramsekera I 1980 A conditioned response model of the placebo effect: Predictions from the model. Biofeedback and Self-Regulation 5:5–18

2

The reality of the placebo response

NIGEL LAWES

Introduction

Placebos are potent therapeutic agents (but see Chapter 4). Until the advent of modern medicine they were the mainstays of medical practice (Benson & McCallie 1979), and in contemporary African medicine placebos are used independently of available pharmacological agents (Okpako 1999). This chapter examines some of the misconceptions of placebos that have led to a denigration of their effectiveness—a self-fulfilling assessment (a nocebo, in fact).

Placebo research has been hampered by the rising tide of ethicalism, which contrasts with the scientific evidence indicating that placebos are effective and legitimate therapeutic agents. This chapter explores mechanisms that might mediate some placebo effects in the hope of raising the acceptance of this marginalised therapeutic strategy.

Conceptions, preconceptions and misconceptions of placebos

A clinician's view of placebo mechanisms identifies their position in the range of conceptions of illness and health. To caricature the extremes, at one end of the range lie absolute materialists who accept only physical concepts and dismiss placebo effects as being 'purely imaginary'. At the other end of the range come those who claim that reality is defined (or even created) entirely by social agreement, so that no conventionally 'organic' process is any more real than a placebo effect, both being the product of verbal convention and social interaction. A third view, seldom defended formally but often held, is that there are two separate entities: one is the 'mind' and the other is the 'body'. Mysteriously, these interact, breaking the laws of physics. Somehow 'mind' acts on 'matter', producing placebo effects. Any discussion between protagonists of these three views is bound to be at cross-purposes.

Placebo effects cannot be discussed productively without making these underlying assumptions explicit. How do such underlying assumptions influence our understanding of placebos?

For those who think that disease is entirely a social process, it would be legitimate to browbeat a patient into re-labelling a symptom with a healthy synonym. Once the patient and clinician agreed that the patient was healthy, the patient would be! Taken to the extreme, attempts to exert social and political pressures to reconstruct reality can lead to consequences as appalling as Stalin's Show Trials and Chairman Mao's Cultural Revolution. Hahn (1985) takes a more moderate and rational position, arguing that beliefs causally influence the reality to which they refer. Some have claimed that 60–90% of somatic complaints are of psychosocial origin (Kroenke & Mangelsdorff 1989). I take the view that natural sciences explore a reality that exists independently of social context, however much the sciences themselves depend on social factors. Despite this position, it is contended in this chapter that the brain events corresponding to beliefs exert objective effects on other parts of the body.

For the extreme materialist, patients' beliefs about their state of health are irrelevant and cannot affect the actual state of their bodies. According to Benson and Friedman (1996), this attitude characterised the medical views of the 1930s. Here, the placebo effect depended on patients only imagining that they were ill, without actually being so. The placebo effect would then be for patients to recover from the illusion of illness and recognise that they were well. Another placebo effect would involve patients actually being ill, but somehow being bamboozled into believing they were not. The disease process would continue unrecognised by the patient, who would simply be in a state of denial. In essence, placebos are assumed to have effects only on subjective perceptions, and to be devoid of any objective effect. It is contended in this chapter that neither of these conceptions describes genuine placebo effects. Instead, it is held that just as the thought of flexing an elbow can lead to the elbow flexing, so the belief in recovery from illness can lead to actual recovery. In both cases, it is argued, there are rational biological explanations linking thought to action. If so, placebo treatments are as ethical as any other treatments, depending on their efficacy.

Clinical practitioners sometimes use these conceptions of the placebo effect to dismiss the claims of some rival school of practice. Similarly, ethics committees are increasingly reluctant to permit placebo control groups because they mistakenly believe that a placebo control is the same as a no-treatment control. For example, some argue that the use of placebos is unethical because it denies patients an effective treatment (Blanz 1990, Rothman & Michels 1994). Direct comparisons of placebo groups with no-treatment groups show that this is not the case (Gelfand et al 1963, Liberman

1964). Those who oppose the use of placebos are presumably unaware that they can be as effective as known therapeutic agents. If, as is extremely likely, all therapies have a substantial placebo component, it is impossible to avoid utilising placebo effects. It will be argued that many effective analgesic procedures operate through the same mechanisms as some placebos. In reality, every treatment has at least three components:

1. The specific biological effect of the treatment
2. The effects mediated by the patient's thoughts about the treatment
3. Other non-specific effects such as spontaneous remission.

It is the contention of this chapter that greater use should be made of the second component. Rather than trying to avoid placebo effects for spurious ethical reasons, we should be trying to maximise them (Benson & Friedman 1996, Oh 1994). To overcome ethical problems, some have advocated openness in the use of placebos. Specifically, we should investigate whether specific and placebo mechanisms are additive or multiplicative. Preliminary investigation has suggested that placebos do not enhance active agents (De Craen et al 2001), but no placebo effect was demonstrated in this study.

For the dualist, 'mind' and 'body' are separate entities that interact. A belief arises in the 'mind' and somehow exerts an influence on the 'body', which actually changes as a result. Placebo effects are then real but inexplicable. Science can investigate and sometimes measure what people say about the content of their minds, because the words used exist in some physical form (such as a sound or written document), but there is no instrument for detecting this dualist version of 'mind' itself. If so, science can only describe the results but not investigate the mechanisms of placebo effects. Any New Age philosophy would be in a better position to pursue the phenomena and we would have to contend with psychic photons or some equivalent agency.

In this chapter it will be assumed instead that there is only one entity, the brain. 'Mind' is then a convenient collective term for those states of brain activity involving awareness, even if we have nothing sensible to say about how such awareness comes about. Any thoughts whatever, including beliefs about health, are already brain states. Under this assumption, the problem of explaining placebo effects is similar to the problem of explaining a voluntary movement: how does a particular state of the brain influence some other part of the body? Although this conception makes no attempt to explain how a particular brain state is associated with awareness or intention, it does at least make all subsequent questions tractable. The problem reduces to this: 'How does activity in the parts of the brain associated with thoughts about health influence those tissues that affect health?' More pragmatically, we can ask: 'How can we exploit and enhance this influence?'

The view that placebo effects are entirely subjective is surprisingly common. This is a misconception (Hennekens & Buring 1987). It implies that placebos can alter only 'functional', not 'organic', illness. Ernst & Abbot (1997) found that a quarter of a group of Australian nurses hold this belief. Placebo effects do not separate psychogenic from organic pain (Bouckoms & Hackett 1991). In the case of chronic pain, a misunderstanding of the processes responsible reinforces such beliefs. In transient and acute pain, there is often an evident cause such as inflammation or traumatised tissue. As the peripheral tissue heals, the acute pain state resolves. In chronic pain, however, plastic changes occur within the central nervous system so that even when the peripheral tissue injury has healed, the central pain state persists. As there is no objective peripheral cause still evident, and as the changes in the central nervous system are typically invisible, it is tempting to conclude that the symptom of pain is somehow 'imaginary'. This formulation is perhaps central to misconceptions about placebo effects in general and pain in particular.

To understand the misconception, consider a subject who is asked to imagine a pink elephant flying from the floor to the ceiling. A scan of their visual cortex would reveal increased activity in the visual cortex. The activity would begin rostrally and dorsally when the 'elephant' was imagined to be on the floor, move caudally as the elephant crossed the centre of the subject's vision, then end up rostrally and ventrally when the elephant reached the ceiling. While most of us would agree that the elephant was imaginary, perhaps not everyone realises that the image of the elephant is an objective event in the subject's visual cortex.

Apply this reasoning to pain. In the case of pain, the experience is not objectively about some event external to the nervous system. Some events involve much tissue damage but are accompanied by little pain, whereas other events creating very little damage are accompanied by intense pain. Pain may therefore purport to signal some external event, but it is actually about our internal reaction to such an event. In acute pain the external event, tissue damage, is evident. In chronic pain, however, the external event is long resolved. Nevertheless, the image of the event, the chronic neural change, is still present. This central change is as real as the image of the flying pink elephant. The difference is that the subject knows that the image of the flying elephant is self-generated and can be terminated at will. The change in chronic pain, by contrast, is generated by the mechanisms of plasticity and people with chronic pain are unable to terminate the activity. If the image of the flying pink elephant were as persistent, the hapless subject might become quite convinced of its external reality. For the patient and some clinicians, the symptom directs investigation towards the site to which the pain is referred (the painful body part), instead of to the site where the pain event is occurring (the central nervous system).

Another misconception is that placebo effects include spontaneous symptom change or remission (Pledger & Hall 1986). Some acute conditions resolve on their own without treatment. Others fluctuate, waxing and waning. In these circumstances, if a patient consults a clinician at the peak of their illness, the condition will resolve on its own, termed 'regression to the mean' (Whitney & von Korff 1992). Some of the apparent effect of placebo may be due to non-specific factors, and not a true placebo effect (Ernst & Resch 1995, but see McQuay et al 1996). These effects should be carefully distinguished from placebo effects, which depend on the patient's perceptions, beliefs and learning from experience.

So far in this chapter, illness is conceived of as real, not merely constructed, and 'mind' is considered to be an attribute of brain activity. Brain activity related to beliefs about illness and health has detectable effects on peripheral tissues and *it is as ethical to manipulate these as it is to use any other efficacious therapeutic agent of process.* The reality of brain states related to a belief is independent of the validity of the belief, so these states must be taken seriously: it is not legitimate to dismiss these as being 'only in the mind'.

The biological reality of placebo effects

A common definition of placebo effects attributes them to the symbolic content of a treatment rather than any pharmacological or physiological process, but how can these be separated? Mounting evidence suggests that they cannot (Stefano et al 2001).

A very interesting effect of suggestion was found in a study of the relaxant effects of carisoprodol versus lactose placebo (Flaten et al 1999). Subjects were given information suggesting relaxation, stimulation or nothing, and they were given either carisoprodol or lactose. Objective measures included the blink reflex, skin conductance responses and serum drug levels. As expected, information that suggested stimulation increased tension, a nocebo effect. Surprisingly, though, the group given information suggesting relaxation showed higher serum levels of carisoprodol than the other groups. Without the serum level changes, this result would have appeared to vindicate a purely 'psychological' mechanism of placebo action, whereas the serum level increase indicates the fundamental inseparability of biological and cognitive processes.

Placebos also influence the levels of endogenous pharmacologically active agents. In one investigation (Stefano et al 2001), 70% of patients with low back pain or sciatica, warm saline injected via lumbar puncture evoked a placebo response and an objective rise in CSF endorphins. In the remaining 30% not exhibiting a placebo response, there was no rise in endorphin. Stefano at al (2001) review similar changes involving adrenalin, nitric oxide and opioids (agents resembling morphine in their actions).

There have been many papers detailing objective biological effects of placebos:

- Using rigorous criteria, placebo was found to improve motor function objectively in all domains of Parkinsonian disability, though favouring bradykinesia and rigidity over tremor, gait, balance and midline function (Goetz et al 2000).
- The placebo effect of ultrasound machines reduced the experience of pain, a subjective measure, but they also reduced swelling induced by extraction of wisdom teeth (Hashish et al 1988).

45

- Placebos compared to cimetidine reduced the size of duodenal ulcers measured on endoscopy by 10–91%, averaging 46% (Moerman 1983).
- Placebos reduced blood pressure by a conditioning mechanism (Suchman & Ader 1992).
- Placebo lowered isolated systolic hypertension (Feldmen et al 2000), but in this study had no significant effects on combined systolic and diastolic hypertension.
- Suggestion can halve the effects of a bronchodilator if the patients are told it causes constriction, relative to the effects of instruction coinciding with its known pharmacology (i.e. relaxation) (Luparello et al 1970).
- Suggestion to asthmatic patients can induce or prevent bronchospasm caused by the inhalation of distilled water (Butler & Steptoe 1986).
- Contractions of the stomach changed in the suggested direction when patients were told that a magnetic pill would increase, decrease or not change their stomach motility (Sternbach 1964).
- Another study indicating the establishment of a placebo effect achieved by conditioning investigated respiratory depression induced by buprenorphine (Benedetti et al 1999). Buprenorphine induces respiratory depression and repeated administration creates a learned association between administration and respiratory depression. No suggestion or information was given to induce an expectation of respiratory depression, nor were the subjects aware of any respiratory discomfort. Nevertheless, after repeated administration of buprenorphine, subsequent administration of placebo also induced depression of respiration. Naloxone completely blocked this effect, demonstrating that it was mediated by endogenous opioids. Thus, although expectation induces an opioid-mediated placebo effect, placebo effects can be induced by opioid conditioning independently of any cognition or motivation.

It could be argued that many of these objective changes are autonomic effects, where responsiveness to emotion has been well documented. In this case, the thought of illness would increase anxiety, which would in turn produce autonomic effects, misinterpreted as evidence of pathology and thereby reinforcing the belief in illness. In addition, anxiety can increase attention to symptoms. By this argument, placebos would then act simply by reducing anxiety and its autonomic consequences.

But placebos alter mortality statistics, an observation that is difficult to brush off merely as misinterpreted autonomic consequences of heightened emotions. Compliance, presumably influenced by the degree of belief of patients in the effectiveness of a placebo, affects such objective measures as mortality (Coronary Drug Project Research Group 1980). Although the overall mortality for placebo groups (21%) was similar to the mortality of patients taking clofibrate for coronary artery disease (20%), *those who adhered to the placebo regime had a lower mortality* (15%) than those who did not comply (28%). This, surely, must be a powerful argument for learning how to harness the potency of placebo effects. If compliance reflected the degree of belief patients had that they were receiving an effective treatment, then belief halved their mortality. There can be few more convincing outcome measures indicating a real biological effect than mortality, after all. Reductions in mortality have also been shown in other trials: the one year mortality of compliant patients receiving placebo in the Beta Blocker Heart Attack Trial (1984) was 3%, compared to a mortality of 7% in non-compliant patients. As the mortality of patients receiving active treatment showed similar effects, *adherence was a better predictor of outcome than the type of treatment received.*

We can now see that placebos have objective biological effects. For example, they alter levels of administered and endogenous chemical signals, smooth muscle activity, and even mortality. Placebo effects should no longer be considered merely subjective, nor should they be regarded as inconsequential or minor.

Characteristics of placebo effects

In line with being a real biological process, placebos have drug-like characteristics such as dose-response curves. One placebo capsule is less effective than two (Blackwell et al 1972). Larger capsules are perceived as stronger than small ones. In 51 trials administering placebo four times a day for the treatment of duodenal ulcer, the healing rate was 44%, whereas in 28 trials administering placebo twice daily, the healing rate fell to 36% (De Craen et al 2000). Not only dose, but also route of administration is important, just as with a conventional drug. Subcutaneous administration of placebo for the treatment of migraine reduced pain in 32% of patients, compared to 26% of patients receiving an oral placebo (De Craen et al 2000a).

The colour of drug influences the placebo effect (De Craen et al 1996). Some colours are associated with specific types of medication, yellow for stimulants and antidepressants and white for analgesics, for example (Buckalew & Coffield 1972). Capsules with coloured contents are more effective than coloured tablets, and white tablets with corners are more effective than round white tablets.

Placebos have identifiable durations of action as well, refuting the commonly held notion that their effects are brief. Sham surgery, for example, improved angina for up to one year (Dimond et al 1960). Placebo effects have been found to last at least four months in a study of pre-menstrual tension (Freeman & Rickels 1999). Placebo effects were found throughout a six month period during a randomised, multicentre placebo-controlled trial of ropinerole for Parkinson's Disease (Goetz et al 2000).

Kaptchuk (1998) has reviewed evidence for the existence of enhanced placebo effects by procedures and devices. Parenteral (injected) administration of placebo was more effective than oral placebo in lowering blood pressure, relieving headache and treating rheumatoid arthritis. The elaborate ritual of topical application of placebo for varicose veins was more effective than oral administration. The enhanced placebo effects of devices may explain the failure of so many studies attempting to demonstrate electrotherapeutic efficacy: the inactive equipment has such a strong placebo effect that the benefits of the active equipment are masked. Such considerations obscure the effectiveness of acupuncture, TENS, ultrasound and epidural steroids. Very high placebo response rates are obtained for surgery, making comparison with medical treatment difficult. After surgical exploration failed to reveal herniated intervertebral discs, 37% of patients with sciatica and 43% of patients with back pain were completely relieved of pain (Spangfort 1972). Kaputchuk (1998) points out that most of the studies were conducted a long time ago and contain methodological problems, but that modern research is hampered by ethical objections.

It has been suggested that if a patient's initial illness is mild, the active drug will have similar effects to placebo, while patients with more severe illness show a greater difference (Benjamin 1963, Fisher et al 1965). The placebo response rate is high in mild depression (Stassen et al 1994) and obsessive compulsive disorders (Montgomery et al 1993), but low in severe conditions.

Turner et al (1994) have reviewed the characteristics of placebo responses. They emphasise the wide variability of placebo response rates, indicate the placebo effects of surgery, outline the 'pharmacokinetics' of placebo responses and discuss factors that improve placebo effects, such as the warmth, friendliness, sympathy, empathy, prestige and positive attitude of clinicians, a positive belief in the treatment, the presence of anxiety, expensive and impressive treatments. They also mention various theories of placebo mechanisms, including reduction of anxiety, expectations of improvement, conditioned learning and endorphins. Turner also enumerates disadvantages of using placebos noting: loss of trust, belief that failure to improve implies greater illness, and nocebo effects.

One of the commonest misconceptions about placebos is that a placebo effect demonstrates a defect in personality. 58% of a group of Australian nurses believe in a placebo personality (Ernst & Abbot 1997). The assumption that there are placebo responders who can be detected and eliminated by 'good' investigators still persists (Montgomery 1999). Patients who are particularly responsive to reassurance are alleged to be placebo responders. Liberman (1964), in contrast, concluded that someone could show placebo responses or not in different situations and that almost everyone might show placebo effects in some circumstances. Voudouris et al (1989) agreed that responders in one situation could become non-responders in another. Shapiro and Shapiro (1984) also concluded that attempts to identify personalities predisposing to placebo responses were unsuccessful. Wickramasekera (1985) agreed that placebo responders could not be identified in advance. The placebo effect on Parkinson's disease does not depend on age, race, religion, level of education, duration of illness or sex (Shetty et al 1999). Placebo effects do not imply psychopathology (Bouckoms & Hackett 1991).

Another misconception is that a fixed proportion of the population, roughly one- third, exhibits placebo effects. This has been refuted many times. Response rates are extremely variable, depending as they do on the behaviour of both the investigator and the patient. Placebo group remission in ulcerative colitis ranges from 4% to 45% (Sutherland et al 1993). Placebo administered for dysthymia induced response rates of 0–72% (Lima & Montcrief 1999). Turner et al (1994) reviewed other variations. Considering the number of patients achieving 50% relief from pain, the range is very large: 15–53% (Beecher 1955), 7–37% (McQuay et al 1996), 0–72% (Moore et al 1997). Figures as high as 100% have also been quoted. Obviously, no treatment could compete against the latter figure! Underestimation of placebo response rates and placebo potency is prevalent among both patients and nurses (Berthelot et al 2001).

Placebo response rates are increasing. Montgomery (1999) suggests that the non-specific support offered to patients may be a contributing factor. Although Montgomery (1999) identified this as undesirable on the grounds that it decreases the difference between placebo and active drug, it does imply that clinicians are improving in their capacity to provide non-specific support. Perhaps the bedside manner of clinicians is better than it was, after all. On the same lines, Montgomery (1999) suggests that investigators in centres producing high placebo response rates need to be retrained. Perhaps, instead, their placebo effectiveness should be encouraged while it is the investigators in centres with low placebo response rates who need to be retrained to improve their effectiveness. Clearly, there is a tension between the requirements for clean research results in clinical trials and the maximisation of therapeutic efficacy. Placebo responses contaminate clinical research but enhance clinical practice. Perhaps grim-faced, unempathic pessimists should conduct clinical trials, whereas clinical practice should be the domain of empathic, enthusiastic optimists.

Sometimes it is not just different centres within one country that display markedly different placebo response rates: whole countries can display a similar effect. Placebo reduction in the size of duodenal ulcers measured on endoscopy varied from 63% in Germany to 23% in Denmark (Moerman 1983). Interestingly, the active drug, cimetidine, did not show the same variation: it reduced the size of ulcers by 75% in trials where it was no more efficacious than placebo, and by 77% in trials in which placebo was less efficacious. Had the trials been conducted solely in Germany, cimetidine would have been rejected, an example of placebo effects obscuring the efficacy of an active drug. More interesting is the question of why this variation of placebo response rates occurred. What is it about German doctors that make them so effective as placebo promoters? What is happening in Denmark?

From the literature it is evident that it is not only the patient's belief that affects the outcome: the investigator's conviction is perhaps as crucial. The clinician's personality, dress, demeanour, voice and body language influence the placebo effect (Bourne 1978). The confidence of the investigators affects the outcome of a clinical trial (Thomas 1987). Concerns about placebo effects undermine the intention of double-blind randomised controlled trials: patients in the placebo arm of a clinical trial may be given additional support (Kienle & Kiene 1997). Even in truly double-blind studies, researchers often know the actions of the active treatment in question, and their expectations of this are subtly conveyed to the experimental subjects, so that even when the subjects receive the placebo treatment, they report the effects of the active treatment. In addition, it is possible that some researchers record only those changes that they know could be attributed to the active treatment.

A frequently cited example of this kind of unblinding was demonstrated by Gracely et al (1983). After dental extraction, patients were assigned to one of two groups. One group was given either saline or naloxone, which is a drug that blocks the effect of natural transmitters resembling morphine. Naloxone is therefore said to be an opioid antagonist. The other group was given saline, naloxone or fentanyl, which is a drug that mimics the effect of morphine-like compounds (an opioid agonist). Both groups were given the same information, so they should have had the same placebo responses. The research was conducted under a double-blind protocol, although the clinicians knew to which of the two groups each patient belonged. Despite the double-blind procedure, however, the clinicians' knowledge that one of the groups could not receive fentanyl was inadvertently conveyed to the patients. The subjects who were given a placebo but could not have received fentanyl had more pain than the subjects who actually were given the same placebo but had a chance of receiving fentanyl instead.

Unwitting communication confers some remarkable properties on placebos. The effect of placebo depends on what the placebo is being compared with (Evans 1985). Placebo has 54% of the effect of aspirin when the two are compared. Against a more potent analgesic, however, placebo had 56% of the effect of morphine. Similar results were obtained with other analgesics. As these were double-blind studies, the conviction of the experimenters when they were unknowingly administering placebo must have been calibrated against the conviction they would have conveyed when administering the active drug.

A further example of subtle, unintended communication to the patients is revealed by so-called run-in single-blind studies. Studies with single-blind placebo run-in periods prior to the formal study indicate that few patients respond at this stage. As soon as randomisation allows the possibility of an active treatment, however, the response to placebo increases (Montgomery 1999). Although the patient is not formally aware of the transition from run-in period to test period, the investigators are aware of the transition and obviously must be communicating this to the patient even if they are not conscious of doing so.

Communication involves not only the semantic content (the meaning of the words), but also the prosodic content (tone of voice, facial expression and body posture, for example). These studies indicate that although the semantic content of communications between investigators and subjects is controlled, the prosodic content clearly differs. There is a possibility that the prosodic content, consisting of largely unconscious alterations in facial expression, posture, tone of voice and general attitude, may well be more relevant to the placebo effect than the semantic content itself.

On the other hand, if the active treatment produces any detectable effect, experimental subjects can distinguish it from the placebo treatment. The more the placebo mimics the treatment, the less the difference in effect between the two (Deyo 1991, Thomson 1982). In neither case is there a truly double-blind design. If patients can detect that they are in the placebo arm of a randomised placebo-controlled trial, they may be more inclined to withdraw. Withdrawal rates of 20–40% are common in psychiatry (Thase 1999), harming the statistical validity of the research.

Early researchers sometimes worried that informing patients of the inclusion of a placebo would reduce the effectiveness of the active drug, perhaps by a nocebo effect. The evidence is conflicting. Informed consent increased the efficacy of both placebo and naproxen (Bergmann et al 1994), simultaneously decreasing the difference between them. Conversely, non-steroidal anti-inflammatory drugs were perceived as less efficacious when a placebo control was included in a randomised controlled trial (Rochon et al 1999). If, on the other hand, there was no placebo control, patients were more likely to withdraw from a trial because of adverse effects. By preventing the inclusion of placebo controls, ethics committees are therefore increasing the reported incidence of adverse effects of drugs, a consideration they might like to include in their ethical deliberations. Similarly, some investigators resort to an 'ethical solution' in encouraging participants to drop out of a placebo-controlled study when there is no efficacy. This 'ethical' solution made little difference to the dropout rate of patients receiving placebo, but it did increase the dropout rate among patients receiving active treatment (Niklson et al 1997). This reduces the detected difference between active drug and placebo, leading to rejection of effective drugs and necessitating increased costs from increased sample size. Once again, a misapplication of 'ethical' considerations leads to a result that is hardly ethical. Analysing the time taken to drop out of the trial may be an alternative (Stassen et al 1993).

Some ethical concerns are well founded, though, and agreeing to participate in a placebo-controlled trial can pose risks. Fifty-nine percent of patients in a placebo group for acute stroke therapy had National Institutes of Health Stroke Scale score of >9 at follow-up one week after a stroke, compared to 15% of control subjects not enrolled on a clinical trial. The difference was attributed to an absence of anticoagulants in the placebo group. It would be hard to justify the omission of a life-saving treatment once its efficacy had been reliably established.

This section shows us that placebos have all the hallmarks of physical agents, including dose-response curves, durations of action and preferred routes of administration. It also shows that there is little to support the widely held misconception that placebos affect only a specific section of the population, particularly a vulnerable sub-section. Widely differing placebo response rates are as likely to reflect differences in the behaviour of investigators as differences in their subjects. This aspect (the behaviour of investigators) deserves considerably more emphasis, particularly if placebo effects are to be exploited therapeutically.

Some mechanisms of placebo analgesia

The complexity of placebo mechanisms is well illustrated by a study comparing conditioning and expectation using opioid (morphine) and non-opioid (ketorolac tromethamine) analgesics (Amanzo & Benedetti 1999).

Expectation alone resulted in a placebo effect that was reversed by naloxone (an opioid antagonist). Thus the belief in pain relief is sufficient to relieve pain by an analgesic system that utilises an opioid transmitter.

Conditioned learning with morphine also generated a naloxone-sensitive placebo effect, so unconscious learning also acts through an opioid analgesic system. Ketorolac (non-opioid) conditioning generated placebo responses that were either naloxone-resistant alone, or partially naloxone-sensitive when combined with expectation. In other words, unconscious learning about the effects of a non-opioid analgesic produces analgesia via a mechanism that does not depend on opioid transmitters. If conscious expectation accompanies this learning, however, a component of the analgesia does now utilise an opioid transmitter. This study emphasises that there is more than one placebo system: if unconscious learning was about an opioid analgesic, an opioid system mediates the placebo effect, but if the learning was about a non-opioid analgesic, then a non-opioid system is responsible instead. It also demonstrates a technique for separating conditioning effects from expectation. Conditioning has had more powerful effects than expectation in some studies (Voudouris et al 1990). Non-opioid placebo mechanisms had previously been found in the treatment of impacted molars (Gracely et al 1983).

Placebo effects could be implemented at multiple levels, from peripheral to central. The remainder of this chapter will focus on placebo analgesia. To appreciate sites at which placebos could operate, pain pathways will be briefly recapitulated.

After an inflammatory event, there is a continuum of change beginning in the peripheral tissues, through the peripheral nerves, the spinal cord, brain stem, the thalamus and finally involving the cerebral neocortex and limbic system. Beginning with the most peripheral site, inflammatory cells release signalling chemicals such as cytokines, serotonin, histamine, bradykinin and neurotropins, all of which have effects on peripheral nerves. Peripheral nerves sensitise by mechanisms including the closure of potassium channels (so that the neurons cannot terminate action potentials as readily), up-regulation of altered receptors (where genes for different receptors are turned on, or up-regulated) and increased release of transmitters, including release into the peripheral tissues as well as into the spinal cord. The peripherally released transmitters, such as substance P and calcitonin gene related peptide, promote the inflammatory response by stimulating leukocytes to release cytokines, creating a positive feedback loop. Spinal cord dorsal horn neurons, which receive nociceptive input from the periphery, also contribute by becoming more responsive and by sending retrograde signals back down the peripheral nerves, inducing them to release more transmitters. Even innocuous mechanoceptors can contribute to pain by inducing synapses from sympathetic nerves to form in the dorsal root ganglion, by increasing the number of sodium channels and by sprouting onto and forming connections with nociceptive neurons in the dorsal horn (see Volume 3 of this series). Consequently, low intensity stimulation of mechanoceptors and activity of the sympathetic nervous system become capable of evoking responses in nociceptive pathways. Allodynia, the perception of normally innocuous stimuli as painful, results.

All these processes enhance pain by mechanisms involving the nervous system. Learning and cognitive processes such as belief can have an effect by neural mechanisms acting at the level of peripheral nerves and their dorsal horn synapses. The field of psycho-neuro-immunology suggests that thoughts, beliefs and emotions can also have effects on peripheral, non-neuronal tissues. Thus, classical conditioning of the immune system has been achieved (Ader & Cohen 1991). Animals have been conditioned to produce delayed hypersensitivity (Bovberg et al 1987), release histamine (Dark et al 1987), modify T-cell ratios (Husband et al 1987), stimulate mast cells (MacQueen et al 1989) and augment killer cell activity (Solvason et al 1988). Human subjects show enhanced immune responses following placebo immunisation (Wasserman et al 1993). Belief in antibiotic efficacy, for example, enhances phagocytosis by leukocytes even after they have been removed from the body. Presumably, the leukocytes are altered by neuroendocrine systems and the nerves innervating lymphatic tissue (Watkins 1994) while they are still in the patient's body, at the time when the patient believes they are receiving treatment.

Continuing along the nociceptive pathways, the dorsal horn cells of the spinal cord become more responsive by phosphorylating existing receptors and by up-regulating the expression of genes for new receptors. The addition of phosphate to receptors (phosphorylation) makes them respond more readily, and for longer, to peripheral input. The up-regulation of receptors increases the number, and possibly the type, of receptors available to respond to input. The dorsal horn cells also release retrograde signals, which include small gasses such as nitric oxide and carbon monoxide, or lipids such as arachidonic acid derivatives. Retrograde signals travel in the opposite direction to conventional signals, passing from post-synaptic to pre-synaptic neurons, where they induce increased synthesis and release of neurotransmitters by the peripheral nociceptors. The dorsal horn cells increase their receptive fields and respond more vigorously to noxious stimulation, producing hyperalgesia (an increased response to a painful stimulus). Although these changes are at a spinal level, they appear to be influenced by the state of the limbic system, via unspecified descending pathways. The posterior cingulate gyrus is involved in the memory of somatosensory events. If the gyrus is anaesthetised prior to a transiently painful event, longer-term noxious activity in the spinal cord is prevented. Emotion and attention can influence activity in the cingulate gyrus, so presumably a patient's beliefs could alter the state of the cingulate gyrus prior to a painful event such as surgery.

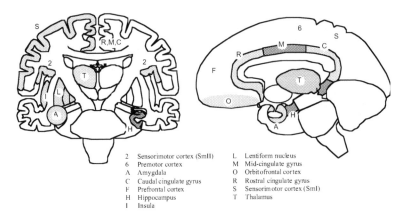

2	Sensorimotor cortex (SmII)	L	Lentiform nucleus
6	Premotor cortex	M	Mid-cingulate gyrus
A	Amygdala	O	Orbitofrontal cortex
C	Caudal cingulate gyrus	R	Rostral cingulate gyrus
F	Prefrontal cortex	S	Sensorimotor cortex (SmI)
H	Hippocampus	T	Thalamus
I	Insula		

Fig. 2.1. Coronal and saggital views of forebrain demonstrating some areas responding to noxious stimulation.

Rostrally, painful stimulation reaches several forebrain areas (Derbyshire et al 1997), each of which could be influenced by cognitive processes and therefore mediate aspects of the placebo response (Fig 2.1). The *amygdala* is involved in fear avoidance and suppression of its activity could enhance behaviour previously avoided because of fear of pain. The *hippocampus* is involved in assimilating contextual cues, some of which could signal danger. The *mid-cingulate gyrus* is involved in response selection during divided attention tasks. The *rostral part of the cingulate gyrus* is associated with affect, eliciting fear and sadness. The *thalamus* is the major route to the cortex. *Medial and anterior thalamic nuclei* responded differentially to higher levels of pain and contribute to the motivational-affective component of pain served by the medial pain system. *Lateral thalamic nuclei* convey sensory information to the cortex. The *thalamus* could act as an active filter preventing painful information from reaching the cortex and also reducing affective responses. The *insula*, receiving input from most nociception-responsive cortical areas and projecting to the amygdala, is well situated to perform a key role in integrating affective and reactive components of pain. The *lentiform nucleus* is associated with planned action and movement, possibly as a component of escape behaviour. Some *prefrontal cortical areas* (areas 10 and 46, and areas 44 and 45) are activated by noxious stimulation. These areas contribute to behavioural planning, attention, working memory and speech. The *inferior parietal area* (area 40) is responsible for preconscious orientation to incoming stimuli. The *premotor cortex* is involved in elaborating movement strategies. Complex changes occur in the *somatosensory cortex*. Treatment strategies that redirect attention, reinterpret painful stimuli and select alternative emotional and behavioural responses could act at any of these levels, as could placebo-inducing techniques. The widespread distribution of responses to pain graphically emphasises the multidimensional nature of the experience and indicates several processes that could be influenced by placebo mechanisms.

It is increasingly clear that chronic painful states have more to do with the central nervous system than with peripheral tissues. Harris (1999) has suggested that some chronic painful conditions could be the result of discordance generated by mismatch between sensory input and motor output. He reviews several lines of evidence, particularly involving phantom limb pain and repetitive strain injury.

By means of a simple mirror box, amputees experiencing phantom limb pain can be shown an image of their intact hand reflected to appear as the missing hand (Ramachandran et al 1996). Visual feedback from the moving intact hand enabled patients to 'move' their apparently restored phantom hand, thereby relieving pain. Thus the belief that the image was of their missing limbs was responsible for the effect, providing an insight into how placebo mechanisms could work through altering cortical representations.

In repetitive strain injury, cortical maps degrade with large overlapping fields of cortical cells representing the hand and loss of discrete mapping of individual fingers. Skilled movements such as typing are usually performed rapidly and without visual monitoring. The degradation of cortical representation may be the result of completion of efferent commands before afferent signals from individual fingers return to the cortex, together with an absence of visual feedback. Afferent activity from the first finger to make contact will still be travelling towards the cortex when efferent activity to the last finger is already on its way to the periphery. The brain then associates the afferent activity returning from the first finger with the efferent activity departing towards the last finger: the difference between fingers becomes blurred. Typically, visual feedback will be missing because a skilled movement is usually performed without visual monitoring: a skilled typist does not look at his or her fingers while typing. As a result, all the feedback relates to all of the efferent commands, corrupting the representation. In humans, there is a corresponding loss of kinaesthesia, stereoacuity and graphaesthesia (Byl et al 1996, Byl & Melnick 1997). The cortical representation of fingers in musicians (Elbert et al 1998) and others (Bara-Jimenez et al 1998) with focal dystonia shows similar overlap to that obtained in monkeys. Harris (1999) has suggested that incongruence between movement and proprioceptive feedback results in pain. As cortical maps can be altered by experience, even in humans (Sterr et al 1998), treatment could be directed towards refining cortical maps, thereby relieving pain (Byl & Melnick 1997, Bara-Jimenez et al 1998). As cortical maps can be activated by imagined movements as well as by real movements, thinking about the involved part might produce similar changes. Thus thoughts about moving a part, perhaps relatively immobilised by pain, could alter its cortical map, relieve the pain and therefore actually permit real movement. Belief that a treatment will work might encourage such thoughts and thereby become self-fulfilling. Beliefs about improved health could possibly improve other aspects of wellness besides movement, if a change in the cerebral areas involved had access to effector systems such as endocrine, autonomic and neuro-immunological targets. This is an area clearly in need of investigation. Which parts of the brain are differentially active when feeling well or unwell, for example?

Flor (2000) has reviewed some quite remarkable studies of reorganisation on cortical maps in phantom limb pain. Using electrical stimulation requiring a discriminative response, her group was able to show changes in cortical sensory maps. Instead of just experiencing stimulation of the stump, subjects had to distinguish one stimulus from another. This discrimination of stimuli requires cortical activity and is crucial to the success of the method; passive sensory experience was insufficient to achieve the effect. In other words, it is the active participation of the cortex in a task, not passive response to an external input, that effects the change; any competent teacher will be familiar with the truth of this proposition when applied to student learning. Flor (2000) also demonstrated the objectively detectable effects of social and psychological interventions on the experience of pain and on cortical maps. These are very convincing studies of the biological reality of psychosocial interventions.

Benedetti and Amanzio (1997) have reviewed the neurobiology of placebo. They review papers indicating that situational anxiety affects placebo-induced tolerance of pain whereas trait anxiety does not. In other words, people who are anxious specifically because of the situation will demonstrate placebo effects, whereas those who are generally anxious regardless of the situation will not. They also cite papers showing that suggestion can alter the effects of adrenaline, amphetamine and other drugs. In particular, they review the interaction between placebo effects, opioid analgesic systems and cholecystokinin (a hormone in the gastrointestinal tract but a neurotransmitter in the nervous system as well). They point out that naloxone, an opioid antagonist, has little effect on low-stress experimental pain, but enhances high-stress pain, which indicates that opioid analgesic systems are activated particularly when there is situational anxiety. Sufficiently complex experimental designs, which include hidden (naloxone or saline) and overt (saline placebo) injections demonstrated that there is an opioid component in placebo analgesia (see also Ch. 1). The opioid analgesic system is antagonised by cholecystokinin. Consequently, proglumide, which blocks cholecystokinin-A (CCK-A) receptors, removes this antagonism and enhances opioid analgesia. It also blocks the anxiogenic effects of CCK-4 and CCK-8. Proglumide, a cholecystokinin antagonist, enhanced the effectiveness of placebo in both experimental ischaemic arm pain and in post-operative thoracotomy pain.

Thus, cholecystokinin evokes anxiety, blocks opioid analgesia and enhances pain. Placebo works best if there is situational anxiety. It works partly through an opioid analgesic mechanism and is to that extent blocked by naloxone. Because cholecystokinin reduces the effect of opioid analgesic mechanisms and opioid mechanisms account for part of the placebo effect, cholecystokinin antagonists enhance placebo effects.

Several analgesic procedures that are effective, but nevertheless comparable to placebo, appear to act through the periaqueductal grey matter (an area in the brain stem). For example, transcutaneous electrical stimulation, acupuncture and hypnosis when administered under stressful conditions are analgesic, as is direct stimulation of the periaqueductal grey matter. Some placebo effects are also achieved through this system. Naloxone is capable of blocking all of these, suggesting that they may all be acting through a common mechanism. Among the areas of the brain known to be activated by painful stimulation, several project to the periaqueductal grey matter, either directly or through the amygdala. Thus, the *orbitofrontal* and *medial frontal cortex*, involved in psychosocial and affective responses; the *insula*, situated en route between sensory regions and limbic regions; the *amygdala*, responsible for fear, anger and associated autonomic and endocrine responses to threat, all have projections to the periaqueductal grey matter. From there, access to descending analgesic systems via the rostral ventromedial medulla and the dorsolateral tracts is well established. It follows that many procedures and factors that are often regarded as rather nebulous and frequently dismissed as ineffective have well-established anatomical routes into bona fide analgesic systems. The nebulous nature and complexity of these factors is probably due to the indiscreet organisation of the medial defence systems, which are anatomically highly interlinked (Lawes 1990). (The nuclei belonging to these peri-ventricular systems all lie in contact with the ventricles; they all connect either directly with each other or via one other member of the group; they are all phylogenetically ancient; and they mediate behavioural escape or avoidance of noxious situations (Lawes 1990)).

The difficulty of demonstrating that the above procedures are more effective than placebo may therefore result from shared mechanisms of action: placebo is another way of activating the same system, so how would much difference arise? *Thus failure to demonstrate superiority over placebo need not imply lack of efficacy; it may imply only similarity of mechanism.* Comparison of such a treatment with placebo would therefore not be a comparison of two mechanisms, only a comparison of their ability to activate the same mechanism, perhaps involving the periaqueductal grey matter, for example. Morphine, perhaps one of the most efficacious of analgesics, works through this system.

It seems that there are multiple mechanisms available to explain the actions of placebos. Expectation, conditioned learning, immunological, endocrine and neurological mechanisms have all been documented. Within the nervous system, effects are detected at spinal, thalamic, neocortical and limbic levels. Some placebo effects are mediated by activation of the analgesic system originating in the periaqueductal grey matter. Interactions between enkephalinergic and cholecystokinin systems deserve attention. Several other analgesic processes including the administration of morphine share the descending analgesic system. This confounds comparison with placebo control groups. Another mechanism of increasing prominence is the change in cortical representation of the body, an obvious target for therapeutic intervention, given the functional plasticity at this level.

Conclusion

In conclusion, although the word 'placebo' took on pejorative connotations when insincere mourners were paid to sing the placebo (church vespers) in the 14th century (Stefano et al 2001), placebo effects are very potent. They are not equivalent to absence of treatment and it is no great defect for an active treatment to be only as effective as placebo. The objections raised by ethicalism to the scientific study of placebos are based largely on misconceptions, rather than on legitimate ethical qualms. Placebos act in a rational manner through the nervous system and have objective, measurable effects on the tissues and systems that promote health. Similarly, nocebo effects impair these systems. Clinicians should become familiar with the factors that promote placebo responses and should openly exploit these mechanisms. As placebos really do work, there is no deception, although *many patients may have to be educated about the potency of their own thought processes as healing agents.* Perhaps a first step in the rehabilitation of placebo strategies would be to change the common definition of placebos—which is that they have no specific effects, hardly applicable in the light of the above evidence. *Perhaps a better definition of placebos is that they are therapeutic agents that achieve their effects through the beliefs of the patients (and their clinicians).*

REFERENCES

Ader R, Cohen N 1991 Conditioning the immune system. Netherlands Journal of Medicine 39:263–273

Amanzo M, Benedetti F 1999 Neuropharmacological dissection of placebo analgesia: Expectation-acitvated opioid systems versu conditioning-activated subsystems. Journal of Neuroscience 19(1):484–494

Bara-Jimenez W, Catalan MJ, Hallett M, Gerloff C 1998 Abnormal somatosensory homunculus in dystonia of the hand. Annals of Neurology 44:828–831

Beecher HK 1955 The powerful placebo. Journal of the American Medical Association 159:1602–1606.

Benedetti F, Amanzio M 1997 The neurobiology of placebo analgesia: From endogenous opioids to cholecystokinin. Progress in Neurobiology 52(2):109–125

Benedetti F, Amanzo M, Baldi S, Casadio C, Maggi G 1999 Inducing placebo respiratory depressent responses in humans via opioid receptors. European Journal of Neuroscience 11(2):625–631

Benjamin LS 1963 Statistical treatment of the law of initial values (LIV) in autonomic research: A review and recommendation. Psychosomatic Medicine 25:556–566

Benson H, Friedman R 1996 Harnessing the power of the placebo effect and renaming it 'remembered wellness'. Annual Review of Medicine 47:193–199

Benson H, McCallie DP 1979 Angina pectoris and the placebo effect. New England Journal of Medicine 300:1424–1429

Bergmann JF, Chassany O, Gandiol J, Deblois P, Kanis JA, Segresta JM, Caulin C, Dahan R 1994 A randomised clinical trial of the effect of informed consent on the analgiesic activity of placebo and naproxen in cancer pain. Clinical Trials and Meta-analysis 29:41–47

Berthelot J-M, Maugers Y, Abgrall M, Prost A 2001 Interindividual variations in beliefs about the palcebo effect: A study in 300 rheumatology inpatients and 100 nurses. Joint Bone Spine 68(1):65–70

Beta-Blocker Heart Attack Trial Research Group 1984 A randomised trial of propranolol in patients with acute myocardial infarction. New England Journal of Medicine 311:552–559

Blackwell B, Bloomfield SS, Buncher CR 1972 Demonstration to medical students of placebo responses and non-drug factors. Lancet 1:1279–1282

Blanz M 1990 Ethical and legal aspects of the use of placebos in research and practice. Fortschritte der Neurologie-Psychiatrie 58:167–174

Bouckoms A, Hackett TP 1991 The pain patient. In: Cassem NH (ed) Massachusetts General Hospital Handbook of General Hospital Psychiatry. Mosby, St. Louis 44–45

Bourne HR 1978 Rational use of placebo. In: Melmon KL, Morelli HF (eds) Clinical Pharmacology: Basic principles in therapeutics. Macmillan, New York 1052–1062

Bovberg D, Cohen N, Ader R 1987 Behaviourly conditioned enhancement of delayed hypersensitivity in the mouse. Brain Behaviour and Immunity 1:64-71

Buckalew LW, Coffield KE 1972 An investigation of drug expectancy as a function of capsule colour and size and preparation form. Journal of Clinical Psychopharmacology 2:245–248

Butler C, Steptoe A 1986 Placebo response: An experimental study of asthmatic volunteers. British Journal of Clinical Psychology 25:73–83

Byl N, Wilson F, Merzenich M et al 1996 Sensory dysfunction associated with repetitive strain injuries of tendonitis and focal hand dystonia: A comparative study. Journal of Orthopaedic and Sports Physical Therapy 23:234–244

Byl NN, Melnick M 1997 The neural consequences of repetition: Clinical implications of a learning hypothesis. Journal of Hand Therapy 10:160–174

Coronary Drug Project Research Group 1980 Influence of adherence to treatment and response of cholesterol on mortality in the Coronary Drug Project. New England Journal of Medicine 303:1038–1041

Dark K, Peeke HVS, Ellman G, Salfi M 1987 Behaviourly conditioned histamine release. Annals of the New York Academy of Science 496:578–582

De Craen AJM, Roos PJ, de Vries AL, Kleijnen J 1996 Effects of colour of drugs: systematic review of perceived effect of drugs and of their effectiveness. British Medical Journal 313:1624–1626

De Craen AJM, Moerman DE, Heisterkamp SH, Tytgat GNJ, Tijsen JGP, Kleijneu J 2000 Placebo effect in the treatment of duodenal ulcer. British Journal of Clinical Pharmacology 48(6):853–860

De Craen AJM, Tijsen JGP, De Gans J, Kleijneu J 2000a Placebo effect in the acute treatment of migraine: subcutaneous placebos are better than oral placebos. Journal of Neuology 247(3):183–188

De Craen AJM, Lampe-Schownmaeckers AJEM, Kraal JW, Tijsen JGP, Kleijneu J 2001 Impact of experimentally-induced expectancy on the analgesic efficacy of tramadol in chronic pain patients: A 2x2 factorial, randomised, placebo-controlled, double-blind trial. Journal of Pain Symptom Management 21(3):210–217

Derbyshire SWG, Jones AKP, Gyulai F, Clark S, Townsend D, Firestone LL 1997 Pain processing during three levels of noxious stimulation produces differential patterns of central activity. Pain 73:431–445

Deyo RA 1991 Clinical research methods in low back pain. Physical Medicine and Rehabilitation 5:209–222

Dimond EG, Kittle CF, Crockett JE 1960 Comparison of internal mammary ligation and sham operation for angina pectoris. American Journal of Cardiology 5:483–486

Elbert T, Candia V, Altenmuller E et al 1998 Alteration of digitial representations in somatosensory cortex in focal hand dystonia. Neurology Report 9:3571–3575

Ernst E, Abbot NC 1997 Placebos in clinical practice: Results of a survey of nurses. Perfusion 10:128–130

Ernst E, Resch KL 1995 Concept of true and perceived placebo effects. British Medical Journal 311:551–553

Evans FJ 1985 Expectancy, therapeutic instructions, and the placebo response. In: White L, Tursky B, Schwartz GE (eds) Placebo: Theory, research and mechanisms. The Guilford Press, New York

Feldmen DC, Spencer CGC, Beevers M, Beevers DG, Lip GYH 2000 Placebo lowers blood pressure in isolated systolic hypertension but not in systolic/diastolic hypertension. American Journal of Hypertension Abstracts 13(4):120A

Fisher S, Lipman RS, Uhlenhuth EH, Rickels K, Park LC 1965 Drug effects and initial severity of symptomatology. Psychopharmacologia 7:57–60

Flaten MA, Simonsen T, Olsen H 1999 Drug-related information generates placebo and nocebo resonses that modify drug response. Psychosomatic Medicine 61(2):250–255

Flor H 2000 The functional organisation of the brain in chroinc pain. Progress in Brain Research 129:313–322

Freeman EW, Rickels K 1999 Characteristics of placebo resonses in medical treatment of pre-menstrual syndrome. American Journal of Psychiatry 156(9):1403–1408

Gelfand S, Ullman LP, Krasner LI 1963 The placebo response: An experimental approach. Journal of Nervous and Mental Disease 136:379–387

Goetz CG, Leurgens S, Ramn R, Stebbins GT 2000 Objective changes in motor function during placebo treatment in PD. Neurology 54(3)710–714

Gracely RH, Dubner R, Wolskee PJ, Deeter WR 1983 Placebo and naxalone can alter post-surgical pain by separate mechanisms. Nature 306:264–265

Hahn RA 1985 A sociocultural model of illness and healing. In: White L, Tursky B, Schwartz GE (eds) Placebo: Theory, Research and Mechanisms. The Guilford Press, New York

Harris AJ 1999 Cortical origin of pathological pain. Lancet 354:1464–1466

Hashish I, Hai HK, Harvey W, Feinman C, Harris M 1988 Reduction of postoperative pain and swelling by ultrasound: A placebo effect. Pain 33:303–311

Hennekens CH, Buring JF 1987 Epidemiology in Medicine. Little Brown, Boston

Husband AJ, King MG, Brown R 1987 Behaviourly conditioned modification of T cell subset ratios in the rat. Immunology Letters 14:91–94

Kaptchuk TJ 1998 Intentional ignorance: A history of blind assessment and placebo controls in medicine. Bulletin of the History of Medicine 72(3):389–433

Kienle GS, Kiene H 1997 The powerful placebo effect: fact or fiction? Journal of Clinical Epidemiology 50:1311–1318

Kroenke K, Mangelsdorff D 1989 Common symptoms in ambulatory care: incidence, evaluation, therapy, and outcome. American Journal of Medicine 86:262–326

Lawes INC 1990 The origin of the vomiting response: A neuroanatomical hypothesis. Canadian Journal of Physiology and Pharmacology 68:254–259

Liberman R 1964 An experimental study of the placebo response under three different situations of pain. Journal of Psychiatric Research 2:233–246

Lima MS, Montcrief J 1999 Drugs versus placebo for the treatment of dysthymia (Cochrane Review). The Cochrane Library Issue 3

Luparello T, Leist N, Lourie CH, Sweet P 1970 The interaction of psychologic stimuli and pharmacologic agents on airway reactivity in asthmatic subjects. Psychosomatic Medicine 32:509–513

MacQueen G, Marshall J, Perdue M, Siegel S, Bienenstock J 1989 Pavlovian conditioning of rat mucosal mast cells to secrete rat mast cell protease II. Science 243:83–85

McQuay H, Carroll D, Moore A 1996 Variation in the placebo effect in randomised controlled trials of analgesics: All is as blind as it seems. Pain 64:331–335

Moerman DE 1983 General medical effectiveness and human biology: Placebo effects in the treatment of ulcer disease. Medical Anthropology Quarterly 14(4):13–16

Montgomery SA 1999 The failure of placebo controlled studies. European Neuropsychopharmacology 9:271–276

Montgomery SA, McIntyre A, Osterherider M, Sarteschi P, Zitterl W, Zohar J, Birkett M, Wood AJ 1993 A double-blind, placebo-controlled study of fluxetine in patients with DSM-III-R obsessive compulsive disorder. European Neuropsychopharmacology 3:143–152

Moore A, Collins S, Carrroll D, McQuay H 1997 Paracetamol with and without codeine in acute pain: A quantitative systemic review. Pain 70:193–201

Niklson IA, Reimitz PE, Sennef C 1997 Factors that influence the outcome of placebo-controlled antidepressant clinical trials. Psychopharmacology Bulletin 33:41–51

Oh VMS 1994 The placebo effect: can we use it better? British Medical Journal 309:69–70

Okpako D T 1999 Traditional African medicine: theory and pharmacology explored, Trends in Pharmacological Sciences 20(12):482-485

Pledger GW, Hall D 1986 Active control trials: Do they address the efficacy issue? Proceedings of the American Statistics Society 1–10

Ramachandran VS, Rogers-Ramachandran D 1996 Synaesthesia in phantom limbs induced with mirrors. Proceedings of the Royal Society London [Biological Sciences] 263:377–386

Rochon PA, Binns MA, Litner JA, Litner GM, Fischbach MS, Eisenberg D, Kaptchuk TJ, Stason WB, Chalmers TC 1999 Are randomised control trial outcomes influenced by the inclusion of a placebo group? A systematic review of nonsteroidal antiinflammatory drug trials for arthrits treatment. Journal of Clinical Epidemiology 52(2):113–122

Rothman KJ, Michels KB 1994 The continuing unethical use of placebo controls. New England Journal of Medicine 33:394–397

Shapiro AK, Shapiro E 1984 Patient-provider relationships and the placebo effect. In: Matarazzo JD, Herd JA, Miller NE, Weiss SM (eds) Behavioural Health: A handbook of health enhancement and disease prevention. Wiley-Interscience, New York 371–383

Shetty N, Friedman JH, Kieburtz K, Marshall FJ, Oakes D 1999 The placebo response in Parkinson's disease. Clinical Neuropharmacology 22(4):207–212

Solvason HB, Ghanta VK, Hiramoto RN 1988 Conditioned augmentation of natural killer cell activity. Independence from nociceptive effects and dependence on interferon-b. Journal of Immunology 140:661–665

Spangfort EV 1972 The lumbar disc herniation: A computer-aided analysis of 2504 operations. Acta Orthopaedica Scandinavia 142(S):1–95

Stassen HH, Delini-Stula A, Angst J 1993 Time course of improvement under antidepressant treatment: A survival-analytical approach. European Neuropsychopharmacology 3:127135

Stassen HH, Angst J, Delini-Stula A 1994 Severity of baseline and onset of improvement in depression. Metaanalysis of imipramine and moclobemide versus placebo. European Psychiatry 9(3):129–136

Stefano GB, Fricchione GL, Slingsby BT, Benson H 2001 The placebo effect and relaxation response: Neural processes and their coupling to constitutive nitric oxide. Brain Research Reviews 35:1–19

Sternbach RA 1964 The effects of instructional sets on autonomic responsivity. Psychophysiology 1:67–72

Sterr A, Muller MM, Elbert T, Rockstroh B, Pantev C, Taub E 1998 Perceptual correlates of changes in cortical representation of fingers in blind multifinger Braille readers. Journal of Neuroscience 18:508–520

Suchman AL, Ader R 1992 Classic conditioning and placebo effects in crossover studies. Clinical Pharmacology and Therapeutics 52:372–377

Sutherland LR, May GR, Shaffer EA 1993 Sulfasalazine revisited: A meta-analysis of 5-aminosalicyclic acid in the treatment of ulcerative colitis. Annals of Internal Medicine 118:540–549

Thase ME 1999 How should efficacy be evaluated in randomised clinical trials of treatments for depression? Journal of Clinical Psychiatry 60:23–31

Thomas KB 1987 General practice consultations: Is there any point in being positive? British Medical Journal 294:1200

Thomson R 1982 Side effects and placebo amplification. British Journal of Psychiatry 140:64–68

Turner JA, Deyo RA, Loeser JD, von Korff M, Fordyce WE 1994 The importance of placebo effects in pain treatment and research. Journal of the American Medical Association 271:1609–1614

Voudouris NJ, Peck CL, Coleman G 1989 Conditioned response models of placebo phenomena: Further support. Pain 38:109–116

Voudouris NJ, Peck CL, Coleman G 1990 The role of conditioning and verbal expectancy in the placebo response. Pain 43:121–128

Wasserman SS, Kotloff KL, Losonsky GA, Levine MM 1993 Immunologic response to oral cholera vaccination in a crossover study: a novel placebo effect. American Journal of Epidemiology 1:988–993

Watkins AD 1994 Heirarchical cortical control of neuroimmunomodulatory pathways. Neuropathology and Applied Neurobiology 20:423–431

Whitney CW, von Korff M 1992 Regression to the mean in treated versus untreated chronic pain. Pain 50:281–285

Wickramasekera I 1985 A conditioned response model of the palcebo effect: Predictions from this model. In:. White L, Tursky B, Schwartz GE (eds) Placebo: theory, research and mechanisms. Guilford Press, New York 255–287

3

Placebo and the therapeutic alliance

MITCH NOON

The interdisciplinary treatment of acute and chronic pain problems has extended the remit of physical therapy and led to the emergence of new roles and skills for physiotherapists. This has important implications for the relationship between physiotherapist and patient. As physiotherapy becomes more explicitly a biopsychosocial process, so the psychosocial skills of physiotherapy require expansion and development.

This chapter examines the notion of the placebo effect and its relationship to the therapeutic alliance. The latter is a term from the psychological literature that is usually associated with psychological therapies. However, in this chapter, I will suggest that the same principles are relevant to the practice of a range of clinical specialties, including physical therapy. The aim is to consider the extent to which lessons learnt from the placebo effect can inform our understanding of the therapeutic alliance, and how this, in turn, can also inform psychosocial aspects of patient care. I will begin with a review of the placebo effect and then consider the implications for the development of a therapeutic alliance between clinician and patient.

The placebo effect

Traditionally, placebos have been used in drug studies as a means of controlling for non-specific factors in treatment. One of the most remarkable characteristics of placebos is how potent they appear to be. Oh (1994) suggests that placebos work best with pain conditions, disorders of the autonomic nervous system, and processes under neurohumoral control. Ross and Olsen (1981) list evidence of efficacy in: '...the treatment of radiation sickness, dental pain, headaches, coughing, asthmas, postoperative pain, multiple sclerosis, the common cold, diabetes, ulcers, arthritis, sea sickness, parkinsonism, and much more' (p. 409). Indeed, such ubiquitous effects have prompted O'Donnell (1995) to make the rather ironic comment that placebo is: 'the most effective medication known to science, subjected to more clinical trials than any other medicament yet (it) nearly always does better than anticipated. The range of susceptible conditions appears to be limitless.'

Shapiro (1961) defines placebo as 'any therapeutic procedure or that component of any therapeutic procedure which is given deliberately to have an effect or unknowingly has an effect on a patient, symptom, syndrome or disease but is *objectively without specific activity* for the condition being treated' (my emphasis). However, the notion of 'objectively without specific activity' contains an ambiguity, and this reflects contrasting views of the placebo found in the literature. On the one hand, without specific activity is often taken to mean *inactive*, and on the other hand it is sometimes taken to refer to a *general* effect; in the latter case, the general effect may not be inactive, but may be very potent. In other words, there are two ways of characterising placebos, both of which are subsumed by the phrase 'without specific activity', and I hope to show that a closer understanding of this ambiguity is instructive.

There are some phenomena that look like the placebo effect, but are not. The placebo effect is not to be confused with fluctuation of symptoms, regression to the mean and spontaneous remission. Many medical conditions have a fluctuating pattern, or vary around some average level, and some conditions improve spontaneously. A placebo effect may sometimes wrongly be inferred from a coincidence of the placebo intervention with these natural patterns. There is also a danger of confusing apparently beneficial but non-specific outcome with compliance or desire to please: 'How are you today Mrs Brown?' 'Oh, very well thank you doctor'! Sometimes a patient in a placebo-controlled trial may be aware of the desired outcome and may, therefore, report benefit where no benefit has occurred. In addition, the placebo is not to be confused with the beneficial effects of additional treatment and/or improved medical care provided during an experimental study. In some research, both the specific treatment and placebo groups may be receiving additional elements to the treatment, such as extra attention or an increased quality of care. Consequently both the specific and placebo conditions comprise more than the standard treatment and comparisons with standard treatment may, therefore, be invalid. Finally, it is important to be aware that in some studies there may be an artefactual effect due to scaling bias in measuring subjective outcomes. Using a scale that has more grades for assessing improvement than for no improvement or worsening, presents a scaling bias. For example, in measuring pain relief from specific and placebo treatments, a common technique has been to use four equally spaced and weighted categories, where 1 = no relief, 2 = slight relief, 3 = moderate relief, and 4 = complete relief. As Tursky (1985) points out, both extreme categories are highly unlikely to apply: 'almost any treatment (real or imagined) will produce at least some indication of slight relief, and complete pain relief is almost never achieved by analgesics' (p. 232). This leaves just the two middle categories and these are not good discriminators of the degree of pain relief. It should not be considered surprising if a larger number of patients receiving the specific treatment score 3. In addition, bearing in mind the nature of placebo, a notable number of patients receiving the placebo treatment will also score 3. The significance of these findings, however, may just be an artefact of the scoring procedure.

Bearing in mind these caveats, the fact remains that, whichever way you look at it, the placebo effect is an extraordinary phenomenon. Ross and Olsen (1981) identify five different trends in the literature on the pharmacological placebo effect. The first is *direction of effect*. It appears that placebos tend to work in the same therapeutic direction as the specific treatment with which they are compared. So, for example, if a specific drug lowers blood pressure then the placebo control drug may also have an effect of lowering blood pressure. Alternatively, if it heightens blood pressure the same directional effect will occur with the placebo. Secondly, there is an *equivalence of strength* so that placebo compared with a strong analgesic such as morphine may provide relatively strong analgesia, while placebo compared with a weak analgesic such as aspirin may have a correspondingly modest effect. Thirdly, there is the issue of *side effects;* it seems that people in the placebo section of a drug trial often report the same side effects as those in the specific drug treatment. So for instance if someone taking the specific drug suffers from stomach problems or nausea or headaches, similar side effects may be reported amongst the placebo group. Fourthly, the *time course* of the placebo seems to mimic the time course of the specific drug. If the specific drug is relatively short lived, the placebo may be correspondingly relatively short lived; if it has a longer effect, so, too, may the placebo. Finally, the *therapeutic window* of the placebo seems to be the same as for the specific drug under comparison. In other words, the frequency with which you have to take a specific drug, to maintain a level within the system that is effective, seems also to apply to the placebo. If, with the placebo, you go outside the therapeutic window that applies to the specific comparison drug, then the placebo effect is less pronounced.

At first sight these are very remarkable characteristics of pharmacological placebos, and I will say more, below, about the explanation that has been proposed to account for these findings. For the time being, it is notable that they appear in many ways to mimic the specific drug for which they are intended as a control; and in this observation is an important element in understanding the nature of placebos: the placebo effect varies depending on the specific treatment with which it is being compared. Surely, if a placebo is simply an inert, inactive, process then it will have the same effect under all circumstances: it would not be expected to vary according to context. However, it is apparent from Ross and Olsen's (1981) observations that the placebo effect is very sensitive to context and *that* observation is extremely important.

Explanations of the placebo

To examine this more fully, we can now consider some of the explanatory models that have been provided for the placebo. In a general statement about explanatory models, Brody (1985) identifies three possibilities for explaining placebo effects.

First of all there is a possibility that the patient got better due to the natural history of the condition. This includes spontaneous remission, fluctuation of symptoms and regression to the mean, as mentioned above. In this case, a placebo effect may sometimes wrongly be ascribed to a coincidence of the placebo intervention with these natural patterns, and the placebo effect is, therefore, an illusion. The second possibility is that the patient got better due to some specific but unknown features of the treatment. We may not know what these are at present, but the placebo effect is a reflection of these undefined features. Accordingly, the task of science is to identify the specific and characteristic features of treatment more fully, and bring them within the ambit of scientific explanation, so that the treatment can be developed and refined. In time science will gain a fuller and clearer understanding of the processes involved and provide an explanation. Thus the ostensible placebo is, in fact, an active but unexplained treatment. The third possibility is that the placebo represents some kind of symbolic effect of treatment. As it stands this is a rather vague proposal. Nevertheless, Brody (1985) suggests that there is something in the treatment itself that has an impact on the imagination, beliefs, or emotions of the person receiving the treatment.

Now if we exclude the first level of explanation, since this is not the placebo effect, then we are left with two levels that are often portrayed as mutually exclusive: the placebo is either potentially objective and, therefore, not really a placebo, or it is 'all in the mind'. Those professionals working in the area of pain will be familiar with this kind of pernicious reasoning. The scientific level is held to be the respectable level of explanation, while the symbolic level is often relegated to the category of artefact. This legacy of mind-body dualism was also implicit in the ambiguity highlighted in Shapiro's definition of the placebo, above. However, an interesting question raised by these alternative levels of explanation is whether, in fact, effective treatment may encompass both levels. If there were a fully explicated and scientifically replicable theory of a particular treatment, would there, nevertheless, be scope for examining the symbolic level of the same treatment? To put it another way, does an understanding of the symbolic level add anything to the theory of the specific treatment? The thesis of this chapter is that an understanding of the symbolic level actually adds a great deal to our understanding of specific treatments, and that these two are not mutually exclusive explanations, but complementary to each other.

As a start, it is useful to consider some of the psychological explanations that have been proposed for placebos, since they address the potential symbolic elements in specific treatments. A number of suggestions have been made for psychological understanding of placebos.

The conditioning model

The basic conditioning paradigm is illustrated in Figure 3.1, and described by Wickramasekera (1985). In this example, an injection of acetylcholine causes lowering of blood pressure (hypotension). The injection is paired with a sound (a bell ringing). After several repetitions of this association, the sound alone is sufficient to elicit the physiological response of hypotension. The remarkable thing about conditioned responses of this kind is that even if the injected substance is then changed to, say, adrenaline, which heightens blood pressure, the conditioned response of hypotension persists. In effect, the physiological response to adrenaline is annulled due to the strong association of the sound and the original injection. This is the process of the generalisation of conditioning effects by *association*.

Analgesia provides a more pertinent example. It is suggested here that when people are given a placebo analgesic and report pain relief, this is not because of the placebo pill, it is because of a variety of different accompanying signs and signals such as white coats, the sounds and smells of the hospital environment, the sight of the stethoscope, an authoritative individual and so forth. These become conditioned in the patient's mind (learned) and associated with pain relief, so that in the same way that Pavlov's dogs began to salivate at the sound of a bell so some patients begin to feel better at the

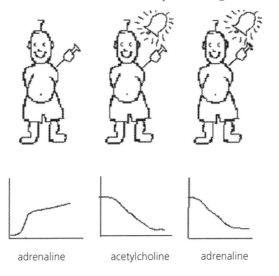

| adrenaline | acetylcholine | adrenaline |

Fig. 3.1 The classical conditioning model. The pictures show increase/decrease in blood pressure following injection of adrenaline/acetylcholine. In the first picture, adrenaline is shown to increase BP. In the second picture, acetylcholine, which decreases BP, is paired with the sound of a bell. After several exposures to this pairing, the sound of the bell would be enough to trigger a decrease in BP. Next, adrenaline is again administered to the same person, but the *decrease* in BP persists due to the learned association of the sound of the bell with decreased BP.

sight and sound and smell of the medical establishment. (Interestingly, some patients report the opposite effect, a nocebo effect, and become anxious and upset by associations of hospitals and medical interventions—for instance, white-coat hypertension.)

Conditioning theories have been much modified over the years (Price & Fields 1997) and in particular the current trends in psychological theory are rather more cognitive than behavioural. Accordingly, conditioning theories have been extended to incorporate cognitive elements such as expectation and motivation. If a patient seeks medical help then there is an expectation, which accompanies the help-seeking. Expectations, in turn, generate beliefs and beliefs can influence the course of healing.

Placebos and the reduction of anxiety

Alongside conditioning, there is the notion of anxiety reduction. This is most clearly illustrated in relation to pain. Pain is defined as: 'an unpleasant sensory and emotional experience associated with actual or potential tissue damage, or described in terms of such damage' (Merskey 1979). Pain can further be distinguished in terms of various dimensions, such as:

- **Sensation**: what the pain feels like (e.g. burning, stabbing, tearing)
- **Intensity**: how strong it is (e.g. VAS score)
- **Reactivity**: how unpleasant it is (e.g. miserable, depressing, unbearable) (Melzak & Torgenson 1971, Tursky 1976).

The broad distinction between sensory pain (sensation) and affective pain (intensity and reactivity) provides the basis for the anxiety reduction hypothesis of placebo. One of the earliest writers on the subject, Beecher (1959), proposed that placebos exert their effect on pain by reducing the emotional distress caused by the pain. Thus, the patient who responds positively to a sugar pill for pain, gains relief by virtue of a reduction in the affective component of the pain. Even if the sensory component remains untouched, the reduction in the affective component amounts to a reduction in the overall level of distress and correspondingly a reduction in symptoms. In addition, with developments in psychoneuroimmunology, we are also beginning to gain an understanding of mechanisms that might be involved whereby changes in emotional function also cause changes at the biological level (e. g. Evans et al 1997, Glaser & Kiercolt-Glaser 1994).

We can now relate this back to the characteristics described by Ross and Olsen (1981) and mentioned earlier. An appreciation of the principles of conditioning and expectancy enables a fuller understanding of the factors underlying the five trends they described. Ross and Olsen (1981) argue that the reason there is such congruence between specific and placebo treatments is that, in both cases, there is explicit or implicit communication between the clinician and the patient. Clinicians in experiments who are blind to the specific or placebo condition will nevertheless be administering both the specific and placebo drug. They may not know which it is at a particular time, however, what they do know is that the specific drug has certain characteristics. It has a time course, it has a therapeutic window, it has side effects, it has strength and potency and so forth and in both the specific and placebo condition they will, explicitly or implicitly, provide cues to the patient about the nature of the specific treatment. Psychological explanations of placebos show how and why the patient is receptive to these cues. This is due to expectations based on past experience of medical treatments, alongside beliefs engendered by the implicit or explicit communication of the clinician.

And here we come to the central point: if you take these characteristics into account, it is possible to see the placebo effect as a result of an interaction between the clinician's and the patient's attitudes and beliefs. If there is a conjunction of shared attitudes and beliefs, then there is more likely to be an active effect, even from a placebo treatment. There is also an interesting corollary to this claim: if a conjunction of attitudes and beliefs can enhance the placebo effect, then a disjunction should *decrease* the probability of a placebo effect and increase the chances of a nocebo effect. There is, in fact, evidence in support of this latter claim. Furthermore, it appears that this may be true not only for placebo treatments, but also for specific treatments.

Evidence from the clinical literature

What is the evidence for the above claim? Here are two examples from the literature that are particularly vivid and interesting in relation to this question. The first addresses the above claim directly, and is to be found in an observation by Freund and colleagues (1971). They undertook a placebo evaluation of a specific treatment for weight loss. Their conclusion was that the specific drug under observation was indeed effective, and reduced weight. However, they also made an additional and very important observation about the circumstances in which the drug was administered. They reported:

> The eight physicians participating in the study were randomly selected from a resident population. They were then 'conditioned' to relate to the patients in a predetermined manner. Nevertheless, even under these standardised conditions, the first week's data demonstrated that the participating physicians were not uniformly capable of producing similar therapeutic results. This supports the long-held belief that physicians differ in the 'art of medicine' and in the quality of the 'bedside manner'…if either Doctor C or Doctor D had been the sole investigator…entirely different conclusions might have been reached as to the effectiveness of the test drug. Apart from the action of the drug and the patient's age, sex, education and social status, the effect of the physician's personality and the manner in which he related to the patients had a significant effect on therapeutic outcome. (p. 177)

Here is dramatic recognition of the importance not only of the drug, nor just of the patient's receptive state, but also of the clinician's attitude and capacity to relate to the patient. As Freund et al (1971) point out, this had a significant influence on outcome. It appears, then, that this supports the view that the presence or absence of shared beliefs between clinician and patient can indeed influence the relative efficacy of a demonstrably active treatment.

A second example, with a slightly different emphasis, comes from a study reported by Benson and McCallie (1979). They describe an investigation of surgery for angina with a technique known as internal mammary ligation. This procedure was originally used in cardiac surgery as a specific treatment for angina and involves re-routing the blood flow by tying one of the arteries. Internal mammary ligation was enthusiastically promoted as the specific treatment of choice for angina and a theoretical rationale was presented in terms of improvements in the blood flow, which reduced ischaemia. Numerous operations were performed with a high rate of apparent success: '...38 per cent found complete relief, and 65 to 75 per cent showed considerable improvement' (p. 1426). Later, however, more sceptical investigators performed the operation with a placebo control in which anaesthetic was given and an incision in the chest wall was made but without the ligation. In order to avoid negative expectancy in the patients, the surgeons maintained a 'reasonably optimistic' attitude when undertaking the placebo intervention. It transpired that the placebo procedure produced essentially the same outcome as the ligation procedure. The conclusion was that the efficacy of internal mammary ligation derived not from any direct physiological or biological changes, but from the enthusiasm of the clinicians undertaking the operation and the belief of the patients receiving it. Once again, the point here is that placebos must be understood in relation not just to patients and their expectations, psychological preparedness and so forth, but also in relation to the clinicians' attitude. This is crucial for the efficacy of both specific and placebo treatments.

The therapeutic alliance

The importance of the attitude and behaviour of the clinician also has a long history in psychotherapy research. Frank (1983) argues that the placebo effect '...contains the necessary, and possibly sufficient, ingredient for much of the beneficial effect of all forms of psychotherapy. This is a helping person who listens to the patient's complaints and offers a procedure to relieve them, thereby inspiring the patient's hopes and combating demoralisation.' (p. 291).

Thus, what has been termed the placebo may also be an important element in successful psychotherapy. But does this mean that psychological therapies are simply 'inactive' placebos? Not at all: Frank (1983) delineates the ingredients of the placebo as consisting of a clinician who is skilled in the art of helping. This, in turn, fosters the patient's receptiveness to the help offered. Bearing this in mind, it is possible to recast the notion of the placebo into alternative terminology. One candidate term would be *therapeutic alliance* (e.g. Luborsky 1988). This term describes the relationship between therapist and patient/client and the ingredients of this relationship. One of the reasons to reframe the notion of placebo within the terms of therapeutic alliance is that it allows us to move away from some of the negative connotations of placebos that have developed over the years.

The therapeutic alliance has been defined by Horvath et al (1993) as:

1. The client's perception of the relevance and potency of the intervention offered.
2. The client's agreement with the therapist on reasonable and important expectations of the therapy in the short and medium term.
3. A cognitive and affective component, influenced by the client's ability to forge a personal bond with the therapist and the therapist's ability to present himself or herself as a caring, sensitive and sympathetic, helping figure.

Horvath et al (1993) were interested in distinguishing between those aspects of psychological therapy that are specific, such as the technique of cognitive therapy compared with the technique of, say, analytic therapy; and those aspects of therapy that are non-specific or general, such as the nature of the relationship between therapist and client (the therapeutic alliance). In a meta-analytic study of a range of psychological therapies, they concluded that 26% of beneficial effects are attributable to the non-specific as opposed to the specific components. Interestingly, this percentage is close to that attributed to the placebo effect in a broad range of other contexts (e.g Beecher 1955). It must be noted, however, that Horvath et al (1993) provide an average effect size that, as with the figure of 33% provided by Beecher, represents a range of individual responses. Nevertheless, the important point for present purposes is that the therapist's belief in the efficacy of the intervention is taken as read. Thus the attitudes both of therapist *and* client are positive and this is the basis for the therapeutic alliance. Note also that in this case, the non-specific element is *not* inactive: quite the contrary.

This raises the question of the extent to which components of the therapeutic alliance can be developed within the realm of general clinical practice. It is important here to be clear about the distinction between specific techniques, which define a particular intervention, and non-specific or general characteristics that are common to a range of interventions. It is the latter characteristics that are relevant to general clinical practice, including the psychosocial aspects of physical therapy. While psychological approaches frequently address the therapeutic alliance explicitly, more traditional medical treatments have depended on the implicit presence of these characteristics: for instance, the perceived authority of the clinician, the patient's expectation of benign help and the power of the institution of medicine (e.g. Balint 1957, Parsons 1951). However, in the past, the emphasis appears to have been on the patient's expectations and receptiveness. The virtue of the therapeutic alliance is that it provides an emphasis on shared expectations between patient and clinician.

The next question is how the ingredients of the therapeutic alliance might be developed. The answer, I believe, is through the deliberate promotion

71

of, and training in, formal helping skills. In fact, it is very difficult in a clinical setting not to use helping skills. The question is not so much whether they are used, but how well. The degree of success of the therapeutic relationship depends not just on the degree of technical skill possessed by the clinician, but also on the extent to which he or she is able to develop an alliance: a collaborative relationship as the basis of treatment. The essential point is that a positive relationship needs to be established in order to maximise the intervention. However, positive relationships do not always happen spontaneously; sometimes they have to be fostered, and helping skills are the means by which a positive relationship can be developed and enhanced. I have described these skills in detail in Noon (1999). Briefly, they consist of:

- Good communication: listening skills, non-verbal communication, problem exploration and clarification.
- The development of trust through collaboration. This requires an understanding of the principles of motivation and the conditions for initiating and maintaining behaviour change (see Rollnick et al 1993).

Each of these, in turn, has a number of aspects that can be learned, practised and developed.

Conclusions

In summary then, let me review the points that have been made. Placebos have, in the past, been defined in two contrasting ways. From one perspective, they are viewed as an artefact of active treatment, in which case they represent a nuisance that needs to be explained away and that complicates our fuller understanding of what really is important, namely the specific ingredients of the treatment. From an alternative perspective, placebos can be seen to represent a non-specific, but active, component of effective treatment. In this case the question is how can we understand them more fully and what can we learn from them? The latter view has been adopted in this chapter. It has been suggested that psychological theories in terms of anxiety-reduction and expectation can help our understanding of the processes that take place within a therapeutic setting. Indeed, it is quite plausible to attribute much of the placebo effect to such variables as expectation of the patient and reduction of negative emotions. However I have also tried to emphasise that this is not just a process of passive conditioning in the patient: there is evidence that the attitude of the clinician too is fundamental to effective therapeutic practice. It has also been suggested that this is true not only in cases of the placebo effect but also in cases where fully explicated specific treatments are involved. The therapeutic alliance was introduced as a means of characterising the non-specific elements of a variety of effective treatments, and links were made between the therapeutic alliance and the placebo effect.

In summary, the therapeutic alliance can be defined as:

1. Non-specific: in the sense of being general to a range of effective treatments.
2. Active: in the sense of consisting of skills that can be learnt and developed.
3. Developed through collaboration, and consisting of a conjunction of the patient's and clinician's attitudes, beliefs and behaviour.

The patient must hold a belief in the potential of the treatment to help, in addition, however, the clinician must also share an equivalent belief and this must be expressed through his or her attitude or behaviour. Both sets of beliefs are founded on collaboration, not deception. The conjunction of these joint belief states gives rise to what elsewhere I have termed the joint *credebo* effect (Noon, 1999a): not 'I shall please', but 'I shall believe'—a requirement of both the clinician *and* the patient.

REFERENCES

Balint M 1957 The doctor, his patient and the illness. Pitman Medical, Tunbridge Wells

Beecher HK 1955 The powerful placebo Journal of the American Medical Association 176:1102–1107

Beecher HK 1959 Measurement of subjective responses: quantitative effect of drugs. Oxford University Press, New York

Benson H, McCallie DP 1979 Angina pectoris and the placebo effect. New England Journal of Medicine 300(25):1424–1429

Brody M 1985 Placebo effect: an examination of Grünbaum's definition. In: White L, Tursky B, Schwartz G E (eds) Placebo: theory research mechanisms. Guilford, New York

Evans P, Crow A, Hucklebridge F 1997 Stress and the immune system. The Psychologist 10(7):303–307

Frank J D 1983 The placebo is psychotherapy. Behavioural and Brain Sciences 6:291–292

Freund J, Krupp G, Goodenough D, Preston LW 1971 The doctor-patient relationship and drug effect. Clinical Pharmacology and Therapeutics 13(2):172–180

Glaser R, Kiercolt-Glaser JK 1994 Handbook of human stress and immunity. Academic Press, London

Horvath AO, Gaston L, Luborsky L 1993 The therapeutic alliance and its measures. In: Miller NE, Luborsky L, Barber JP, Docherty JP (eds) Psychotherapy Treatment Research: a handbook for clinical practice. Basic Books, New York

Luborsky L, Crits-Christoph P, Mintz J, Auerbach A 1988 Who Will Benefit From Psychotherapy? Basic Books, New York

Melzak R, Torgerson WS 1971 On the language of pain. Anaesthesiology 34:50–59

Merskey H 1979 International Association for the Study of Pain. Pain terms: A list with definitions and notes on usage. Pain 6:249–252

Noon JM 1999 Counselling and helping carers. British Psychological Society Books

Noon JM 1999a Placebo to credebo: The missing link in the healing process. Pain Reviews 6:133–142

O'Donnell M 1995 Our oath is hypocritical. Monitor Weekly 1:44

Oh VMS 1994 The placebo effect: can we use it better? British Medical Journal 309:69–70

Parsons T 1951 The Social System. Free Press, New York

Price D, Fields H 1997 The contribution of desire and expectation to placebo analgesia: implications for new research strategies. In: Harrington A (ed) The Placebo Effect: an interdisciplinary exploration. Harvard University Press, Cambridge MA 117–137

Rollnick S, Kinnersley P, Stott N 1993 Methods of helping patients with behaviour change. British Medical Journal 307:188–190

Ross M, Olsen JM 1981 An expectancy attribution model of the effects of placebos. Psychological Review 88(5):408–437

Shapiro AK 1961 Factors contributing to the placebo effect: Their implications for psychotherapy. American Journal of Psychotherapy 18:73–88

Tursky B 1976 Development of a pain perception profile. In: Weisenberg M, Tursky B (eds) Pain: New perspectives in therapy and research. Plenum, New York

Tursky B 1985 The 55% analgesic effect: real or artefact? In: White L, Tursky B, Schwartz GE (eds) Placebo: Theory research mechanisms. Guilford, New York

Wickramasekera I 1985 A conditioned response model of the placebo effect: predictions from the model. In: White L, Tursky B, Schwartz GE (eds) Placebo: Theory research mechanisms. Guilford, New York

4

The powerful placebo: hit or myth?

RICHARD SHORTALL

...a good myth is immune to attack.

Wall (1992) referring to the myth of personality defects in placebo responders

Introduction

I brought a bias for a number of ideas to the writing of this chapter. The first is that placebos have considerable power. This power has been demonstrated in many thousands of clinical trials and recounted in innumerable clinical anecdotes. Many of the modalities and techniques I use in my daily practice have failed to surpass placebos in clinical trials. Therefore much of my treatment effect might actually be the placebo effect and the modalities, props. Further, irrespective of the treatment used, patients derive great benefit from the inherent qualities of some clinicians—their personality, their 'bedside manner', their *modus operandi* seem to have some special curative properties.

Researching and writing this chapter has caused me to rethink these assumptions and to look at research that has measured or calculated the size of the placebo effect. I began to wonder whether the 'powerful placebo' is really as powerful as some argue, whether we should take a more critical look at the way authors select and cite evidence to support their positions on placebos, and to ask if the way scientific evidence is being used in rehabilitation medicine is sound.

The aims of this chapter are:

1. To present recent evidence that the therapeutic effect of placebos, *regardless of how they are defined or explained theoretically*, may not be as large as placebo proponents seem to believe.

2. To argue that if the placebo effect is clinically important then it deserves to be investigated properly and arguments for it supported by high quality trials specifically designed to investigate it.
3. To show that there are problems with the way authors and investigators of placebo effects select and cite evidence to support their arguments.
4. To suggest that authors should cite a small amount of high quality evidence rather than a large number of poorer quality articles.

Definition

We need to define what a placebo is and what it is not to ensure that the following discussion on placebo literature makes sense. Gøtzsche (1994) proposed the following definition:

> Placebo is an intervention that is believed to lack a specific effect—i.e., an effect for which an empirically supported theory exists for its mechanism of action—on the condition in question, but which has been demonstrated to be better than no intervention.

There seems to be some confusion about the word *specific*. Administration of a placebo to a given patient may appear to have a very specific effect, e.g. elevation of blood pressure, the production of a skin rash or elevation of the levels of a specific neurotransmitter, but the *same* sugar pill given to another patient, or even to the same patient in another context, is likely to have completely different 'specific' effects. Irrespective of how 'specific' the effect seems to be in a particular patient, it is difficult to defend the argument that a pill that has different effects on different people in different contexts has a 'specific' effect.

Shapiro and Shapiro (1997) defined placebos as follows:

> A placebo is any therapy (or that component of any therapy) that is intentionally or knowingly used for its *nonspecific*, psychological, or psychophysiological, therapeutic effect, or that is used for a presumed specific therapeutic effect on a patient, symptom, or illness but is *without specific activity for the condition being treated*.
>
> A placebo, when used as a control in experimental studies, is a substance or procedure that is without specific activity for the condition being treated.
>
> The placebo effect is the nonspecific psychological or psycho-physiological therapeutic effect produced by a placebo.

According the Shapiros' definitions placebos may be either inert or active but they must be inactive in respect of the condition being treated. The definition does not elaborate on the difficulties inherent in proving that 'placebo effects' witnessed or felt after the administration of a placebo are really attributable to the placebo—a problem discussed later in more detail. This definition is quoted in its entirety because it separates the placebo (a thing or procedure) on the one hand from its *effect* and its *mechanism* of effect on the other. This distinction is important because many writers contend that the therapeutic effect of placebos is considerable (e.g. see Wall 1994, Spiro 1986, Shapiro & Shapiro 1997). The results of placebo controlled trials and their derivative meta-analyses are often cited in support of elaborate theoretical explanations for this effectiveness. Shapiro and Shapiro (1997) do not specify the mechanism of placebo action in their definition because, in their own words: 'None of these mechanisms [cited specifically as expectation, transference, conditioning, mobilization of hope, faith etc.] have been experimentally verified' (1997 p. 37).

Spiro (1986 pp. 12–13) differentiated between a *trial* placebo given to keep both blinded patient and blinded clinician in ignorance of the nature of the intervention and the *clinical* placebo given to a patient as part of therapy. This is an important distinction, as it is likely that the 'powerful placebo' administered by clinicians in the field is more likely to consist of social interaction with the patient and the psychological effects this interaction has on the patient rather than a 'dummy pill' or a sham procedure (see Box 4.1).

Box 4.1. Events in the patient-clinician interaction

Patient's condition requires attention
—Patient visits clinician

The 'psychosocial placebo'
—a component of all clinical interactions
—independent of whether pill is real or 'dummy'
- Opportunity to give history
  - Conditioned responses elicited
- Clinician's concern
- Patient's expectations
- Clinician's knowledge
  - Response to clinician's explanation and expertise
- Anticipation of improvement in condition

Intervention options
- 'Active' medication
- Advice and education
- None (refer on)
- Surgery or other 'active' intervention
- Placebo or 'dummy pill' (considered to be pharmacologically inert)
  - Treatment believed to be active by clinician

Outome
- No change
- Change in patient's condition
  - Is change clinically relevant?

Outcome partition
—? Proportion of the outcome
- Attributable to administered substance/procedure?
- Attributable to social interaction?
- Attributable to 'disease variation' and related factors?

The term 'dummy pill' is used synecdochically throughout this chapter. It should be taken, in context, to mean sugar pills, injections of saline, so-called 'placebo-surgical procedures', acupuncture needles not placed on acupuncture points, or ultrasound or laser machines that have been surreptitiously disconnected or otherwise rendered therapeutically impotent.

Some of the placebo literature is imprecise because it fails to clarify the events of the patient/clinician interaction and separate this interaction from the placebo itself. In Box 4.1 I have separated the act of administering an actual treatment or placebo to a patient from all the other events of the clinician/patient interaction. The opinion here is that much of what we regard as the placebo effect takes place separately from the actual administration of any treatment and is probably not dependent on whether the treatment is 'real' or a placebo. The contention here is that the 'dummy pill' does not represent the essence of the placebo—the interaction with the clinician does. The dummy pill (and possibly even the real treatment in many cases) is a prop. In Box 4.1 I have given the effects of the patient/clinician interaction the label 'psychosocial placebo' and the effects of the administration of a placebo the label 'dummy pill'. The psychosocial placebo is important but its elements are poorly understood. They need to be researched systematically in high quality experimental and clinical trials. Picking apart the psychosocial placebo is likely to yield much clinically useful information. If we can identify the active components of the patient/clinician interaction, measure them, isolate them, and utilize them effectively in our consultations, we can maximize the effectiveness of our treatments.

Utilizing dummy pills allows us to focus on the importance of the qualities and skills of the clinician to the patient's progress and to separate these effects from those attributable to the chemical properties of a particular drug. The clinician is present whether the treatment is 'real' or 'dummy' so placebos can be used to help us to identify which clinician qualities and behaviours are best. Research that optimizes clinical skills is likely to have far-reaching and positive effects on patients. We can obtain much more useful information by using dummy pills to investigate clinicians than by marvelling at the observation that some patients have improved while taking pharmacologically inert substances.

The effect of a placebo

Examiners of a clinical effect should meet the following four requirements:

1. Establish that the effect really exists.
2. Try to work out its mechanism of action.
3. Measure or at least estimate its size.
4. Investigate whether the effect produces clinically relevant changes in patients' conditions.

The present chapter deals mostly with requirements 3 and 4. I have chosen to discuss the first and second requirements briefly as they are discussed in detail elsewhere in this and other volumes.

Does the effect really exist?

If we think of the placebo effect as the observation of improvement in patients who have been given a dummy pill then this effect has been demonstrated adequately in the literature. Some recent meta-analyses below illustrate this.

- Ferrari et al (2001) reviewed seven randomised controlled trials (RCTs) into the efficacy of rizatriptan for acute migraine headache. 71% of patients who received active treatment (rizatriptan) said their pain and other associated symptoms were reduced from 'severe' or 'moderate' to 'mild' or 'none', compared to 38% of placebo subjects (p<0.001).

- In another meta-analysis investigating the efficacy of various types of antidepressants for the treatment of chronic headache, Tomkins et al (2001) found that patients on 'active' treatments were twice as likely as patients taking placebos to report relief of headache (rate ratio[1] 2.0; 95% CI[2] 1.6–2.4). Treated patients also consumed significantly less analgesic medication.

- Browning et al (2001) reviewed the efficacy of the muscle relaxant, cyclobenzaprine hydrochloride for treating back pain. Patients treated with cyclobenzaprine were nearly 5 times (odds ratio[3] 4.7; 95% CI 2.7–8.1) as likely to report symptom improvement by day 14 as were those treated with placebo. The magnitude of this improvement was modest, (effect size of 0.38 to 0.58 in all 5 measured outcomes: local pain, muscle spasm, tenderness to palpation, range of motion, and activities of daily living).

- McQuay et al (1996) carried out a systematic review of antidepressants in the treatment of neuropathic pain. Patients with diabetic neuropathy who received active treatment (rather than placebo) were 3.6 times more likely to report significant improvement (>50% reduction in pain; odds ratio 3.6; 95% CI 2.5–5.2). In the post-herpetic neuralgia and atypical facial pain trials the corresponding odds ratios were 6.8 and 4.1. The authors concluded: 'Treatment would be improved if we could harness the dramatic improvement seen on placebo in some of the trials.'

In all of these meta-analyses the patients receiving placebos showed clinical improvement. However, rigorous critical thinking is just as important when making decisions about the efficacy of placebos as it is in decisions about the efficacy of 'active' treatments. Improvements observed *after* administration of a placebo are not necessarily attributable to the placebo. It is desirable to exclude all other possible explanations for observed improvements whether the intervention is 'active' or a 'dummy pill'. When we automatically assume that observed changes are due to treatments given, our thinking resembles superstitious thinking processes more than scientific ones.[4] In particular, clinicians enthused by the power of placebos should take care not to apply lower standards of critical thinking to their observations of placebo effects than they would to observations of the efficacy of 'active' treatments.

Three things can be said about the results of these meta-analyses:

1. Some patients improve while they are taking placebos—sometimes dramatically. Proponents of placebos should resist the temptation to attribute this solely to the placebos.

2. Not surprisingly, treatment with drugs containing active ingredients designed to target a specific disease seems generally to be more effective than treatment with placebos. A proportional relationship between active and placebo effects has even been proposed. Wall (1994 p. 1303) cited a review by Evans (1974) that found that the placebo response in analgesic trials was a fixed 55–60% of the active drug response—the stronger the drug, the greater the placebo response, even in so-called blinded trials. This means when patients are aware that the drug being investigated in their trial is a 'strong' drug they experience stronger analgesic effects after ingesting placebos in that trial compared to patients who participate in trials investigating drugs considered to be 'weaker'. Such is the power of suggestion. Wall (1994) concluded that placebo and 'therapeutic' effects are difficult to isolate from each other. McQuay et al (1995) however, attributed this apparent relationship to a statistical artefact caused by using an inappropriate measure of central tendency (the mean) for patient analgesic and placebo responses that are not normally distributed. These authors suggested the median as a more correct descriptor and found no significant relationship between the median 'drug' scores and median 'placebo' scores in their sample of trials.

3. The trials in these meta-analyses, like many similar trials used to support placebo theories, were designed to investigate the efficacy of drugs, not the efficacy of placebos.

Much placebo theorizing is supported by evidence derived from drug studies. There are two problems with citing these trials. First, they are trials of drugs—they are not specifically designed to test the efficacy of the placebos administered for control purposes. This is not optimal use of evidence to support theory. Secondly, these trials usually comprise two or more groups of patients all of whom are equally likely to have benefited from the mechanism outlined in Box 4.1 (the 'psychosocial placebo'). According to this mechanism, as both groups of patients have similar social interactions with clinicians, both groups have received what is substantially a 'placebo' treatment. It is generally agreed that the power of placebos lies in the elements of the 'psychosocial placebo' (see Box. 4.1). We have no reason to believe that 'dummy pills' have any intrinsic pharmacological effects. An inert pill hidden in a subject's food is only likely to have an effect if the subject knows about it and this effect may differ according to what (s)he has been told about the pill, how the information interfaces with the sum total of their life experiences, and even who is telling them and how they relay the information. We cannot hold the position that the psychosocial mechanism works only in the placebo arms of trials, when these elements are just as likely to be present in the 'active' treatment arms. Similar interaction is just as likely to occur between the patient and the clinician whether a pill is real or a 'dummy' one. In fact this is why placebo arms are mandatory in modern clinical trials. We need to learn more about the skills necessary to maximize the power of this interaction. To do this, we need to investigate the components of the 'psychosocial placebo' properly. More urgently we need to stop citing drug studies as if they were 'placebo studies'. Most placebo-controlled clinical trials that we encounter have not investigated the effects of placebos and their results are not the best evidence to support (or estimate) the placebo effect. This includes all the trials that were reviewed for the four meta-analyses cited above.

So called 'dummy pills' have been shown to bring about measurable physiological changes in patients (de la Fuente-Fernandez et al 2001, Kirsch & Weixel 1988, Lansky & Wilson 1981, Briddell et al 1978, Blackwell et al 1972). My opinion is that the true value of placebo research is not likely to be found here. It is likely to be found in the systematic investigation of the interaction between patient and clinician. If we wish to argue that the placebo effect is clinically significant and to develop explanatory theories that will withstand the test of experimentation, we need to develop placebo-controlled trials of treatments that 'control' for the treatment *and* the placebo. It follows from this argument that trials that specifically investigate the placebo effect (rather than the efficacy of a so-called 'active' treatment) and systematic reviews derived from these trials contain valuable information for placebo proponents and theorists. Some of these are outlined later. A simple experimental model for investigating placebos is to perform a drug study with matched groups who have equal contact with and standardized advice from health professionals. The study arms could comprise an 'active treatment' group, a 'placebo' group, and a third group that received no pill. The next phase of trials would identify those components of the clinician/patient interaction likely to affect clinical outcomes and manipulate these in controlled situations. Basically, you keep the 'drug' and the 'placebo' constant and vary the clinician. A study like this was carried out in the 1980s to investigate whether the doctor's 'positive' attitude (an attitude of optimism, reassurance that the treatment would help the patient) has an effect on treatment outcomes (Thomas, 1987). The placebo debate needs more studies like this.

Identify the mechanism of placebo action

Most clinicians have probably seen improvement in patients or trial subjects who received 'dummy' pills. As the placebo is 'inert' with respect to the condition being investigated or treated, the mechanism is likely to be of a psychosocial rather than a pharmacological nature. This is likely to be true even if the placebo induces physiological effects that closely resemble those of the 'real' drug being investigated. Another explanation is that humans display a highly heterogeneous set of responses to sugar!

Theorists attribute the placebo effect to a variety of psychosocial mechanisms activated by the interplay between clinician and patient (e.g. see Pollo et al 2001, Benedetti et al 1998). These mechanisms facilitate the establishment of a 'therapeutic alliance' between the clinician and the patient. They may involve conditioned responses (Vourdouris et al 1989, 1990, Montgomery & Kirsch 1997), patients' and clinicians' expectations (Wall 1994 p. 1304, Fillmore et al 1994, Turner et al 1994, Gracely et al 1985), behavioural mechanisms, learned behaviour or conditioned responses (Spiro 1986 p. 213, Amanzio & Benedetti, 1999), wellness behaviour, symbolism (Spiro 1986 p. 217), transference and the formation of a dyadic bond between the patient and the clinician (see also Chs 1–3).

Measurable physiological changes accompany these interactions that could explain the improvements so often observed in patients who have received placebos. But the placebo effect is not the sole property of purveyors of placebos. Clinicians who give their patients pharmacologically active treatments ('non-placebos') are no less likely to establish therapeutic alliances with them, to develop expectancies and conditioned responses in their patients, or to activate the powerful mechanisms attendant on the placebo effect. Thus these psychosocial mechanisms are not placebo mechanisms— they are 'treatment' mechanisms. It is likely that many are activated long before any treatment (real or dummy) is administered (see Box. 4.1) and continue to modify the treatment effect during and after its administration. In what must be a marvellously complex performance, the patient is the participating audience, the clinician is the performer, and the pill is the prop.

However placebo is defined, or its effects explained, it is unlikely to be simple. Spiro (1986) cites evidence that placebo effects differ between countries (Gudjonsson & Spiro 1978), between different geographical regions in the same country (MacDonald et al 1981), between clinicians (Sarles et al 1977), and even within the same clinician in different hospitals in the same city (Littman et al 1977). The inclusion of a placebo group in double-blinded clinical trials has even been shown to affect the rate at which subjects experience side effects and withdraw from a trial—even if they have received a placebo (Rochon et al 1999).

Estimate the size of the placebo effect

Thus, the powerful placebo turns out to be a fiction.

Kienle and Kiene 1997

Until recently, arguments about the effectiveness of placebos lacked definitive literature reviews. The New England Journal of Medicine recently published a systematic review of articles involving placebos (Hróbjartsson & Gøtzsche 2001). In an editorial on the paper, Bailar (2001) suggested the placebo effect may be a myth and likened it to the story of the Wizard of Oz. The Wizard was a myth because his power lay solely in people's belief that he was powerful. In reality, there was just an old man, with no supernatural powers, behind a curtain pretending to be a Wizard. Perhaps he goes too far in declaring the placebo effect a myth, but the evidence cited below supports the notion that some overestimation has occurred.

The statement that placebos are 30–35% effective has attained the status of self-evident truth (although estimates of placebo effect have soared as high as 75–80%, even 100%: Enserink 1999, Kienle & Kiene 1996).

Harrington (1997 p. 3) refers to the 'widely cited statistic 30–40%' of placebo responders, Morris (1997, cited in Harrington p. 188) warns us of a 'widespread myth that one-third of all patients are placebo responders'— Spiro (1986 p. 91) concurs. According to McQuay et al (2001), 'Medical folklore has it that the amount of relief obtained with placebo is one-third of the maximum possible (and does not vary) and that one-third of patients respond to placebo'. They then went on to demonstrate that even in high-quality double blind studies the placebo response (and response rate) varies considerably.

The 'one-third' estimate was quoted to me several times during my undergraduate education; each time accompanied by unabashed belief in its truth but unaccompanied by supporting research. The source of this number appears to be a 1955 article by Beecher (Kienle & Kiene 1996, Wall 1992). Beecher published a review of 15 studies investigating the effect of placebos on complaints such as the common cold (Diehl 1953), pain (Jellinek 1946), cardiac pain (Greiner et al 1950), antitussives (Hillis 1952), and toxic drug reactions (Wolf & Pinsky 1954). It is important to examine Beecher's (1955) review because it is probably the most frequently cited article in placebo literature. It is difficult to find a textbook chapter or review of placebo literature that does not cite this article. Scrutiny of Beecher's original article reveals three problems with his review:

1. None of these articles specifically investigated placebos or the placebo effect.
2. All the articles measured *differences from baseline* status of the patient's or subject's condition after administration of a placebo. Beecher attributed these changes to treatment or placebo interventions. None of these articles accounted for other possible explanatory factors.
3. He divided the number of patients who improved with placebo treatment by the total number of patients and came up with a 'percentage efficacy' for placebo. This does not account for subjects whose conditions deteriorated during the course of the reviewed trials. The average effect of placebo must be less than that estimated in these trials.

I have discussed the first point already with respect to placebo research in general.

With respect to the second point above, it is incorrect to attribute all changes of a patient's condition to clinical interventions[5] as it fails to take into account changes in the subjects' conditions that occur during a trial or between treatments (see Boxes 4.2 & 4.3) that are not attributable to the treatment. The design used in Beecher's reviewed trials could not differentiate between placebo effect and other uncontrolled effects such as the natural course of the condition and regression to the mean.[6]

83

Box 4.2 Beecher's evidence to support the 'Powerful Placebo' (from Kienle & Kiene 1997

- 35% of patients who received placebos in a placebo controlled trial of common cold treatment felt better within 6 days (2 days after placebo administration).

- Patients in 4 trials of post-operative pain had diminishing pain in the first few days after surgery whether they received placebos or not.

- In a placebo-controlled trial of angina pectoris medication, 72% of the placebo-treated patients deteriorated and 20% of the placebo-treated patients improved. A 20% placebo effect was claimed.

- He reported a 61% placebo effect in a trial of a hypertension drug in spite of the fact that there was no observed change in the blood pressure of the placebo group. However, 61% of the patients said they 'felt better'.

- In many of the trials the patients were known to be receiving other treatments in addition to both the active treatment being investigated and the placebo.

- In one morphine trial patients were treated alternately with placebo and morphine. Unsurprisingly, the placebo 'effect' diminished gradually with repeated administrations of placebo.

- In one of Beecher's own studies (Lasagne et al 1954) of severe post-operative pain he inferred a strong dose response relationship between placebo administration and 'wound pain'. Unfortunately, this was an inverse relationship: patients who received more doses had *less* reduction in pain.

Kienle and Kiene (1997) carried out a detailed re-evaluation of Beecher's methods and conclusions. They found *no* evidence in *any* of the original articles to support claims of a placebo effect. The observed outcomes in *all* the source trials could be 'fully, plausibly, and easily explained without presuming any therapeutic placebo effect' (Kienle & Kiene 1997).

When a change is seen which is thought to be a placebo effect we must differentiate the real placebo effect from the perceived placebo effect. In order to do this, the researcher (or clinician) must account for, or at least consider, *all other probable factors* that could have contributed to the subject's (or patient's) improvement (Ernst & Resch 1995). Once the effect of these factors (Box 4.3) has been subtracted, the true placebo effect is likely to be considerably smaller than the perceived placebo effect. Physiotherapists should include these factors in their clinical thinking algorithms when they are trying to explain improvements in their patient's condition. The related factors, regression to the mean and spontaneous variation of symptoms over time, probably influence this error most (Whitney & VonKorff 1992, McDonald & Mazzuca 1983).

Box 4.3: The difference between the true and the perceived placebo effect. Factors likely to cause a false impression of a placebo effect in the trials reviewed by Beecher (1955). Adapted from Kienle and Kiene 1997

Natural course of a disease
- Spontaneous improvement of symptoms
- Fluctuation of symptoms over time regardless of intervention
- Regression to the mean
- Habituation

Additional treatments obtained by the patient

Observer bias
- Patients switched from placebo to treatment group as symptoms changed
- Scaling bias. In some trials the rating scales had two or more categories to denote improvement and only one to denote deterioration
- Poor definition of drug efficacy

Irrelevant response variables

Subsiding toxic effect of previous medication—interpreted as improvement while taking placebo

Patient bias
- Answer of politeness and experimental subordination
- Conditioned answers
- Neurotic or psychotic misjudgment

No placebo given at all in trial
- Psychotherapy
- Psychosomatic phenomena
- Voodoo medicine

Uncritical reporting of anecdotes as evidence

Misquotation by reviewer or original author

False assumption of toxic placebo effects created by:
- The observance of everyday symptoms and attributing them to placebo administration: e.g. dry mouth, drowsiness, headache
- Misquotation of original trial results (Beecher misquoted 10 of the original 15 trials)
- Persistence of original symptoms interpreted as toxic placebo effects

---

With respect to the third problem: the calculation of the likely size of placebo effect in Beecher's article. McDonald and Mazzuca (1983) used statistical methods to find out how large the placebo effect is likely to be when regression to the mean has been taken into account. They made a random sample of 30 placebo-controlled RCTs from *Index Medicus* and calculated the expected contribution of regression to the mean[7] to the change in patients' condition and compared it to the actual change attributable to placebo. They found a median improvement with placebo of 0.3% in the sample of trials. They concluded that the most reasonable explanation for the observed improvement in patients' conditions was statistical regression and that placebo effect was negligible.

Beecher (1955) inadvertently supported the notion that 'placebo effect' comprises mostly regression to the mean. He stated that placebos do not work equally well on all individuals, they tend to work better on more severe symptoms and are more effective on subjective outcomes than objective outcomes. These are all characteristics of regression (McDonald & Mazzuca 1983).

Some examples of observations that led Beecher to infer a placebo effect are given in Box 4.2. The reader is referred to the reviews of Kienle and Kiene (1996, 1997) for a full exposition. By failing to acknowledge the possibility that factors other than 'the powerful placebo' had brought about the observed outcomes, Beecher misinterpreted the evidence in the 15 trials he reviewed. He also misquoted 10 of the 15 articles (Kienle & Kiene 1996). That Beecher attributes all changes in the patients' conditions to medical intervention ('about 17% *were made better*' Beecher 1955 p. 1603) perhaps reflects the elevated position of physicians in 1955 and a pervading belief that the patient's physiology only functions at the behest of the physician. The claims of a corresponding review from the German literature (Netter et al 1986) lauding the 'powerful placebo' were refuted by Kiene (1996) in a re-examination of 800 source placebo articles. They found no reliable demonstration of a specific placebo effect.

Further evidence of overestimation came from a recent systematic review of 130 randomized, controlled clinical trials (Hróbjartsson & Gøtzsche 2001). Using a published meta-analysis protocol based on the Cochrane standards to estimate the placebo effect, these writers carried out a blinded systematic overview in several international data-bases and five languages to extract 727 candidate articles from the literature. They excluded 597 trials because of methodological flaws and examined the placebo effect in the remaining 114 articles that met all the inclusion criteria. The final selection of articles contained information on the effect of placebo on 8525 patients with over 40 clinical conditions. In 32 trials with binary outcomes (e.g. cessation of smoking) placebos had no effect. In the 53 trials with continuous objective outcomes (e.g. blood pressure) placebos had no significant effect. In 29 trials with subjective continuous outcomes (e.g. pain scales) placebos had a statistically significant effect on outcomes when *compared with no treatment*. The calculated effect of placebo on pain corresponds to a reduction of 6.5mm on a 100mm VAS, or approximately 15% reduction in pain.

This finding raises several important points:

- The calculated average placebo effect on pain (6.5mm on a 100mm VAS) was smaller in larger trials. This may have been caused by reporting bias or publication bias (Bailar 2001) and suggests that the effect in clinical situations is probably less than 6.5mm.
- The failure of placebos in trials with objective outcomes suggests that *reporting bias* is a factor in the subjective trials. This is especially likely

when placebo is compared to no treatment. Patients in the untreated group know they are receiving no treatment. The results of such trials are subject to *expectation bias*.

- This 15% (or 6.5mm) average improvement includes an estimate of the effect of placebo administration *plus* unaccounted for factors such as spontaneous remission, reporting bias and regression to the mean (Box 4.3). The average placebo effect is 15% *at best*: but the real effect is likely to be considerably less than this estimate.

- The 15% was calculated from trials in which experimenters were blinded in order to preserve the integrity of any placebo effect. Clinicians are not so blinded and a reduction of the effect seen in clinical trials is likely in the clinical situation. If subtle non-verbal cues from a clinician to a patient can enhance a treatment or placebo, then if a clinician knows they are administering an 'inert' placebo these cues are more likely to reduce than enhance the effect on the patient. This is the principle reason for double-blinding.

Establish the clinical significance of an observed effect

The statistical significance of an observed difference is relatively easy to establish and interpret. Unfortunately statistical significance and clinical significance (or importance) are often considered synonymous. A change in VAS of just over half a centimeter after a course of treatment for pain may be statistically significant but it is not a particularly impressive clinical outcome. I would not regard such a small improvement as clinically significant (and neither, I suspect, would many patients.) There is some recent evidence to support this opinion. Some authors (van Walraven et al 1999) have suggested an arbitrary cut-off of 50% reduction in pain as a clinically important (or significant) outcome. This is a 50mm reduction on the standard 100mm VAS scale. Clearly, this is considerably greater than the 6.5mm average improvement with placebos calculated by Hróbjartsson and Gøtzsche (2001) and the 0.3% median improvement measured by McDonald and Mazzuca (1983) but it is arbitrary and does not ask patients what they consider a significant reduction in what is after all *their* pain. Another option is to ask an expert to observe patients and decide when their behaviour suggests they have had significant pain relief. However, second parties do not accurately quantify patients' pain (Grossman et al 1991). Todd and Funk (1996) proposed that an absolute minimum of 18mm change in VAS scores in clinical trials should be observed before the change is considered to be clinically important. Even this minimum recommendation is almost three times that measured by Hróbjartsson and Gøtzsche's (2001) meta-analysis.

To determine the point at which patients felt they had obtained clinically significant analgesia Farrar and co-workers (2000) utilized the data from the titration phase of a previous multiple-crossover, randomized, clinical trial of oral transmucosal fentanyl citrate in the treatment of cancer-related breakthrough pain. Adequate analgesia was defined operationally. When patients chose *not* to request a second, 'rescue dose' of opiate medication this was interpreted as an instance of adequate analgesia from the first dose. Patients perceived they were enjoying a clinically significant reduction in pain when their pain was reduced by 35%. This corresponded with VAS reduction of 20mm on the standard 11-point scales. The authors replicated these results for chronic pain patients in a later (Farrar et al 2001) article. Clearly, 6.5mm also falls short of this cut-off point for clinical significance.

The sum of a course of treatment with placebo and numerous unmeasured and unaccounted for factors seems to be capable of bringing about an average VAS pain improvement of 6.5mm on a 100mm scale. This means that half of the patients in Hróbjartsson and Gøtzsche's (2001) trial had improvements in pain that were *less* than this. Bearing in mind that VAS scores are subjective reports and they are likely to be influenced by a number of extenuating factors (Box 4.3) it is reasonable to assert *on the basis of this evidence* that placebos have a very small, possibly negligible effect on pain. It is therefore irrelevant that Hróbjartsson and Gøtzsche's (2001) review found statistically significant improvements in pain after administration of placebos. Superficially, these estimations of the placebo effect seem to be at odds with the evidence of the meta-analyses cited above and the considered opinion of respected writers on the subject such as Wall and Shapiro. However it is important to restate that these estimations allowed for extraneous factors such as those listed in Box 4.3. These factors are not controlled for in standard research, clinical practice or anecdotal evidence.

Therapists should not be swayed by the statistically significant gains made on pain by placebos. One of the major drawbacks of the meta-analytical method used by Hróbjartsson and Gøtzsche (2001) is that they greatly increase the number of subjects. Clinically insignificant differences may reach statistical significance. Readers of meta-analyses need to examine the clinical importance of statistically significant results more carefully than in individual trials (Feinstein & Horowitz 1997, Farrar et al 2001).

The so-called placebo effect is a myth born of misperception, mis-understanding, mystery and hope.

Roberts 1995

There can be no doubt that the extent and frequency of placebo effects as published in most of the literature are gross exaggerations.

Kienle & Kiene 1997

Standing, or falling, on evidence

The philosopher of science Sir Karl Popper (Popper 1974, in Bolles 2000 p. 43) complimented great scientists such as Galileo, Kepler, Newton, Einstein and Bohr for their principle of deliberately and actively seeking evidence *refuting their own theories.*

....these are men of bold ideas, but highly critical of their own ideas; they try to find whether their ideas are right *by trying first to find whether they are not perhaps wrong*. They work with bold conjectures and *severe attempts at refuting their own conjectures*.

In my opinion there is a considerable amount of writing on the subject of placebos that does not seem to aspire to this standard. Perhaps it is human nature to leave the boat un-rocked or to shelter on common ground. This preference makes us more likely to accept or even actively seek out evidence that supports what we already believe. These are not modern problems produced by the unmanageable volumes of research articles. In 1620, Francis Bacon (Bacon in Bolles 2000) described our tendency for flawed thinking and weak analysis like this:

For what a man had rather were true he more readily believes. Therefore he rejects difficult things from impatience of research; sober things, because they narrow hope; the deeper things of nature, from superstition; the light of experience, from arrogance and pride, lest his mind should seem to be occupied with things mean and transitory; things not commonly believed, out of deference to the opinion of the vulgar. (p. 91)

and publication bias in these terms;

...it is the peculiar and perpetual error of the human intellect to be more moved and excited by affirmatives than by negatives. (p. 89)

and our predilection for superstitious thinking thus;

The human understanding, when it has once adopted an opinion (either as being the received opinion or as being agreeable to itself) draws all things else to support and agree with it...And such is the way of all superstition...men...mark the events where [their preconceptions] are fulfilled, but where they fail, though this happen much oftener, neglect and pass them by. (p. 89)

The editorial committees of our scientific journals are just as subject to the foibles of human weakness. There is a significant bias towards positive results in the literature, and articles producing statistically significant, or non-controversial results are more likely to be published (Vickers et al 1998, Goetzche 1987, Easterbrook et al 1991, Dickersin et al 1992). Seeking out contradictory evidence is not 'human nature' but it is essential for producing good research and powerful, robust, explanatory scientific theories. We need to apply this standard to the reading and writing of the placebo literature.

Some problems with citation

Evidence-based clinical professions seek to examine accepted thinking incisively and aggressively and to question current practice. The aim is to discard unsatisfactory treatments and adopt better ones in order to improve patient care. We use the evidence of scientific publications to support our statements and to direct our practice. Entering into this relationship with evidence creates problems for the clinician. Once we use scientific evidence to support our positions we must be prepared to accept it when the same mechanism for generating evidence shows that we might be wrong. We have to accept that a hierarchy of evidence sources exists and the balance of evidence shifts inexorably in favour of higher quality trials and reviews and away from more pedestrian research. It is not unknown for two lines of research of comparable quality to yield conflicting conclusions. The evidence-based resolution of differences of opinion is the harder, not the easier, option. This process requires us to be acquainted with important evidence that is relevant to our chosen field. Furthermore, we need to be capable of sorting good evidence from bad and be willing to do so even if, or rather *especially if,* the poor quality evidence supports our point of view. In short we cannot just 'cherry pick'.

All evidence is not created equal: it is organized hierarchically according to its methodological quality (Cook et al 1992, Hadorn et al 1996). Irrespective of which evidence one prefers or which supports one's preferred theory, the evidence yielded by higher quality research prevails. This distinction is not evident in the pattern of citation in the placebo literature. Seldom do writers evaluate and criticize the research they cite. Notable exceptions to this are Wall's (1994 p. 1302–03) critique of a 1979 article (Levine et al 1979) that concluded that placebo responses are produced by endogenous opiates and Spiro's (1986) critical review of placebo literature. This 'reference bias' is not uncommon (Gøtzsche 1987), but clinical scientists should acknowledge this bias and account for it when considering where the weight of evidence lies. In evidence-based practice the persuasiveness of a statement lies not in the number of citations following it or in the reputation of the writer (*eminence-based practice*). It is much more important that the statement is supported by high quality evidence that has been replicated.

In his chapter on the placebo effect, Wall (1994 Ch 71, p. 1300) described two anecdotes of the 'powerful placebo' at work to illustrate its power. He referred to a detailed review of almost 1000 articles related to placebos (Turner et al 1980) but did not evaluate it. It was unfortunate to have missed this opportunity because what is needed in the placebo literature and in conversations among proponents of placebo, is fewer anecdotes, interesting and stimulating though they are, more high quality research directed specifically at the placebo effect, and especially, more aggressive evaluation of the research cited. Aggressive research evaluation is particularly important for those articles that are most often cited that have become part of 'placebo folklore' (e.g. Beecher 1955, Cobb et al 1959, Dimond et al 1958, Lasagne et al 1954).[8] Published standards exist to help authors and readers evaluate research literature (Chalmers et al 1981, Cook et al 1995, de Vet et al 1997, Dickersin et al 1994).

Clinical anecdotes should act as a stimulus for research; they should not supplant it.

> In clinical practice, the personal experience of patients and clinicians who observe improvement after initiation of treatment should be regarded as an unreliable guide to treatment efficacy due to regression to the mean.
>
> *Whitney & vonKorff 1992*

Social psychologist WJ McGuire (Harrington 1997) described the three stages in the life of an artefact: 'First is it ignored; then it is controlled for its presumed contaminating effects; and, finally, it is studied as an important phenomenon in its own right.' The present status of the placebo effect among placebo theorists does not seem to belong in any of these three stages. It seems to be lying in a fourth stage that lies somewhere between the second and third. Specifically, it is being considered for use for its curative, restorative and palliative powers but *before* it has been studied properly as a phenomenon in its own right.

Examples of faulty citation of evidence

Kirsch (in Harrington 1997; p167) cited 21 articles[9] to support the assertion that 'placebo analgesics, tranquilizers, stimulants and alcohol have been found to produce effects beyond those observed in untreated control conditions.' The implication is that these trials had investigated the placebo effect by including a 'no-treatment' group and had established that placebos could significantly alter baseline physiological parameters. This is relevant to the present chapter because the literature cited above (Hróbjartsson & Gøtzsche 2001, Kienle & Kiene 1996, Kienle & Kiene 1997) suggests that, irrespective of the physiological events that may follow placebo administration, *placebos do not bring about significant clinical improvements.* Ten of the 21 trials cited by Kirsch were not readily available for review by the present author, but of the 11 that were available, 8 (73%) did not include an adequate control group in their design (identified by an asterisk* in the endnote). When making inferences about the placebo group or when investigating the placebo effect, the placebo group in a drug trial cannot be regarded as the control group. Similarly, the drug group is not the control for the placebo group. Without adequate controls one cannot say that these trials established that placebos significantly altered baseline physiological parameters.

In only a small segment of their chapter *The placebo: is it much ado about nothing?*, titled 'Present-day placebo effects', Shapiro and Shapiro (Harrington 1997 Ch. 1) cited 230 articles, some of which were published as early as 1910, to support some very high estimates of the placebo effect. The authors did not reveal any methodological faults in any of these articles. This suggests that none of the 230 articles had faults worthy of mention, or the authors did not evaluate the methodology sections of the articles they cited. Alternatively they may have evaluated the articles and, disregarding any faults, chosen to cite them because they supported the notion of the 'powerful placebo'. Selection and citation bias is frequently seen in narrative reviews, particularly in textbook reviews (Mulrow 1987, Gøtzsche 1987).

The authors finished the section by stating that placebos do not perform well in tightly controlled scientific studies and fare best 'for the treatment of diseases *that do not exist* and in illnesses whose *symptoms wax, wane, fluctuate, and spontaneously remit,* as do most symptoms and illnesses. Although the *percentages* (of patients relieved by placebos) *decrease for serious illness with infrequent spontaneous remissions,* they still appear in *anecdotal* reports and placebo controls in studies, even for malignancies' (p. 22, my italics). Three things can be said about this segment and the many other similar examples of this type of citation in the literature:

- Perhaps unintentionally, this is good evidence that much of the placebo effect is actually a combination of regression to the mean, the natural history of illness and spontaneous remission. As they take place without the administration of placebos, many of the observed effects are not placebo effects. We need to know how much of the observed improvement in a patient's condition is due to placebo administration and how much to these other factors.
- When attempting to establish the actual value of placebos it is preferable to cite articles that have reached pre-determined methodological standards. Supporting claims for the efficacy of placebos with bad evidence only serves to weaken arguments irrespective of the number of bad articles cited.
- There seems to be considerable citation bias in the placebo literature.

In a footnote Shapiro and Shapiro (1997 p. 40) caution the reader about the dangers of basing inferences on studies done on 'the personality of the placebo reactor' during the 1950s as 'methodology was in a relatively primitive state when these studies were done.' However, when studies from this and earlier periods are cited throughout the book and inferences made from them to support the 'powerful placebo' the warning, though just as valid, is not repeated.

Discussion

There is now persuasive evidence that the size of the placebo effect may be less than many authors may have asserted. Some may find the small size of the estimations of placebo effect in this chapter perplexing. In many thousands of clinical trials, some of which were reviewed in this chapter, administration of placebo treatments preceded significant improvements in patients' conditions. Elaborate theoretical models have been developed to support the placebo effect. However, theories are based on observations and measurements, not the other way around. Once a measurement is made one cannot reject it because it does not fit in with one's beliefs or theories—especially if the measurement is replicated. When this happens it is time to develop new theories more descriptive of observed phenomena and to alter ones beliefs. Researchers have been charged with being too 'reductionist'. This suggests a prevailing belief that the placebo effect is so complex that measuring it using methods that control for extraneous or confounding factors (such as regression to the mean and spontaneous recovery) displays a lack of understanding of placebos. The opinion here is that these measurements and statistical estimates of the placebo effect are the best we presently have. They represent important knowledge, newly added to the debate on placebos. Defending reductionism Dennett (1995 p. 82) made a statement that is pertinent to this kind of response to new information:

> We might learn some surprising or even shocking things about these treasures, but unless our valuing these things was based all along on confusion or mistaken identity, how could increased understanding of them diminish their value in our eyes?

He explains (p. 82) that the pejorative use of the term 'reductionism' is motivated by the fear that it will not only explain a valued phenomenon but 'explain it away', and that 'by our own misguided efforts, we might come to discard or destroy something valuable' (p. 83). Reductionism does not lead inexorably to the scientific destruction of cherished monuments. The proper reductionist explanation of phenomena 'leaves them still standing, but just demystified, unified, placed on more secure foundations' (Dennett 1995 p. 82). It seems likely that the more passionate one is about the placebo effect, the more convinced one is of its value; the more one would want this.

There are problems with evidence and citation practices in the placebo literature. This problem is not exclusive to writing on the placebo effect (Gøtzsche 1987) but when an observed effect is as controversial as the placebo effect (Wall 1992) its proponents should seek out and present supporting evidence that is as close to unimpeachable as possible. There is a vast amount of literature that shows that patients taking placebos improve, but much of it is drug research, not placebo research. Many authors use the information derived from trials designed to investigate drugs (and not placebos) to make *post hoc* inferences about the efficacy of placebos or to augment theories about placebos. This information should stimulate specific placebo research not replace it. We cannot attribute clinical improvement in patients who have received 'dummy pills' in placebo-controlled trials solely to 'placebo power'. This is because we usually neglect to consider all the other factors that may have had some impact on the patients' conditions (see Box 4.2). Cited research is generally unevaluated by authors and is frequently cited inappropriately.

We need to stop using scientific evidence as a 'straight-man' that we trot out when our beliefs and pronouncements need support. The more rigorous habit of actively seeking evidence that tests our statements and exposes weaknesses in our theories should be encouraged. This is more important when the topic being discussed is, as Patrick Wall put it 'unpopular' (Wall 1992). It is tempting to 'cherry pick' in the literature for evidence that seems to agree with us but the result is a house of cards—with no inherent stability, as it grows its collapse becomes inevitable. When seeking to make a persuasive argument we need to site strong, persuasive evidence. Persuasion does not lie in repeating the same weak evidence over and over again. Adding more weak evidence to the argument is also ineffective.

Many of the factors responsible for the placebo effect are not exclusive to placebo administration. It is likely that they accompany and empower all therapeutic interventions and they are often activated before any treatment, real or 'dummy' is administered (see Box 4.1). In this author's opinion two

93

strands of placebo research may yield important information: the first comprises placebo research that focuses on identifying and investigating the components of the 'psychosocial placebo'; the second consists of studies that measure changes in the concentration of specific neurotransmitters or other endogenous substances after placebo administration. An example of this is the study by de la Fuente-Fernandez and co-workers (2001) who found that dopamine levels in Parkinson's patients increased after placebo ingestion. The research reviewed in this chapter on effect sizes associated with placebos suggests that these changes may not necessarily precede significant clinical or functional improvements. For the reasons outlined above, experiments that show that some patients in the placebo arms of drug studies improve are less useful and less persuasive. Investigation of placebos could help us to measure the role played by factors such as the clinical consultation, patient education, previous experiences, re-assurance, expectancies, conditioned responses and faith in the clinician in the final clinical outcome. The opinion here is that it is in our interpersonal skills, our ability to optimize the patient/ therapist interaction that our true power probably lies—not in our ultrasound head, whether it is turned on or not. *This belief helps one to reconcile the small size of the placebo effect, as measured by the studies reviewed above, with the belief that the psychosocial factors allied to the placebo effect are more influential than whatever 'dummy pill' is administered.* Research using placebos could help us to identify the particular set of qualities, techniques or social skills a clinician needs to develop if he or she is to optimize patients' recovery.

The evidence reviewed in this chapter suggests that the placebo effect may be small. This does not mean it is not potentially important. In order to facilitate understanding and research, medicine and science have tended to divide the socially functioning human 'mature organism' artificially into manageable compartments. Perhaps much of the subtlety and richness of the overall picture has been lost by this process. Patients are fully integrated— both within themselves and within society. It is likely that clinical outcomes are regulated by social, psychological, physiological and pharmacological and possibly even spiritual factors. Placebos stand at the margin between the personal and the interpersonal. The manipulation of placebos may be an important tool for unifying psychosocial influences on the one hand with psychoneuroimmunological ones on the other. Placebo research is a tool for studying interpersonal medicine: to explain what happens when a patient, a socially functioning human being, with a unique set of motivations, expectations and experiences, comes to a clinician for help. The placebo effect may be small; but it may be a small key to a large and important door.

If everyone believes a thing, it is probably untrue.

W. Arbuthnot Lane (in Macnab & McCulloch 1994 p. 369)

ENDNOTES

1 Rate ratio: this is the ratio of the rate of an event in a group to that event in the comparison group. Here, the rate is the number of persons with improved symptoms in a group divided by the total number of persons in that group. More generally, such rates may be expressed as decimal fractions, percentages, or per 1000 persons. A rate ratio is calculated by dividing the rate of an event by the rate of a second event. If two events have equal rates of occurrence the rate ratio is 1.0. The patients in the treatment group in the cited meta-analysis (Tomkins et al. 2001) reported a higher rate of headache relief (almost twice as high) than the patients in the untreated group. This ratio is statistically significant because the confidence interval does not contain the value 1.0.

2 CI: confidence interval

3 Odds ratio: this is the ratio of the odds that an event occurs in a group (circumstance) to the odds of that event occurring in the comparison group (circumstance). An odds ratio of 1.0 indicates that there is no difference between the two groups and the events are equally likely. An odds ratio of 2.0 means the first event is twice as likely as the second to occur—the patients in the treatment group in another meta-analysis example cited above (Browning et al 2001) were almost five times as likely as those in the untreated (placebo) group to report symptom improvement. This ratio is statistically significant because the confidence interval does not contain the value 1.0.

4 For example, retrospectively attributing a period of bad luck to a mirror broken just prior to its onset.

5 The mechanism of a 'No Intervention Group' helps to control for natural variation over time although in some modern studies there may be ethical objections to this model and indeed to the use of 'Placebo Intervention' groups also (Rothman & Michaels 1994).

6 Statistical regression describes a tendency of extreme measures to move closer to the mean when they are repeated. Regression to the mean predicts that patients selected for abnormalcy will, on the average, tend to improve (McDonald & Mazzuca 1983, Galton 1885-86)

7 The authors made a conservative estimate of the magnitude of regression.

8 The same standard applies to the pillars of the 'traction' folklore, the 'McKenzie' folklore, and the 'muscle imbalance' folklore.

9 Abrams & Wilson 1979,* Baker & Kirsch 1993, Blackwel et al 1972,* Briddell et al 1978,* Brodeur 1965, Buckalew 1965, Camatte et al 1969, Fillmore et al 1994, Frankenhaeuser et al 1963, Frankenhaeuser et al 1964, Gelfand et al 1963, Kirsch & Weixel 1988, Lang et al 1975,* Lang et al 1980,* Lansky & Wilson 1981,* Liberman 1964, Lyerly et al 1964, Montgomery & Kirsch 1997, Morris & O'Neal 1974,* Ross et al 1962, Wilson & Abrams 1977, Wilson & Lawson 1976*

REFERENCES

Abrams DB, Wilson GT 1979 Effects of alcohol on social anxiety in women: Cognitive versus physiological processes. Journal of Abnormal Psychology 88(2):161–173

Amanzio M, Benedetti F 1999 Neuropharmacological dissection of placebo analgesia: Expectation-activated opioid systems versus conditioning-activated specific subsystems. Journal of Neuroscience 19(1):484–494

Bailar J C 2001 The powerful placebo and the Wizard of Oz. Editorial, New England Journal of Medicine 344(21):1630–1632

Baker SL, Kirsch I 1993 Hypnotic and placebo analgesia: Order effects and the placebo label. Contemporary Hypnosis 10:117–126

Beecher H K 1955 The powerful placebo. Journal of the American Medical Association 159:1602–1606

Benedetti F et al. 1998 The specific effects of prior opioid exposure on placebo analgesia and placebo respiratory depression. Pain 75:313–319

Blackwell B, Bloomfield SS, Buncher C 1972 Demonstration to medical students of placebo responses and non-drug factors. The Lancet 19:1279–1282

Bland JM, Altman DG 1994 Some examples of regression towards the mean. British Medical Journal 309:780

Bolles EB 2000 Gallileo's Commandment—An anthology of great science writing. Abacus, London

Briddell DW et al 1978 Effects of alcohol and cognitive set on sexual arousal to deviant stumuli. Journal of Abnormal Psychology 87(4):418–430

Brodeur DW 1965 The effects of stimulant and tranquilizer placebos on healthy subjects in real-life situation. Psychopharmacologia 7:444–452

Browning R, Jackson JL, O'Malley PG 2001 Cyclobenzaprine and back pain: A meta-analysis. Archives of Internal Medicine Jul 9 161(13):1613–1620

Buckalew LW 1965 An analysis of experimental components in a placebo effect. The Psychological Record 22:113–119

Camatte R, Gerolami A, Sarles H 1969 Comparative study of the action of different treatments and placebos on pain crises of gastroduodenal ulcers. Clinical Therapeutica 49:411–419

Chalmers T, Smith H, Blackburn B et al 1981 A method for assessing the quality of a randomized controlled trial. Controlled Clinical Trials 2:31–49

Cobb LA, Thomas GI, Dillard DH, Merendino KA, Bruce RA 1959 An evaluation of internal mammary artery ligation by a double-blind technique. New England Journal of Medicine 20:1115–1118

Cook D, Guyatt G, Laupacis A, Sackett DL 1992 Rules of evidence and clinical recommendations on the use of anti-thrombotic agents. Chest Supplement 102(4):305S–311S

Cook D, Sackett D, Spiter W 1995 Methodologic guidelines for systematic reviews of randomized control trials in health care from the Potsdam Consultation on Meta-Analysis. Journal of Clinical Epidemiology 48(1):167–171

de la Fuente-Fernandez R, Ruth TJ, Sossi V, Schulzer M, Calne DB, Stoessl AJ 2001 Expectation and dopamine release: mechanism of the placebo effect in Parkinson's disease. Science 10 August 293:1164–1166

Dennett DC 1995 Darwin's dangerous idea. Evolution and the meanings of life. Penguin Books. London

de Vet HC, de Bie RA, van der Heijden GJ, Verhagen AP, Knipschild PG 1997 Systematic reviews on the basis of methodological criteria. Physiotherapy 83(6):284–289

Dickersin K, Min Yuan-I, Meinert C 1992 Factors influencing publication of research results. Journal of the American Medical Association 267(3):374–378

Dickersin K, Scherer R, Lefebvre C 1994 Identifying relevant studies for systematic reviews. British Medical Journal 309:1286–1291

Diehl HS 1953 Medicinal treatment of the common cold. Journal of the American Medical Association 101:2042–2049

Dimond EG, Kittle CF, Crockett JE 1958 Evaluation of internal mammary ligation and sham procedure in angina pectoris. Circulation 18:712–713

Easterbrook P, Berlin J, Gopalan R, Matthews D 1991 Publication bias in clinical research. Lancet 337(8746):867–872

Enserink M 1999 Can placebo be the cure? Science 284:238–240

Ernst E, Resch KL 1995 Concept of true and perceived placebo effects. British Medical Journal 311:551–553

Evans F J 1974 The placebo response in pain reduction. In: Bonica JJ (ed). Advances in Neurology Vol 4. Raven Press, New York. 289–296

Farrar JT, Russell K, Berlin JA, Kinman JL, Strom BL 2000 Defining the clinically important difference in pain outcome measures. Pain 88:287–294

Farrar JT, Young JP, LaMoreaux L, Werth JL, Poole MR 2001 Clinical importance of changes in chronic pain intensity measured on an 11-point numerical pain rating scale. Pain 94:149–158

Feinstein AR, Horowitz RI 1997 Problems in the 'evidence' of 'evidence-based practice'. Special Article. The American Journal of Medicine 103:529–535

Ferrari MD, Loder E, McCarroll KA, Lines CR 2001 Meta-analysis of rizatriptan efficacy in randomized controlled clinical trials. Cephalalgia 21(2):129–136

Fillmore MT, Mulviill LE, Vogel-Sprott M 1994 The expected drug and its expected effect interact to determine placebo responses to alcohol and caffeine. Psychopharmagology 115:383–388

Frankenhaeuser M, Jarpe G, Svan H, Wrangsjo B 1963 Physiological reactions to two different placebo treatments. Scandinavian Journal of Psychology 4:245–250

Frankenhaeuser M, Post B, Hagdahl R, Wrangsjo B 1964 Effects of a depressant drug as modified experimentally-induced expectation. Perceptual and Motor Skills 18:513–522

Galton F 1885-86 Regression towards mediocrity in hereditary stature. Journal of the Anthropological Institute of Great Britain and Ireland 15:246–263

Gelfand S, Ullmann P, Krasner L 1963 The placebo response: an experimental approach. Journal of Nervous and Mental Disease 136:379–387

Gøtzsche P 1987 Reference bias in reporting of drug trials. British Medical Journal 295:654–656

Gøtzsche P 1994 Is there logic in the placebo? Lancet 344:925–926

Gracely RH, Dubner R, Deeter WR, Wolskee PJ 1985 Clinicians' expectations influence placebo analgesia. Lancet 1:43

Greiner TH, Gold H, Cattell M, Travell J et al 1950 A method for the evaluation of the effects of drugs on cardiac pain in patients with angina of effort. A study of khellin (visammin). American Journal of Medicine 9:143–155

Grossman SA, Sheidler BR, Swedeen K, Mucenski J, Piantadosi S 1991 Correlation of patient and caregiver ratings of cancer pain. Journal of Pain and Symptom Management 6:53–57

Gudjonsson B, Spiro HM 1978 Response to placebos in ulcer disease. American Journal of Medicine 65:399-402

Hadorn DC, Baker D, Hodges JS, Hicks N 1996 Rating the quality of evidence for clinical practice guidelines. Journal of Clinical Epidemiology 49:749–754

Harrington A 1997 The Placebo Effect—an interdisciplinary exploration. Harvard University Press, Cambridge , Massachusetts

Hillis BR 1952 The assessment of cough-suppressing drugs. Lancet June21:1230–1235

Hróbjartsson A, Gøtzsche P 2001 Is the placebo powerless? An analysis of clinical trials comparing placebo with no treatment. New England Journal of Medicine 344(21):1594–1602

Jellinek EM 1946 Clinical tests on comparative effectiveness of analgesic drugs. Biometrics 2(5):87–91

Kiene GS 1996 Placebo effect and placebo concept: A critical methodological and conceptual analysis of reports on the magnitude of the placebo effect. Alternative Therapies in Health and Medicine 2(6):39–54

Kienle GS, Kiene H 1996 Placebo effect and placebo concept: A critical methodological and conceptual analysis of reports on the magnitude of the placebo effect. Alternative Therapies 2(6):39–54

Kienle GS, Kiene H 1997 The powerful placebo effect: fact or fiction? Journal of Clinical Epidemiology 50(12):1311–1318

Kirsch I, Weixel LJ 1988 Double-blind versus deceptive administration of a placebo. Behavioural Neuroscience 102(2):319–327

Lang AR, et al 1975 Effects of alcohol on aggression in make social drinkers. Journal of Abnormal Psychology 84:508–518

Lang AR et al 1980 Expectancy, alcohol, and sex-guilt as determinants of interest in and reaction to sexual stimuli. Journal of Abnormal Psychology 89(5):644–653

Lansky D, Wilson GT 1981 Alcohol, expectancies, and sexual arousal in males: An information processing analysis. Journal of Abnormal Psychology 90(1):35–45

Lasagne L, Mosteller F, Felsinger JM, Beecher HK 1954 A study of the placebo response. American Journal of Medicine 16:770–779

Levine JD, Gordon NC, Fields HL 1979 The mechanisms of placebo analgesia. Lancet 2:654–657

Lieberman R 1964 An experimental study of the placebo response under three different situations of pain. Journal of Psychiatric Research 2:233–246

Littman A, Welch T, Fruin et al 1977 Controlled trials of aluminium hydroxide gels for peptic ulcer. Gastorenterology 73:6–10

Lyerly SB et al 1964 Drugs and placebos: the effects of instructions upon performance and mood under amphetamine sulphate and chloral hydrate. Journal of Abnormal Psychology 68:321–327

Macnab I, McCulloch J 1994 Neck Ache and Shoulder Pain. Williams and Wilkins, Baltimore

McDonald AJ, Peden MR, Hayton R et al 1981 Symptom relief and the placebo effect in the trial of an antipeptic drug. Gut 22:323–326

McDonald CJ, Mazzuca SA 1983 How much of the placebo 'effect' is really statistical regression? Statistics in Medicine 2:417–427

McQuay HJ, Carroll D, Moore A 1995 Variation in the placebo effect in randomized controlled trials of analgesics: All is as blind as it seems. Pain 64:331–335

McQuay HJ, Tramer M, Nye BA, Carroll D, Wiffen PJ, Moore RA 1996 A systematic review of antidepressants in neuropathic pain. Pain 68(2-3):217–227

Montgomery GH, Kirsch I 1997 Classical conditioning and the placebo effect. Pain 72:107–113

Morris LA, O'Neal E 1974 Drug name familiarity and the placebo effect. Journal of Clinical Psychology 30:280–282

Mulrow C 1987 The medical review article: state of the science. Annals of Internal Medicine 106:485–488

Netter P, Klassen W, Feingold E 1986 Das Placeboproblem. In: Dolle W, Muller-Oerlinghausen B, Schwabe U (Eds) Grundlangen der Arzneimitteltherapie—Entwicklung, Buerteilund und Anwendung von Arzneimitteln. Mannheim Wien, Wissenschaftsverlag, Zurich 355–366

Pollo A, Amanzio M, Arslanian A, Casadio C, Maggi G, Benedetti F 2001 Response expectancies in placebo analgesia and their clinical relevance. Pain 93:77–84

Roberts AH 1995 The powerful placebo revisited: The magnitude of nonspecific effects. Mind/Body Medicine March:1–10

Rochon PA, Binns MA, Litner JA Litner GM, Sischbach MS, Eisenberg D, Kaptchuk TJ, Stasnon WB, Chalmers TC 1999 Are randomized control trial outcomes influenced by the inclusion of a placebo group? A systematic review of non-steroidal anti-inflammatory drug trials for arthritis treatment. Journal of Clinical Epidemiology 52(2):113–122

Ross S, Krugman AD, Lyerly AB, Clyde DJ 1962 Drugs and placebos: a model design. Psychological Reports 10:383–392

Rothman KJ, Michaels KB 1994 The continuing unethical use of placebo controls. New England Journal of Medicine 331(6):394–398

Sarles H, Camatte R, Sahal J 1977 A study of the variations in response regarding duodenal ulcers when treated with placebo by different investigators. Digestion 16:289–292

Shapiro AK, Shapiro E 1997 The placebo: is it much ado about nothing? In: Harrington A (ed) The Placebo Effect—an interdisciplinary exploration. Harvard University Press, Cambridge Massachusetts

Shapiro AK, Shapiro E 1997 The Powerful Placebo. From ancient priest to modern physician. The Johns Hopkins University Press, Baltimore

Spiro HM, 1986 Doctors, Patients and Placebos. Yale University Press, New Haven

Thomas KB 1987 General practice consultations: Is there any point in being positive? British Medical Journal 294:1200–1202

Todd KH, Funk JP 1996 The minimum clinically important difference in physician-assigned visual analog pain scores. Academic Emergency Medicine 3:142–146

Tomkins GE, Jackson JL, O'Malley PG, Balden E, Santoro JE 2001 Treatment of chronic headache with antidepressants: A meta-analysis. American Journal of Medicine 111(1):54–63

Turner JL, Gallimore R, Fox-Henning C 1980 An annotated bibliography of placebo research. Journal Supplemental Abstract Service of the American Psychological Association 10(2):22

Turner JA, Deyo RA, Loeser JD, von Korff M, Fordyce WE 1994 The importance of placebo effects in pain treatment and research. Journal of the American Medical Association 271(20):1609–1615

van Walraven C, Mahon L, Moher D, Bohm C, Laupacis A 1999 Surveying physicians to determine the minimal important difference: implications for sample-size calculation. Journal of Clinical Epidemiology 52:717–723

Vickers A, Harland R, Goyal N, Rees R 1998 6th Annual Cochrane Colloquium Abstracts, October 1998 (in Baltimore)

Vourdouris NJ, Peck CL, Coleman G 1989 Conditioned response models of placebo phenomena. Pain 38:100–116

Vourdouris NJ, Peck CL, Coleman G 1990 The role of conditioning and verbal expectancy in the placebo response. Pain 43:121–128

Wall PD 1992 The placebo effect: an unpopular topic. Pain 51:1–3

Wall PD 1994 The placebo and the placebo response. In: Wall PD, Melzack R (eds) Textbook of Pain. 3rd edn. Churchill Livingstone, Edinburgh 1297–1307

Whitney CW, von Korff M 1992 Regression to the mean in treated versus untreated chronic pain. Pain 50:281–285

Wilson GT, Abrams D 1977 Effects of alcohol on social anxiety and psychological arousal: cognitive versus pharmacological processes. Cognitive Therapy and Research 1:195–210

Wilson TG, Lawson DM 1976 Expectancies, alcohol, and sexual arousal in male social drinkers. Journal of Abnormal Psychology 85(6):587–594

Wolf S, Pinsky RG 1954 Effects of placebo administration and the occurrence of toxic reactions. Journal the American Medical Association 155:339–341

5

The information we give may be detrimental

CAROLINE HAFNER

Editor's note

This chapter stems from a Masters research dissertation that investigated, on the one hand, what patients with a chronic pain condition had been told about their pain condition by doctors and Consultants and, on the other, what it actually meant to them. It is included in this section on placebo and nocebo because it highlights the potential negative impact on outcome of some forms of clinician-therapist information giving—part of a possible 'nocebo' effect (see Chapters 1 & 2 in this volume).

Introduction

Beliefs associated with chronicity and disability

In attempts to reduce the rise in chronicity and disability associated with low back pain, researchers and clinicians have been exploring the secondary prevention of low back pain. Secondary prevention refers to interventions that aim to prevent the development of long-term problems.

It is suggested that the ever increasing resources being channelled into chronic pain may be spent more effectively on identifying risk factors involved with chronicity and eliminating them with early and effective primary care management (Linton 1998). This appears to be a controversial area with competing theories and ideas. Indeed, Frank et al (1996) likened the quest to identify risk factors to the quest for the Holy Grail. Gatchel et al (1995) observed that the search for pre-chronicity predictors has been limited in the United States because of the time and cost involved in conducting the necessary prospective trials. However, they note that some studies have identified pain intensity and personality factors together with compensation and gender issues as predictors of chronicity (Frymoyer 1991, von Korff & Saunders 1996). In order to confirm these findings, Gatchel et al (1995) carried out a study on 421 acute low back pain patients to determine whether a comprehensive evaluation of their psychosocial characteristics could significantly predict those who would subsequently develop chronic disability. Their results suggested 'the presence of a robust psychosocial disability factor' associated with those patients who are likely to develop chronic problems. Gatchel et al (1995) and Frymoyer (1991) make no suggestion that health professionals could be implicated in the development of chronic problems.

As well as identifying these factors, studies from Europe, New Zealand and Australia have also examined the way in which patients' belief systems may be contributing to chronicity. Fear of damage, fear-avoidance and fear of (re)injury are hypothesised to contribute to distress and activity restriction (Vlaeyen et al 1995, Klenerman et al 1995, Hill 1998). There are indications in some clinical literature of possible iatrogenic causes of chronicity arising from misinformation and inappropriate advice regarding low back pain (Harding & Williams 1995, Rose 1998). As a result, increasing importance is given to the de-medicalisation of back pain and to fundamental changes in beliefs systems. There appears to be a growing awareness that the beliefs of both the patient and the physician may influence the path towards chronicity (Rose 1998, Kendall et al 1997). Zusman (1998) explains the situation cogently:

> Decades of conditioning have bred a convinced and expectant lay public who, abetted by medical professionals of all types, tend to believe that pain is evidence of some potentially correctable structural/biomechanical impairment of the spine...and that normal function is impossible or at best dangerous.
>
> *(Zusman 1998 p. 200)*

In the United States, some physicians are implicating the medical system and health professionals in the development of chronicity (Loeser & Sullivan 1995).

In a recent report from an international forum for primary care research on low back pain (Borkan et al 1998), there is an acknowledgement that more emphasis should be placed on identifying predictors and risk factors for chronicity and disability. This report also notes that more emphasis should be placed on patient self-management, on physicians' education about low back pain, and on qualitative studies. However, the suggestion that health professional are involved in the development of chronicity and iatrogenesis comes mainly from specialists working in chronic pain management (e.g. Rose et al 1993, Kouyanou et al 1997), and from the few qualitative studies exploring patients' own views of their low back pain (Borkan et al 1995, Skelton et al 1996, Osborn & Smith 1998). Thus it appears that health professionals are not widely recognised as being associated with chronicity or iatrogenesis in this condition.

Recent research studies suggest that the first three months appear to be a critical period in the natural history of low back pain (Klenerman et al 1995). Kendall et al (1997) see the early assessment and management of psychosocial factors as a vital process in the prevention of chronicity. They recommend assessment within the first 2–4 weeks of onset of acute low back pain. In support, Waddell (1998) argues that psychosocial factors are more important in explaining disability arising from low back pain than medical variables such as evidence of musculoskeletal damage. The recognition of the importance of psychological factors in the management of low back pain has been acknowledged in Clinical Guidelines produced both here and in the United States (Rosen 1994, AHCPR 1994). However, in routine medical practice, psychological assessment is not normally employed. Clinical judgement is based primarily on physical examination and symptomatic reports of pain (Main & Burton 1995).

It should be noted that an appreciation of the role of psychological factors in the assessment and management of early low back pain are comparatively recent. Indeed, Roland and Morris (1983) were adamant that psychological issues only arose as a result of long-standing pain.

The prevalent medical management approach to low back pain, focusing on bed rest, restrictions of activity and analgesia, has been criticised, not only because it is often ineffective, but also because it is considered harmful (Rosen 1994, Indahl et al 1995, Kouyanou et al 1997). Research suggests that taking into account patients' own beliefs and understanding is important in the provision of more effective management (Linton 1998). From the qualitative studies that are available, there is a wealth of information to be gained about the personal meanings of pain and about how patients feel their condition has been managed (Borkan et al 1995, Osborn & Smith 1998, Skelton et al 1996). There do not appear to be any studies that explore what patients are actually told about the causes and implications of their low back pain. This chapter reports on an exploratory study that was designed to examine this particular area.

The study

The purpose of the study was two-fold: first, it aimed to find out what patients with chronic low back pain have been told about the causes of their pain. Secondly, it aimed to determine the patients' understanding of the explanation given to them. In order to do this, 38 patients with chronic low back pain were asked two open-ended questions:

1. What have you been told about the cause of your pain?
2. What is your understanding of this explanation?

The study took place at a residential pain management centre based in a rural community hospital. The centre runs pain management programmes for chronic non-malignant intractable pain conditions. The majority of referrals come from within 100 miles of the centre and are referred via pain clinics, orthopaedic or neurosurgical consultants, rheumatologists, general practitioners and other health professionals such as physiotherapists and occupational therapists. The centre is staffed by a multidisciplinary team comprising a clinical psychologist, a clinical nurse specialist, an occupational therapist, a physiotherapist and an administrator.

Patients attend an assessment interview prior to acceptance on a programme so that their suitability for the pain management programme can be evaluated. At the assessment interview the patient is examined by a consultant anaesthetist who takes a detailed medical history to confirm or establish the patient's diagnosis, their medical stability and their suitability for the programme. The patient then has a psychosocial assessment carried out by one or more of the multidisciplinary team.

The study took place between May and September 1998 and data were obtained from all patients attending the initial assessment interview during this period. All patients were asked the two study questions concerning their chronic pain and their responses were recorded verbatim by the interviewer, in his/her own handwriting. Only those responses obtained from patients with chronic low back pain were used in the study.

Chronic low back pain was chosen for study because of the recognised medical and socioeconomic problems attributed to it. Furthermore, patients with chronic low back pain make up 73% of attendances at this particular pain management centre. Low back pain is also the most widely researched musculoskeletal pain problem. The responses obtained from patients with other chronic pain conditions were retained for future study purposes.

Results and findings

Of the 38 patients in the sample, 23 were males and 15 were females. A breakdown of their age and pain duration characteristics is shown in Table 5.1.

Table 5.1. Patient age and pain characteristics

Attribute	Female	Male	Overall
Age (years)			
Range	61–28	59–22	61–22
Mean	45.40	42.65	43.73
Duration of pain (years)			
Range	34–1	30–1	34–1
Mean	12.06	9.34	10.68

Patients' responses

Most patients seemed to have no difficulty in responding to the two questions, appearing to report simply what they remembered being told. For example:

> The specialist who operated said that all the discs were very badly worn.
>
> (Patient 18, age 49)

Many of the responses consisted of traditional textbook, biomedical causes of low back pain, together with simplistic jargonised descriptions. For example:

> I've been told by orthopaedic doctors that I have degenerating back muscles, wear and tear and arthritis.
>
> (Patient 9, age 49)

Some responses were very brief whilst other gave very detailed information. The patients appeared to believe what they had been told, perhaps because the explanations given fit within a common 'folk model' of pain.

From an analysis of the responses a variety of themes were identifiable. Most were understandably orientated around the biomedical model of pain which attributes causes to musculoskeletal damage and/or deterioration. The responses gathered in the study reflected the experience of this author with previous patients over several years. Although there is no way of authenticating the responses, there are no reasonable grounds to assume that they do not reflect the information that patients have received about their low back pain and their understanding of it.

The themes

Maintaining the medical model

The medical profession's understanding and interpretation of low back pain appears to have become established as fact in the minds of health professionals and the general public. The biomedical model used indicates that all low back pain arises from damage to the spinal apparatus and requires rest, protection or surgery.

The responses from the two questions indicate that health professionals are continuing to give a message which confirms that low back pain is arising from spinal damage, that the spine is vulnerable, and that damage can be made worse. Thus, patients appear to have been told that their pain is a symptom of damage or structural fault in the spine. For example:

> The orthopaedic surgeon said that there was deterioration in my spine with the discs narrowing. I was told this usually happens in someone much older.
>
> (Patient 5, age 39)

and

> *I was told nerve damage and they said I had a couple of discs to*
> *remove and some scar tissue.*
> (Patient 31, age 42)

Following on from this indication of damage, patients have been told to rest. This may cause them to be fearful of making the problem worse:

> *I rested because I...was fearful of making things worse.*
> (Patient 7, age 53)

A comment here is that these responses indicate a stereotypical and reductionist explanation of their low back pain. There appears to be an assumption that what is seen on an X-ray or in other investigations represents the cause of the pain. This situation could be seen as a process by which the patients' own inaccurate beliefs and misconceptions are confirmed rather than challenged. Sadly, by the style and type of information giving, patients seem to be encouraged to remain prisoners to misinformation and myths about spinal degeneration, with the result that their pessimism is reinforced and their vulnerability enhanced. The responses do not indicate that the patients have been empowered to investigate strategies for self-management of their pain or that they have been treated from a biopsychosocial perspective.

Spinal degeneration

A consistently strong theme to emerge from the responses was that the patients appear to have been told that their pain was caused by some kind of degeneration or deterioration in their spine.

> *I have been told by doctors that I have arthritis...in the base of my*
> *spine and that I have degenerative discs.*
> (Patient 2, age 49)

The term degeneration is widely used by health professionals to describe skeletal changes. It has been customary to label normal age-related changes in the spinal apparatus as features of degenerative joint disease. It appears from many of the responses that degenerative changes have been given as the main cause of pain. For example:

> *I was told that my pain was caused by degenerative disc disease.*
> (Patient 7, age 53)

'Degenerative changes' could be interpreted as a negative descriptive term by the lay person. Patients may associate it with an inevitable decline especially when it is linked with the word 'disease'. It is possible that feelings of anxiety or fear may be reinforced by the use of these descriptive terms.

> *He said the base of the spine was worn out and it sounded pretty*
> *hopeless to me.*
> (Patient 3, age 36)

According to these responses, it would appear that the descriptions which focus upon degenerative discs and spinal deterioration have been given great significance as a cause of pain.

There is a varied selection of descriptive medical terminology appearing in the patients' responses. Terms include: severe disc degeneration, spinal deterioration. severe spinal stenosis. prolapsed discs, osteoarthritis, spondylitis, ossification, and fusing of bones.

The use of these terms by health professionals in explaining low back pain may inadvertently cause patients to become fearful of their condition. The seeds of physical dysfunction may be sown at a very early stage of back pain, causing unfortunate interactions between the patients' attitudes and beliefs with fear and anxiety about the future. The medical explanations are often mixed with more overtly non-medical descriptions, such as: crumbling discs, badly worn, wearing away, come to the end of its life, or worn discs.

Spinal degeneration is a typical element in the reports that patients make of their exchanges with their health professionals. It appears to be poor medicine in both a diagnostic and a rehabilitative sense, as it suggests an inevitable decline in physical stability and strength.

Enhancing vulnerability

The more it hurt the more it was wearing away.
(Patient 8, age 37)

Many of the responses appear to suggest that health professionals could be reinforcing the belief that pain means spinal deterioration. The patients' understanding of some of the explanations given to them suggest that they feel their spines are vulnerable, causing them to lose confidence in the structural integrity of their musculoskeletal system.

I've got a picture that my spine is crumbling and breaking down.
(Patient 12, age 34)

This could be interpreted as giving a disturbing image of spinal vulnerability which may have a significant effect upon a patient's coping ability. For the patient quoted above pain may be a clear indication that he must rest to preserve what is left of this 'crumbling' mess. Furthermore, if sticks, crutches, collars, corsets and wheelchairs are also offered in a situation such as this, the health professional is encouraging and indulging these erroneous beliefs and misconceptions.

A fear that further damage is a major risk is identified in some responses.

...and the Professor said it was ossification and fusing. I was told
this would not get better and will get worse.
(Patient 21, age 58)

...I was frightened of being paralysed.
(Patient 32, age 59)

It is difficult to believe that anxiety and fear will not have a serious effect upon physical functioning. Indeed, the patients frequently report just how abnormal a lifestyle they can now expect.

> *To me it is my body telling me that I can't do this.*
> *(Patient 36, age 28)*

> *I thought…that it was a fairly hopeless situation.*
> *(Patient 5, age 39)*

> *All I could imagine was that I would walk bent over crippled and eventually be pushed around in a chair.*
> *(Patient 14, age 41)*

From these responses the health professional appears to promote the fear that the spinal apparatus is vulnerable and will inevitably get worse. In these circumstances it is not surprising that patients feel they have to be careful and protect their tissues as much as possible from further harm.

On the other hand, it is difficult to find in the responses any advice to the patient to remain active. The following kind of advice is rare:

> *In the very beginning I was told not to move around, but after the third operation I was encouraged to move.*
> *(Patient 30, age 50)*

Giving inaccurate or inappropriate information

Examples of inaccurate information emerge very clearly from the responses:

> *I was told that my pain was caused…because my discs had crumbled.*
> *(Patient 7, age 53)*

Crumbling means 'breaking into crumbs or falling apart'. This is clearly incorrect in terms of what is actually happening to the spinal apparatus.

> *My discs are starting to crumble.*
> *(Patient 23, age 52)*

> *…And I was told that my spine was crumbling…and that I would end up in a wheelchair.*
> *(Patient 14, age 41)*

One patient was told,

> *You've got the body of a seventy year old.*
> *(Patient 18, age 49)*

This is unhelpful information. What use could the patient make of this observation? In these circumstances, how could he reasonably conclude that his body had the resilience to allow him to have a normal lifestyle? What constraints are placed upon him? What hope is he entitled to?

> *He told me to stay in bed for six weeks…the doctor told me it was spinal degeneration.*
> (Patient 14, age 41)

It seems likely that many health professionals are unaware of the impact that their diagnosis and explanations may have upon the patient. The previous examples cannot be considered as appropriate or helpful information. Indeed, they are likely to be confirming the misconceptions about the causes and management of back pain.

Lack of information

One unhappy alternative to inappropriate or inaccurate information is no information at all. It may be debated as to which is worse. Patients may become worried and anxious by a dearth of information about their pain.

> *The doctor hasn't said much really.*
> (Patient 33, age 48)

> *Not a lot…not sat down and said what's the matter. Not told why it keeps happening.*
> (Patient 37, age 33)

Along with misinformation and no information, contradictory or inconsistent diagnoses may be confusing and worrying. For example:

> *I've been told that many things…*
> (Patient 29, age 55)

> *I was told that my pain was caused by childbirth…my imagination…a slipped disc…degenerative disc disease…because my discs have crumbled.*
> (Patient 7, age 53)

Although many of the patients in the sample had experienced their pain for over 10 years and had longstanding contact with health professionals, they appeared still to be uninformed about their problem, and did not know what they could do to help themselves.

> *The doctor just said that I would always have it. It's something to do with the pain and the vertebrae but they couldn't find anything wrong.*
> (Patient 25, age 55)

> *All I knew was that I had a lot of pain in my legs.*
> (Patient 31, age 42)

As is commonly said, ignorance may breed fear. Fear may serve to restrict the patient and promote a view that all of the normal risks that attend life are enhanced. It is important to point out that in the instances in which the patient did feel informed, some relief and satisfaction was expressed.

> *I understood a bit about slipped disc because it was explained by the registrar who also showed me the MRI scan.*
> *(Patient 7, age 53)*

> *The most helpful explanation came from the neurosurgeon who showed me the MRI scan and pointed out the facet joints that had degenerative changes. I was given a reason for my pain and this was helpful. I was relieved that it wasn't more sinister.*
> *(Patient 9, age 49)*

From the entire set of responses, these are the only two that showed the health professional offering some meaningful explanation. However, even here there was a tendency to maintain the misinformation about 'slipped discs and degenerative changes' and to base diagnoses on the results of scans and X-rays.

Pessimistic prognoses

Many of the responses indicated that patients had been given poor prognoses regarding their condition.

> *My wife asked what that meant and he said that I would end up in a wheelchair.*
> *(Patient 14, age 41)*

The wheelchair must be the most potent image indicating decline and disability. Unfortunately health professionals appear to resort to it in consultations. Whilst the health professional may, in his or her mind, be issuing nothing more than a warning, the patient may feel he is being sentenced to a future of invalidity. Sometimes the prognosis is confirmed as inevitable. As one patient said so simply:

> *I was told I would end up in a wheelchair.*
> *(Patient 11, age 37)*

Even when the health professional does not paint the future outcome as pessimistically as this, there is often very little to look forward to in the way in which their condition is described.

> *My spine was worn...come to the end of its life.*
> *(Patient 3, age 36)*

> *...suggested I go home and live with it.*
> *(Patient 8, age 37)*

> *I remember that when the GP filled in my monthly form, on the back was 'prognosis', and he always put 'poor'.*
> *(Patient 29, age 55)*

> *The damage is too great, it might paralyse you. I can't help you.*
> *(Patient 32, age 59)*

Health professionals should, perhaps, be concerned that low back pain appears to be singled out for this profound pessimism without any reasonable diagnostic foundation.

Disempowering the patient

An analysis of the responses highlights a theme of disempowerment conveyed from health professionals to patients, maintaining the latter's passive role in the understanding and management of their condition.

> *I wasn't told anything.*
> (Patient 3, age 36)

> *The doctor...suggested that I go home and live with it.*
> (Patient 8, age 37)

Taken overall, the responses from this sample of patients gave no indication that the health professionals proposed advice which may have enabled a belief that the patient could help themselves in some way. The study appears to suggest that some of these patients have come to regard their situation as hopeless, and as one in which there was nothing that they can do to change things.

> *I asked how long I would be mobile for and he said 'How long is a piece of string?'*
> (Patient 11, age 37)

> *I thought the bones were rubbing together and that it was a fairly hopeless situation.*
> (Patient 5, age 39)

> *...anything physical I thought I couldn't do.*
> (Patient 31, age 42)

The use of metaphor and red herrings

Contained within the responses are examples of the use of language by health professionals which may create unhelpful images of pain problems.

> *The consultant...said that my spine was worn out. He said it was the same as a car you didn't service, it would just go clunk and that's what had happened to my back—come to the end of its life.*
> (Patient 3, age 36)

How may this analogy be of help to the patient? It is inaccurate, it is punishing in that the patient appears to have been chastised for not 'servicing' his back, and it indicates a vulnerable and irreversible condition. The fact that a description resonates with a patient's own understanding does not mean that it is either accurate or helpful. For example,

111

> *I thought the osteopath gave me a good explanation about a*
> *prolapsed disc — a bit like pastry being rolled out and overlapping at*
> *the edges.*
> (Patient 8, age 37)

However much the patient liked this explanation, it did not provide a useful understanding of it:

> *When I felt it rubbing I thought it was the bones touching and*
> *wearing away. The more it hurt the more it was wearing away.*
> (Patient 8, age 37)

When health professionals use metaphor or analogy rather than evidence-based explanation, there is a risk that the patient will develop images that constrain normal behaviour,

> *You've got the body of a seventy year old.*
> (Patient 18, age 49)

> *...and I was told my spine was crumbling.*
> (Patient 14, age 41)

This may produce images of poorly packed digestive biscuits, or possibly cliffs crumbling away into the sea. If health professional use analogy or metaphor, it may be more helpful to use positive images. Language can be powerfully constructive. It may be more useful to say, 'Although you have pain, your spine is strong—just like the Pennines, the backbone of England.'

Congenital structural abnormalities are offered to patients as causes or contributory causes of their problem. They may be 'red herrings.' While it may be reasonable for patients to know about these findings, their presence in a great many people who do not suffer pain or movement disability suggests that it is quite unreasonable to label them as being responsible.

> *I was told...that I had a couple of bits missing off the vertebrae.*
> (Patient 1, age 61)

> *...and a curve in my spine which was causing spasm.*
> (Patient 12, age 34)

> *There is a problem with one of my vertebra which is deformed. I've*
> *got muscle deterioration and possible curvature of the spine.*
> (Patient 24, age 47)

> *The doctor told me that my X-ray was such a mess at the base of my*
> *spine it looked like TB.*
> (Patient 8, age 37)

What can patients do with this information, apart from using it as further evidence that their spine is irrevocably damaged?

Discussion

The effective management of low back pain has been the subject of considerable study. As yet there is no consensus about the precise causes of chronicity and the disability that can arise from it. The role of health professionals has been implicated in a number of ways but there is little specific and detailed research about precisely how.

The data obtained during this study suggest that, however inadvertently, health professionals may be contributing to chronicity through their information giving. In this study the biomedical model remains paramount.

This study appears to confirm Waddell's observation that patients and health professionals continue to interpret and to treat pain through a biomedical model of ongoing tissue damage (Waddell 1996). Many of the responses obtained suggest that the patients' low back pain has not been explained to them in any way other than damage and deterioration. The responses also suggest that patients have been made fearful of a benign, self-limiting condition, and have not been given ways to facilitate possible recovery, or shown how to manage their problem effectively. Much of the literature indicates that the understanding and management of low back pain requires a paradigm shift to incorporate its multi-factorial nature (Borkan et al 1998) However, the importance of this shift away from the biomedical model, whilst first recognised thirty years ago (Engel 1977), is yet to be universally acknowledged (Cherkin 1998).

One of the main issues to emerge from the study responses was the tendency of health professionals to suggest that 'degenerative changes' identified by X-rays and scans were the direct source of the patient's pain. There is accumulating evidence from the literature that this is unhelpful, over-simplistic and, at worst, iatrogenic (Rosen 1994, Abenhaim et al 1995, Kouyanou et al 1997).

This diagnostic form of information giving is recognised as a problem in a number of different ways. Most significantly, it appears to promote misconceptions, fear and avoidance behaviour (Waddell et al 1993, Symonds et al 1996). Although the patients in the study were not directly asked about 'fear', they did convey many misconceptions and a number of their responses appeared to indicate that they were fearful of making their condition worse. It also appeared that few of the patients had been given reassurance that their condition was benign and that normal activity was possible and would be beneficial. Approaching low back pain in a way that avoids 'diagnostic labelling' and that encourages accurate information and early activity has been demonstrated to be more effective than traditional medical treatment (Indahl et al 1995, Ryan et al 1995). The literature indicates that there is no direct link between pain and degenerative signs seen in investigations. Thus the use of these signs as the cause of pain and incapacity is inaccurate and serves to perpetuate misconceptions and medical myths (Harding 1998).

It is important to bear in mind that people search for meanings to help them understand their illness, and having a diagnosis is hypothesised as enabling patients to have some control over their condition (Petrie et al 1996). However, attributing chronic low back pain to damage has been shown to affect physical functioning and quality of life adversely (Jensen et al 1996).

Some of the responses suggested that patients had not been given a diagnosis that made sense to them. If chronic pain remains mysterious, research suggests that the patient will have a poor outcome (Kouyanou et al 1997). We have no way of reliably knowing what these patients were originally told, but there appears to be an area of information giving, or lack of it, that requires further study.

Prognostic judgements from health professionals demonstrate another problem area within the responses. They indicate that patients had become fearful and negative about their future and it might be assumed that their expectations had been influenced inappropriately. Self-efficacy expectations are regarded as an important part of the self-management of chronic conditions. Indeed, these cognitions have been shown to be more powerful than actual behaviour change (Lorig et al 1993). Little investigation has been done to explore how health professionals influence self-efficacy by their prognostications in relation to low back pain. Bandura (1997) confirms that prognostic judgements can affect patients' beliefs in their physical efficacy and that health professionals can also influence beliefs by their attitudes and the way they treat the patient.

In this study there was very little indication that the patients had been made aware of any self-management strategies other than rest, reliance on continuing medical care and learning 'to live with it'. However, one of the main targets of chronic pain management programmes is to encourage self-reliance and a sense of personal control. If this approach can be helpful in long-standing pain (Williams et al 1993), there is good reason to believe it could be useful earlier in the understanding and management of low back pain.

How patients interpret what they have been told during consultations is not, of course, straightforward. Many other recognised psychosocial factors may affect patients' responses to their back pain (Kendall et al 1997) The need to assess these factors is now being recognised as fundamental in the prevention of chronicity, but much research remains to be done (Gatchel et al 1995, Klenerman et al 1995).

There are limitations in this study. In the design of the study, there is only a small amount of information from each patient. However, this is an exploratory study, and constructed so as to be unobtrusive in its method of data collection. Also the sample of patients came from a specialist area of medical treatment—chronic pain management. Thus the sample is not representative of the general population or of primary care patients. Another limitation refers to the reliance on patient recollection of information and advice received previously, gained from Question 1. There is no scientific way to judge the accuracy of the patients' recollections of what had been said to them over the years they have been in pain. Their previous medical records were not available and in any case may not contain what was said in consultations. *However, it is what the individual patient remembers and interprets that is important, and this is an area that appears to require further investigation.*

It is noteworthy that the responses appear similar to verbatim responses gained from other chronic pain patients and recorded in other literature on low back pain (Rose et al 1993, Harding & Williams 1995, Rose 1998). The judgement of what may be considered inappropriate diagnosis, information or advice is arbitrary, but there is some evidence that a consensus is forming about what kind of information giving is unhelpful (Waddell 1987, Rosen 1994, Zusman 1998).

Another limitation is researcher bias. Are the particular themes chosen by the researcher completely justified by the data or to some extent a reflection of personal interpretation? In order to minimise this bias, the transcripts were subjected to a content analysis by an independent rater.

Conclusions and recommendations

This study suggests that patients' understanding of their low back pain can be inaccurate and unhelpful and that doctors and other health professionals could be contributing to this misunderstanding. It highlights an area in which patients' beliefs and expectations may be shifted unnecessarily towards a vulnerable future and a pessimistic outcome. It also indicates that a rehabilitative model of pain is rarely applied during medical consultations regarding low back pain.

It appears that information giving in relation to low back pain may be contributing to chronic incapacity. Therefore health professionals need to be made aware of this influence and encouraged to develop a more positive rehabilitative approach. It seems clear that the whole area of information giving by health professionals requires investigation. Some of this investigation might profitably focus on the extent to which the role of the health professional contributes to chronicity, and so build upon the tentative findings of this study.

Recent clinical guidelines (Agency for Health Policy and Research 1994, Rosen 1994, Kendal et al 1997) concerning low back pain present a way forward in managing this condition more effectively. The guidelines emphasise the importance of evidence-based advice and information that should promote normal activity and ultimately prevent chronicity. Accurate and up-to-date information should be provided in primary care so that the problem is managed well early on and not allowed to fester while waiting for specialist opinions. Pain management classes and appropriate booklets and videos for patients may well help to dispel pervasive misconceptions and myths.

A paradigm shift away from the medical model of pain is required by society in general so that people are encouraged to remain active with back pain. Specific health education information could be given regularly in the media and advertised on posters. This approach has already been adopted in Australia but results have not yet been evaluated.

There is a need for consensus about how clinical guidelines are implemented. Introducing a different management approach will require time, education and monitoring as health professionals are unlikely to suddenly change their practices. Low back pain appears to have become over-medicalised with subsequent neglect of sociocultural influences. To most patients and health professionals low back pain means 'injury' or 'damage' requiring protective treatment. The evidence suggests that current diagnoses and treatment approaches are flawed, and that incentives for self-management are few and far between.

Psychosocial factors are considered to have a major role (Kendal et al 1997, reviewed in detail in Volume 2 of this series) in the prediction of chronicity, but there is no consensus on what these factors are and no standard way of assessing them. Kendall et al (1997) formulated a psychosocial screening questionnaire for use in primary care in New Zealand, but this has yet to be evaluated in the UK (see Volume 2 of this series). At the time of writing psychosocial assessments are rarely carried out in primary care. The ability to assess patients accurately in a more holistic manner requires not only training and practice but also time (see chapters in Volumes 2 and 3 of this series for guidance). Physiotherapists may well be the most useful clinicians to carry out many of the clinical guideline recommendations. Training and working within a biopsychosocial model of management and assessment could be combined with an already sound knowledge of musculoskeletal functioning and rehabilitation.

The self-management of low back pain should be encouraged (see all volumes in this series). Health professionals need to empower the patient by giving useful information and enhancing self-efficacy beliefs, and this should be carried out in the acute stage of low back pain rather than when chronicity and disability have developed.

ACKNOWLEDGEMENT

I would like to acknowledge that this study was done as part of the MSc Degree in Pain Management at University of Wales College of Medicine, Cardiff.

REFERENCES

Abenhaim L, Rossignol, Gobeille D, Bonvalot Y, Fines P, Scott S 1995 The prognostic consequences in the making of the initial diagnosis of work-related back injuries. Spine 20 (7):791–795

Agency for Health Policy and Research 1994 Acute low back problems in adults. Clinical Advice Guidelines Number 14. Washington DC: US Government Printing Office

Bandura A 1997 Self-efficacy and health behaviour. In: Baum A et al (ed) Cambridge Handbook of Psychology, Health and Medicine. Cambridge University Press, Cambridge

Borkan JM, Koes B, Reis S, Cherkin DC 1998 A report from the second international forum for primary care research on low back. Spine 23 (18):1992–1996

Borkan JM, Reis S, Hermoni D, Biderman A 1995 Talking about the pain: A patient centred study of low back pain in primary care. Social Science and Medicine 40 (7):977–988

Cherkin DC 1998 Primary care research on low back pain. The state of the science. Spine 23 (18):1997–2002

Engel GL 1977 The need for a new medical model: A challenge for biomedicine. Science 196 (4286):129–136

Frank JW, Brooker AS, DeMaio SE, Kerr MS, Maetzel A, Shannon HS, Sullivan TJ, Norman RW, Wells RP 1996 Disability resulting from occupational low back pain. Spine 21(24):2918–2929

Frymoyer JW 1991 Predicting disability from low back pain. Clinical Orthopaedics and Related Research 279:101–104

Gatchel RJ, Polatin PB, Mayer TG 1995 The dominant role of psychosocial risk factors in the development of chronic low back pain disability. Spine 24:2702–2709

Harding V, Williams C De C 1995 Extending physiotherapy skills using a psychological approach: Cognitive behavioural management of chronic pain. Physiotherapy 18(11):681–688

Harding V 1998 Cognitive-behavioural approach to fear and avoidance. In: Gifford LS (ed) Topical Issues in Pain 1. Whiplash—science and management. Fear-avoidance beliefs and behaviour. CNS Press, Falmouth 173–192

Hill P 1998 Fear-avoidance theories. In: Gifford LS (ed) Topical Issues in Pain 1. Whiplash—science and management. Fear-avoidance beliefs and behaviour. CNS Press, Falmouth 159–166

Indahl A, Velund L, Reikeraas O 1995 Good prognosis for LBP when left untampered. Spine 20(4):473–477

Jensen MP, Romano JM, Turner JA, Good AB, Wald LH 1996 The survey of pain attitudes: Further evidence of validity. Abstract, 8th World Congress on Pain. IASP Press, Seattle

Kendall NAS, Linton SJ, Main CJ 1997 Guide to assessing psychological yellow flags in acute low back pain: risk factors for long term disability and work loss. Accident Rehabilitation and Compensation Insurance Corporation of New Zealand and the National Health Committee, Wellington, NZ

Klenerman L, Slade PD, Stanley IM, Bennie B, Reilly JP, Atchison LE, Troup JDG, Rose MJ 1995 The prediction of chronicity in patients with an acute attack of low back pain in a general practice setting. Spine 20(4):478–484

Kouyanou K, Pither CE, Wessely S 1997 Iatrogenic factors and chronic pain. Psychosomatic Medicine 59:597–604

Linton SJ 1998 The socioeconomic impact of chronic back pain: is anyone benefiting? Pain 75:163–168

Loeser JD, Sullivan K 1995 Disability in the chronic low back patient may be iatrogenic. Pain Forum 4:114–121

Lorig KR, Mazonson PD, Holman HR 1993 Evidence suggesting that health education for self-management in patients with chronic arthritis has sustained health benefits while reducing health care costs. Arthritis and Rheumatism 36(4):439–446

Main CJ, Burton AK 1995 The patient with low back pain: who or what are we assessing? An experimental investigation of a clinical puzzle. Pain Reviews 2:203–209

Osborn M, Smith JA 1988 The personal experience of chronic benign lower back pain: An interpretative phenomenological analysis. British Journal of Health Psychology 3:65–83

Petrie KJ, Weinman J, Sharpe N, Buckley J 1996 Role of patients view of their illness in predicting return to work and functioning after myocardial infarction: Longitudinal study. British Medical Journal 312:1191–1194

117

Roland M, Morris R 1983 A study of the natural history of back pain. Part I Spine 8:141–144

Rose MJ 1998 Iatrogenic disability and back pain rehabilitation. In: Gifford LS (ed) Topical Issues in Pain 1. Whiplash—science and management. Fear avoidance behaviour and beliefs. CNS Press, Falmouth 167–172

Rose MJ, Reilly JP, Pennie B, Slade PD 1993 Chronic low back pain: a consequence of misinformation? Employee Counselling Today 5(1):12–15

Rosen M 1994 Report of a Clinical Standards Advisory Group Committee on Back Pain. London, The Stationery Office

Ryan WE, Krishna MK, Swanson CE 1995 A prospective study evaluating early rehabilitation in preventing back pain chronicity in mine workers. Spine 20(4):489–491

Skelton AM, Murphy EA, Murphy RJL, O'Dowd TC 1996 Patients' views of low back pain and its management in general practice. British Journal of General Practice 46:153–156

Symonds TL, Burton AK, Tillotson KM, Main CL 1996 Do attitudes and beliefs influence work loss due to low back trouble? Occupational Medicine 46(1):25–32

Vlaeyen JWS, Kole-Snijders AMJ, Boeren RGB, Van Eek H 1995 Fear of movement/ (re)injury in chronic low back pain and its relation to behavioural performance. Pain 62:363–372

Von Korff M, Saunders K 1996 The course of back pain in primary care. Spine 21 (24):2833–2839

Waddell G 1987 A new clinical model for the treatment of low back pain. Spine 12(7):632–644

Waddell G 1996 Low back pain: A twentieth century health care enigma. Spine 21(24):2820–2825

Waddell G, Newton M, Henderson I, Somerville D, Main CJ 1993 A Fear-Avoidance Beliefs Questionnaire (FABQ) and the role of fear avoidance beliefs in chronic low back pain and disability. Pain 52:157–168

Waddell G 1998 Diagnostic triage. In: Waddell G (ed) The Back Pain Revolution. Churchill Livingstone, Edinburgh 22

Williams ACdeC, Nicholas MK, Richardson PH, Pither CE, Justins DM, Chamberlain JH, Harding VR, Ralphs JA, Jones SC, Dieudonne I, Featherstone JD, Hodgson DR, Ridout KL, Shannon EM 1993 Evaluation of a cognitive behavioural programme for rehabilitating patients with chronic pain. British Journal of General Practice 43:513–518

Zusman M 1998 Structure-oriented beliefs and disability due to back pain. In: Gifford LS (ed) Topical Issues in Pain 1: Whiplash—science and management. Fear avoidance beliefs and behaviour. CNS Press, Falmouth 199–213

118

6

An introduction to evolutionary reasoning: diets, discs, fevers and the placebo

LOUIS GIFFORD

Foundations

In the ground-breaking book *Evolution and Healing. The new Science of Darwinian Medicine*, Randloph Nesse and George Williams (1994) make a passionate plea for the integration of evolutionary reasoning into the practice of everyday medicine. This is a stance that is argued for here, in particular for use by physiotherapists working with patients in pain.

While evolutionary reasoning may raise as many questions as it answers, what it does best is to promote a paradigm of thinking that is at once open-minded, uncluttered, quite logical and, above all, easy to follow. The opinion here is that it will first, be beneficial for our patients in the long run, and secondly, provide an alternative broad reaching and open-minded umbrella approach to reasoning that will aid clinical management and also be very helpful for framing more productive research questions.

In order to be able to reflect and reason from an evolutionary perspective we need to accept and appreciate a number of propositions. The first is that man, like all other animals and plants is the product of an evolutionary process—and as such is, just like all of them (from bacteria, to brambles, to bullfrogs and bristlecone pines), a successful and remarkable 'replicating machine.' We just happen to be here, we're very new to the scene, and it's been very much a chance thing that we exist.

Further, while producing what often appears to be an exquisite design, evolution also produces frailties and flaws that make all organisms vulnerable to dysfunction and disease. As Nesse and Williams put it, our bodies are a 'bundle of careful compromises'—they work well enough to allow our continued survival and successful reproduction, but along the way many of us may suffer as a result of this vulnerability. For evolution, and for those who have not succumbed to extinction, an organism's success is self evident, these careful compromises have worked, and it's just tough on a given individual if they suffer!

Of course, all organisms are vulnerable. Perhaps the least vulnerable, smartest and best adapted, are those that have been around the longest. Thus respect is due to organisms like bacteria and to sharks, examples of creatures that evolved so successfully that they have changed very little over an incredibly long time and have witnessed a great many environmental changes and challenges.

We live today in conditions that are very different from those of our 'hunter-gatherer' ancestors. Or as Charlton (1996) has expressed it, 'Humans have been designed for a historical situation, not for contemporary society.' In other words, evolutionary forces operated to produce advantages for life and survival in those conditions—not in the very recent modern day ones. In order to better understand the way we are, and the way we act and react, it is often informative to think in terms of a hunter-gatherer type of existence, and the likely implications of, or consequences from, those times for the issues we are contemplating.

Ponder the following question, for example: Why is it that we crave the very foods that are bad for us (fats, salt and sugars), but have less desire for pure grains and vegetables? Could it be simply because the tastes and food preferences we have today evolved long ago when fat, sugars and salt were always in short supply? In the words of Nesse and Williams (1994): 'Almost everyone, most of the time, would have been better off with more of these substances, and it was consistently advantageous to want more and to try and get it. Today most of us can afford to eat more fat, sugar and salt than is biologically adaptive, more than would ever have been available to our ancestors of a few thousand years ago.' It seems that conditions in the past never required the evolution an effective biological 'stop button' that prevents our over-indulgence and self destruction.

Nesse and Williams (1994) warn their reader to be wary of romantic concepts of life being better back then. While modern life has its disadvantages, it also has advantages—for example, lower mortality rates in early life. Fewer people die from smallpox, appendicitis, childbirth complications and hunting accidents, and therefore many of us in Western style civilisations live a lot longer. But, as a result, we suffer the consequences of ageing, and vulnerability to age-related afflictions such as heart disease and cancer. 'The price of not being eaten by a lion at age ten or thirty may be a heart attack at eighty' (Nesse & Williams 1994). One contemporary problem is that many are unwilling to accept this notion, resulting in strong, arguably unreasonable, pressures on the governments of the day to provide cures for these diseases, or to take responsibility to prevent them happening. In part, if we understand our background, we can be better informed to be able to tackle and prevent these afflictions in ourselves.

Nesse and Williams (1994) provide a powerful example:

Cancer rates are increased substantially by high-fat diets. Much diabetes results from the obesity caused by excess fat consumption. Forty percent of the calories in the average American diet come from fat, while the figure for the average hunter-gatherer is less than 20 percent. Some of our ancestors ate lots of meat, but the fat content of wild game is only about 15 percent. The single thing most people can do to most improve their health is to cut the fat content of their diets.

They go on...

One of us once met with three others early one morning to travel to a hearing on claims that agricultural uses of pesticides were endangering the health of nearby suburban residents. A stop at a diner for breakfast yielded a vivid memory. One of the eaters lamented the likelihood that the wheat and eggs in his pancakes were no doubt contaminated with unnatural pesticides and antibiotics that might give him cancer ten or twenty years later. Perhaps so, but these toxins were a minor danger to his future health compared to the grossly unnatural fat content of his sausage and buttery pancakes, and the enormous caloric value of the syrup in which everything was bathed. The cumulative effect of that kind of eating is surely more likely to cause future health problems than are the traces of exotic chemicals.

(As an aside, the above is an excellent example of a reasoning error based on insufficient evidence or failing to take all the available evidence into account in an unbiased way. We need to reflect that very often, our reasoning, and that of our patients too, is ill-informed and sometimes shockingly 'un'-reasonable!)

We need also to appreciate that successful evolution/survival requires variation and variability. For guaranteed species success in the future, we all need to be slightly different while at the same time having stable 'core' attributes for everyday existence and successful reproduction. Some of us are tall, some short, some thin, some big, some athletic some lethargic, some witty, some fiery and so forth. Attributes vary—and in some environmental conditions some of us are at an advantage. I'm thin and wiry, I can move about quickly, have good balance and can pull myself up with my arms with ease—I have a sure advantage over my overweight, slothful friend when out hunting or when fleeing a rival tribe or threatening beast. However, in times of scarce food resources, he has it over me by far. When times get tough, the one with the best attributes for the prevailing conditions will be the one whose genes are preserved for the next generation.

Variation applies to every attribute any investigator cares to examine—from the physical to the psychological and behavioural. For example, relevant to pain, it is now well established that different varieties of rat respond differently to identical experimentally produced nerve lesions. Researchers term the pain behaviour observed in animals *autotomy*—a condition where

121

the rat self mutilates the limb affected by a nerve lesion, and thought to represent a reaction to neuropathic pain following denervation (see Devor & Seltzer 1999). 'Lewis' strains of rat appear quite oblivious to the injury, showing no or very little pain behaviour. In contrast to 'Lewis' rats, 'Sabra' rat strains show marked autotomy behaviour. The underlying reason for this variation is likely a single recessive gene (Devor 1990, see also Mogil 1999, Mogil et al 1999, Mogil et al 1999a, Lariviere et al 2002).

Astonishingly, some genes seem to be preserved through evolution even though they confer apparent disadvantages, like this susceptibility to chronic neuropathic pain and hypersensitivity. Appreciate, however, that genes that are found responsible for apparently negative effects are likely to confer some benefit in other ways elsewhere. Those who have studied genetics know that a single gene can have more than one effect (pleiotropy). Thus, the gene responsible for autotomy behaviour following nerve injury may well confer advantages that are yet to be revealed. Evolutionary reasoning dictates that traits tend to remain because their advantages on balance will always outweigh any disadvantages. The sickle cell trait (see Allison 1997) is probably the best known example—here, individuals with the trait (herterozygous for the sickle cell gene) suffer from malaria less often and less severely than those without the trait. The sickle cell gene is thus vital for survival in regions where malaria is rife; the unfortunate cost, though, is sickle cell disease (those who are homozygous for the gene).

Let us return to diet. As already noted, there is a huge variation in our fatness and thinness, and some of us are more prone to the effects of dietary overdosing than others. Some of us can eat and eat and change little, while others only have to look at food to put on weight!

In their attempts to relieve chronic malnutrition of the Pima Indians of Arizona, researchers inadvertently caused an epidemic of obesity and diabetes (see Nesse & Williams 1994, p. 129). The researchers concluded that the affected individuals had what they called a 'thrifty phenotype'—a genetically derived attribute that provided the ability to store food energy as fat with great efficiency. Thus, what to us would be considered a reasonably normal and modest diet gets quickly stored away as fat in these Indians, leading to obesity and detrimental consequences like diabetes. From an evolutionary perspective this food storage efficiency can be applauded. What better way to survive conditions where famine is commonplace? Evolution has endowed the Pima Indians, and many of us, with highly efficient food to fat metabolism—we put on weight rapidly in times when food is in good supply, and then we lose it very slowly in more pressing times. Clever stuff, but we pay the price now. No wonder it is so easy to put on weight, yet so difficult and slow to lose it. Famine-adapted individuals unfortunately get fatter and fatter in conditions where food shortages never occur and where low physical activity and low energy expenditure is the norm.

Finally, evolution endows us with an innate laziness. The biological rule is that for best survival, use the least amount of energy possible and don't waste it. Always take the easy, most efficient route and hence preserve precious resources at all costs. For many, it takes a great deal of will power to do something physical in a way that uses more energy than is necessary. This thinking may well be applied to the pointless, boring, dull and frequently unrewarding exercises that physiotherapist often prescribe!

From an evolutionary perspective all behaviours can be narrowed down to two fundamental purposes. First, behaviours that can be classified as preventing death and which promote staying alive—fighting, fleeing and feeding etc., and secondly, behaviours orientated to passing genes on successfully to the next generation—finding a partner, having sex and nurturing offspring until they can exist independently. You cannot have the second without the first. Ultimately, the forces of nature that lead to an organism's success rely on selfishness (try reading Watson 1995).

Two types of reasoning

Good reasoning when applied to the understanding of any presenting observation, or condition involves two perspectives: An evolutionary perspective asks the simple question 'Why?' and a more traditionally scientific perspective asks the questions 'What?' or 'How?' about structure and mechanisms. The 'what' and 'how' reasoning perspective is termed a *proximal, or near* explanation of cause for a given observation. In medicine, proximal explanations address how a body works and why some people get a disease and others don't. Evolutionary or *ultimate* explanations show why humans, in general, are susceptible to some diseases and not to others (Nesse & Williams 1994).

An amusing general example is given by Jared Diamond in his excellent book *The Rise and Fall of the Third Chimpanzee* (Diamond 1991). In it, he asks, 'Why to skunks smell bad?'

A chemist or molecular biologist might answer:

It's because skunks secrete chemical compounds with certain particular molecular structures. Due to the principles of quantum mechanics, those structures result in bad smells. Those particular chemicals would smell bad no matter what the biological function of their bad smell was. (Diamond 1991)

An evolutionary biologist would reason:

It's because skunks would be easy victims for predators if they didn't defend themselves with bad smells. Natural selection made skunks evolve to secrete bad-smelling chemicals; those skunks with the worst smells survived to produce the most baby skunks. The molecular structure of those chemicals is a mere incidental detail; any other bad smelling chemicals would suit skunks equally well. (Diamond 1991)

From the pain perspective our question might be: 'Why does tissue injury cause pain?'

A **proximal** explanation might run along the following lines. Injury produces physical and chemical stimulation of sensory nerve endings that relay messages into the central nervous system. The spinal cord and brain, via complex electrochemical processing mechanisms, then reacts to the incoming messages, which may then give rise to pain.

An **evolutionary** explanation might provide another answer. Because pain generates behavioural and physiological responses that are compatible with best recovery of the tissue injured, overall function of the organism, and ultimately improves the injured organisms survival chances.

We all know this, but do we act on it in clinical practice? The following section looks at a very common pain problem—back and leg pain.

Back and leg pain

When physiotherapists observe patients we seek answers to what we observe. We most often use a proximal style of reasoning whose very nature is wedded to a biomedical, mechanistic view. We don't often use evolutionary thinking, and even less often act on an evolutionary reasoned management strategy. For example, why does a patient with back and left leg pain of one week duration so often flex and side-shift to the right? How should the presentation be managed?

Proximal reasoning

Many might offer the following 'proximal' style of explaining the patient's problems: 'Because she probably has a disc problem and the disc problem has lead to irritation of the sciatic nerve.' Proximal reasoning with regard management might go: 'Reduce disc problem, manipulate its structure in some way, overcome the problem which has mechanical origins and hence relieve patient of the pain.' Or similar thinking involving a different pathway: 'Correct the abnormal posture, get normal movements back, again, fix problem.'

Evolutionary reasoning

An evolutionary perspective might consider the following issues before formulating an answer:

- The pain and resultant physical tension produced help her to avoid doing something that might be injurious or slow adequate healing. In another sense, pain can be seen to promote behaviours that provide the best conditions for healing and recovery.
- Her posture and movements warn other community members to avoid her and be very careful when approaching her.
- The posture and the behaviours generated by pain help her to gain favourable attention and receive protection.
- Having pain can be associated with rewards.
- Postures, gestures, words and actions that indicate suffering foster acts of kindness within the social group.

Symptoms help speed healing and prevent further damage

The pain and resultant physical tension produced help her to avoid doing something that might be injurious or slow adequate healing, as well as help speed healing. Tension and pain are useful for early physical recovery. Pain demands cautious movements. Pain may 'request' inactivity and stiff fixed postures. But, if you think about it, pain may also demand, quite the opposite, regular *activity* of the injured part, too; patients are frequently physically restless, often shifting, wriggling and moving with their pain.

Pain helps generate self-care, vigilance and the feeling of vulnerability. The implicit message might run: 'I'd rather not go out gathering food today if you don't mind, and I'm not at all keen on having sex.' Pain also generates a need state (see also Ch. 1 and Introductory Essay this volume) that requires help and protection (see placebo section of this chapter later). Pain often generates a quick temper—anyone who gets a bit too close or appears to be clumsy or in the least bit threatening gets bawled at.

Posture may send protective warning signals

Her posture and movements warn other community members to avoid her and be very careful when approaching her—again helping to provide best healing conditions by not disturbing vulnerable recovering tissues with sudden movements. The fact that an animal that is moving awkwardly or abnormally in some way labels them as weak and hence an easy meal is dealt with in the placebo section later. Thus, the buffalo that limps is soon picked out and killed by hunting lions, wild dogs or hyenas. In some circumstances, pain and the behaviours and postures it can produce are worth concealing.

Pain postures generate sympathetic attention

The posture and the behaviours generated by pain help her to gain favourable attention and receive protection from those who know her, are close to her and value her. Feeling protected and cared for may be important for best healing (see placebo section below).

Pain can be associated with rewards

Having pain can be associated with rewards, more especially if you have some status in the group in which you live. If you are deemed to be important by your peers, you get a lot of attention and protection; you get out of working and doing chores that you dislike doing, you are given more time to heal, which may be a good deal more than that given to others of lower ranking. High ranking individuals in a hunter-gatherer community may have vital knowledge and skills in relation to things like security and well being of the group. Without that skilled and/or knowledgeable individual, the community is potentially more vulnerable (see Diamond

1991). Evolution (continued species survival) often demands cruel efficiency and thus endows some higher social mammals with behaviours and emotions that say, effectively. 'Look after those who are valuable, take less time and care with those who are not or who are a burden.' Think about it, and it becomes quite obvious that even though we try to suppress them, these deep-rooted sentiments and prejudices still persist today. They are not necessarily nice, but they are acts of evolutionary wisdom that must be applauded because they have contributed to our being here today. In the reality of our day to day clinical practice, one has to be a very strong willed therapist not to give 101% of our skills and time to a client who is a celebrity of some kind.

Visible signs of suffering foster kindness

Postures, gestures, words and actions that indicate suffering foster acts of kindness within the social group. If you are in a hunter-gatherer community you may get a few days off from hunting and gathering. In modern society you can get paid by the social services and have drinks bought for you by sympathetic friends down at the pub (recall the innate laziness rule discussed earlier.) The fact that having more than a few days off is now being shown to be detrimental to recovery seems hardly surprising. What use are you if you are unproductive? No wonder our sympathy for those in our midst who are unwell, don't 'get going in a reasonable time', or are disabled soon wears thin.

Perhaps these are uncomfortable thoughts, but if you're thinking from an evolutionary perspective it starts to help explain and make sense of a great many issues that can often 'leave a lot to be desired' when viewed from more cultural, civilised, and social perspectives. Our animal instincts were valuable; if we appreciate them and accept them we are more likely to bear judgement on them with greater insight and understanding.

Before addressing management and bearing the above points in mind, the next important part of reasoning like this is to ask if the presentation (the pain, the postures and the observed behaviour in its context) can be considered to be useful or 'adaptive'—and therefore to be respected—or of no use whatsoever and, hence, 'maladaptive'. Or, finally, is the observation some kind of imperfection or defect?

We tend to think that we are in a healing profession and the pressure is on us to provide a cure. Evolutionary reasoning invites a shift of thinking to consider that this flexed and deviated posture in the patient example, might be a very adaptive response and one not to be meddled with? Would you ever consider saying to a patient: 'Don't worry about your flexed and shifted posture, it's very useful and protective at the present time—it will get better as your problem gets better, and at the appropriate time I will help you to gradually overcome it. If we attempt to correct the way you stand and move too quickly, we may actually prolong your problem.'

In other words, if the pain and posture are adaptive, what right do we have to get rid of them? If we do deem such a posture and pain to be adaptive, evolutionary reasoning would predict that too early a resolution of the pain, or too rapid a correction of the posture might not be a good thing, may prolong recovery and lead to more episodes later on. This is a very useful type of research question that is challenging to several physiotherapy methods—and which needs answering.

Clearly, whenever we examine a patient it is important to reason whether what we observe can be viewed as adaptive, maladaptive, or an imperfection/defect. On the one hand we need to consider millions of years of success, yet on the other, we ought to consider that the phenomenon we are observing, and deeming 'abnormal' in some way, may not have been at all obstructive to success. The pain and posture adopted by our patient are of little consequence to the passage of genes from one generation to the next. Eventually, especially if you are ignored, with or without a spinal shift, pain or no pain, you have to get on with life, fend for yourself and your community, or you get (adaptively) ignored and may die!

The opinion here is that not all acute pain is necessarily useful pain in the sense that it is adaptive and should therefore command respect. An example is the early severe pain that is often the result of minor nerve injury (Gifford 2001). The pain is often out of all proportion to the injury sustained. While the pain level can be incredibly high, continuous, extremely distressing and debilitating, the actual injury to a nerve may be minimal with the nerve's ability to conduct normally hardly affected, if at all. It could be argued then, that most neurogenic or neuropathic pain is maladaptive pain, or an imperfection/defect related pain, even in its acute stages, and hence should be subdued as quickly and efficiently as possible without ill effect later on.

Pain and deformity may be an unfortunate by-product of the healing chemistry or related to genetic factors as already discussed. The fact that there are many people who suffer nerve injury, or who have squashed, compressed or fibrotic nerves without ever getting any pain is in part, testament to this 'maladaptive' imperfection/defect perspective for neurogenic pain. An alternative reasoning perspective is proposed in the next section however.

A major problem for patients *and clinicians* is that high levels of pain are often interpreted in terms of seriousness, which then generates understandable fear—leading to inappropriate inactivity/rest and/or inappropriate medicalisation. A high level of pain, or at least the witnessed distress and suffering, is scary to clinicians—but remember, high intensity pain is *not* a 'red flag'(for red flags, see Waddell 1998, Roberts 2000).

There is a dire need for research to inform us as to whether common severe acute nerve pains like acute sciatica and brachialgia are adaptive or maladaptive in nature. If indeed, the pain is maladaptive from the beginning, it will surely help reduce clinicians' fears, which are so often implicitly or explicitly passed on to patients to their detriment.

When clinicians ask themselves whether a problem is adaptive or maladaptive it is important to think beyond just the physical dimension. Consideration as to whether psychological, behavioural, social, work, and cultural responses are adaptive or maladaptive needs reasoning, too.

127

Whatever we decide, whether adaptive or maladaptive, evolutionary perspectives should also be accompanied by thoughts about 'costs'. This balances the reasoning process but, unfortunately for those who like clear-cut black and white answers, leads to frustration! In terms of our patient with back and leg pain we need to address the question: 'If the patient maintains this posture for some protective or other reason—what are the costs?' There are a number of possibilities:

- It might cause more discomfort and pain by straining other structures—which might lead to secondary problems there. Ongoing poor movement and postural habits may be being set up or 'conditioned' into the organism as normal when they needn't be (see Gifford 1998).
- If they keep going round like this, it's pretty obvious they're injured—they'd be an easy target for any predator! If you look vulnerable, you are easy prey. Thankfully nature has endowed us with responses that can extinguish pain and deformity in an instant (see placebo section below).
- The sufferer might be unable to fend properly for themselves, or their family—they are unable to work effectively, they may suffer financially, they may feel very frustrated and upset and lose their self esteem, they may feel very embarrassed or distressed by it and so forth. The long term consequences of pain and disability are well described. (See chapters in this and other volumes in this series. Also, Waddell 1998, Main & Spanswick 2000.)
- They are likely to be poor at chasing the opposite sex (usually relevant to males) or keeping them off (usually relevant to females!) and hence there are unsatisfactory reproductive consequences. 'She' may end up being saddled with a child she can ill afford to bring up, and 'he' just wallows in the misery of an unfulfilled sex drive and, to a lesser extent, reproductive failure. Or, because they move awkwardly and look weak and unpleasant (hence poor stock or poor parental capabilities) they may receive little attention from the opposite sex, or may only get it from others similarly afflicted.

Having dissected our 'disc' and nerve problem by raising a few issues on either side of the evolutionary adaptive/maladaptive argument, the reader may well be left thinking, 'What should I do with the next problem I see like this—should I tell the patient it's OK to be in pain and be awkwardly immobile, or should I try to correct the problem and lead them back to normal function?' The stance advocated here is to provide a balance of both—meaning, avoid the 'fix it/correct it now' style of approach, engender a graded recovery period similar to that for other strains and sprains but with awareness that the added nerve dimension may take a bit longer, and reassure the patient that what they are experiencing is normal and common to all, though annoying, but will lessen given some time and an appropriate recovery programme. Also provide and explain that early and effective pain relief is a great advantage for best outcome and the prevention of ongoing incapacity (see Linton 1997, Watson 2000). This means that just as drugs should work, so should physiotherapy treatments aimed at reducing pain.

If it works do it, if it doesn't work, for goodness sake, keep trying different things until you find something that is effective! A good message here for the patient is that pain relief may actually speed up healing and recovery—rather than the common belief of 'dull the pain...lose the protection and hence promote further injury', which is how most react to the suggestion of using pain killers.

So far, questions have been raised about the value of the back and leg pain and the resultant deformity. Evolutionary reasoning on the one hand suggests that since this pain and posture are common occurrences, they are likely to have evolved for very good reasons. The other side of the coin is that what we see and what the individual feels represents an unfortunate quirk, suffered as a consequence of imperfections that have been of no major consequence to successful survival.

But, why does the disc bother to hurt?

Previously we made an assumption that a disc injury is a possible precipitating cause of the patient's problem. If it is a disc—what *proximal* explanation might be used? We know a disc has an innervation (albeit a poor one), we know it is a collagenous structure and that, when injured, collagenous structures mount a healing response that begins with inflammation. Inflammation can lead to pain. Disc extrusions and protrusions can physically and chemically irritate nearby sensitive structures to produce pain too.

But, why should the disc itself bother to hurt in terms of its own health or that of the organism? Pain created by injury usually provides a background for behaviour that promotes best healing and recovery—usually guarded movement and opportunistic rest for an appropriate time. This reasoning is problematic since the disc is a metabolically sluggish structure, for example, biological turnover rate of the glycosaminoglycan in discs of dogs is said to be about 500 days and collagen is even longer than this (Adams & Hutton 1983). Collagen in a disc may not change itself for nearly two years! Very little biological activity seems to go on inside a disc and the healing potential is known to be very poor. One perspective based on the work of Osti and colleagues (Osti et al 1990) actually shows that, once injured, discs tend to 'fall apart'—*whether they are immobilised or not*. Pain and subsequent immobility appear to provide little help and may well be yet another example of maladaptive pain and the potential for prolonged maladaptive immobility.

The findings provided by Osti and colleagues (Osti et al 1990) are worthy of some scrutiny. These researchers investigated the effects of surgically producing a 5mm long and 5mm deep cut in the anterolateral aspect of young and otherwise normal lumbar discs of sheep. They lesioned 3 discs in each of 21 sheep and culled and examined them at different times after producing the experimental wound. They found:

- The lesion lead to a progressive failure of the inner annulus which occurred between the 4th and 12th month in the majority of animals.

129

- As early as the first 1–2 months there was evidence of nuclear degeneration, nuclear displacement, the presence of clefts, and the early loss of definition between outer nucleus and inner annulus in several of the discs. These features were present in all discs examined at 12 months.
- Narrowing of the disc space was observable in most discs by 8 months and was moderate or marked in all discs by 18 months.
- Osteophytes were apparent in some after 4 months and in all discs by 8 months.
- Marked changes over the whole length of the end plates were also observed.
- The actual incised area of the annulus did show healing capability, however. By 1–2 months the outer one-third of the cut area was filled with granulation tissue and this tissue was markedly vascularised.
- The deeper regions of the cut were never bridged by healing tissues.
- By 8–12 months collagenised scar tissue bridged the thin outer region of the defect and this tissue remained modestly vascularised in many of the discs.
- Some remodelling of collagen lamellae in the healed outer annulus was observed.

The research group went on to reason that degeneration following the artificial annular tear may be a result of continued movement in the vicinity of the lesion and that plate fixation may prevent such dramatic changes. They therefore repeated the experiments but included plate fixation across some of the injured discs to prevent movement. Interestingly, their work showed that the plate fixation had no effect on the degenerative process (Moore et al 1994).

The conclusion is that the disc barely seems to heal, it takes ages to change and immobilising it seems to have little effect on the end result. Since pain usually prevents movement it seems unhelpful here. From the 'selfish' perspective of the disc tissue, producing pain for a healing defence seems utterly pointless.

The message from this line of reasoning is that since the pain is useless, get rid of it and get on with life as soon as you possibly can. Symptomatic treatment and restoration of range and posture as quickly as possible seem justified. The pain is a quirk related to disc innervation and really has little value in creating best outcome, it may even, according to mounting current evidence, have quite a negative impact on us modern day humans and the societies we live in.

But, flexed and shifted, so often away from the painful side, and with movements towards the painful side being far more limited than those that are away from it, are such a common presentation. Why are there such stereotyped responses? Surely they wouldn't have evolved without good reason.

Consider the relationship of the disc to the nervous system (reviewed in Gifford 1997). In the radicular canal and intervertebral foramen the lumbosacral nerve roots lie in close proximity to the disc. Any change in disc size or in the local environment will potentially threaten the nerve's integrity and put it at risk. I have discussed the effect of movement and posture on the nerve roots in detail elsewhere (see Gifford 1997, Gifford 2001 for discussion and further literature). For the purposes of the arguments here, it is enough to state that spinal flexion plus deviation towards the contralateral side tends to increase the size of the spinal and radicular canals, and movement towards the opposite direction, i.e. extension plus ipsilateral deviation/rotation side flexion, tends to reduce their size. It would be a wise action for an individual with a disc bulge or extrusion (or even the potential for one), or oedema/swelling in the area adjacent to a nerve root, to adopt a posture that puts the least pressure or strain on the nerve—i.e. flexion and deviation away from the affected side. Any threat to the nervous system is a potential disaster for the future efficiency of those afflicted. Far better, and more efficient to, whenever possible, adapt to a new posture that protects the nervous system, than to injure the nerve and suffer the consequences of neuropathy. A weak calf muscle, or a numb foot is likely to be a serious impairment for an active hunter-gatherer.

The observations that follow support the 'adaptive' nature of the early flexed shifted posture for the health of adjacent emerging nerve roots.

In my clinical experience it is common to see patients who have developed sciatica and often some neurological deficit following spinal manipulation or regimes of management that encourage repeated extension for simple acute low back pain. This observation is pure anecdote: while it may have happened anyway, it is something well worth researching; it is quite reasonable, it is commonly agreed upon by other clinicians, and has to have some explanation. What is noticeable in these patients is that there is often a delay of anything from several hours to 2–3 days or longer after the treatment or exercise is performed and before the problem worsens. Research showing prolonged delays of onset for hyperexcitability following experimental nerve injury supports this clinical observation (see Devor & Seltzer 1999).

Knowledge like this highlights *the dangers of accepting an immediate change in pain response to a movement procedure as an indicator of helpfulness*. It also adds weight to an approach to management that requires graduated progress rather than instant success or instant change. 'I walked in bent double and walked out straight' may not be such a good thing after all.

An evolutionary style of reasoning, based on the proposals above might predict the following (all potentially valuable research questions):

- Disc injury that does little to threaten nerve roots is likely to hurt less or not hurt at all. Discs do not need pain because immobility is of no advantage to any recovery. There may be literature that refutes this, if so, it needs to be presented to balance the argument.
- A disc (or any tissue) that is in a vulnerable state, and which has the potential to injure or irritate the nervous system may provide some helpful pain. This may be long lasting and lead to permanent changes in flexibility and posture, or it may be very brief and very intense with particular movements or postures.

131

- Nociceptive innervation density should be higher in parts of the disc adjacent to the nervous system. Logically, dura and root epineurium most likely to be affected by disc material should have a more dense innervation too. Certainly the dural innervation anteriorly is far more profound than posteriorly, where there is virtually no innervation (Groen et al 1988).
- Some prolonged pains, altered movement patterns, muscle imbalances, disc degeneration, osteophytes and motion segment stiffening associated with the consequences of disc injury, are very adaptive processes in that they may well be nervous system and vertebral column protective. Medically these findings are viewed as 'pathological' when they may well be highly adaptive biologically. Could we be inadvertently over-treating and putting too much emphasis on some of these impairments we skillfully observe and try so hard to change? Could it be that it may be appropriate to teach patients to adopt antalgic movement patterns and postures in order to for them to remain active and productive?

As already argued, our eagerness and our obligation to overcome pain, correct deformity and restore range of motion as quickly as possible, may actually be prolonging recovery. Clinical anecdote sometimes supports this—for example, many patients having been on treatment for long periods, go on holiday, stop their exercises, stop treatment, and feel a great deal better. The patients put it down to the weather, the doctors to rest or relief from stress, and physios to the daily swimming. This may be so, but we ought to realise that stopping what we have given them to do, or what we have been doing to them, are also factors to consider.

Fever for an infection—an evolutionary masterpiece!

The reader may find this section interesting, considering it an interlude before the final section perhaps, but what it really spells out is how important evolutionary thinking can be in our clinical reasoning.

A patient has a streptococcal infection; symptoms include headache, painful throat, fever, anaemia, and the impaired speech of laryngitis. Should any of these be considered good symptoms? The answer is yes, all of them, except the speech impairment.

- The headache makes you want to relax and avoid stress, a good strategy to hasten recovery from an illness.
- The sore throat means you will not try to shout or talk too much, and will be careful about what you swallow.
- The fever and anaemia are things *you are doing to the bacteria*, not what they are doing to you. The high temperature hastens and facilitates immunological responses, and the anaemia deprives the bacteria of a needed nutrient (iron) as the body hides its iron in the liver.

According to Nesse and Williams (1994), if we get an infection the body releases a chemical called leukocyte endogenous mediator (LEM) which both raises the temperature and greatly reduces the availability of iron in the blood. Iron absorption by the gut is also decreased during infection. Even our food preferences change. In the midst of a bout of influenza, such iron-rich foods as ham and eggs suddenly seem disgusting; we prefer tea and toast. Remember that blood letting—perhaps not so daft—reduced iron levels! Iron supplements may harm patients who have infections (only 11% of doctors and 6% of pharmacists know this).

Fever is an adaptive 'host' response to infection that has persisted throughout the animal kingdom for hundreds of millions of years. For example, even lizards benefit from fever; when infected they actively seek places that will warm their bodies by 2°C. Blocking fever in animals increases their likelihood of dying (Nesse & Williams 1994).

What about costs and benefits?

Considering fever—if a higher temperature prevents infections having their way, why isn't our body temperature 40°C all the time? A moderate fever has costs: it depletes nutrient reserves 20% faster, and it causes temporary male sterility. And a higher fever causes delirium, possible seizures and lasting tissue damage.

When considering any observation a balanced approach is necessary. We should always think about the potential costs and benefits of interventions. For example, reducing an 'adaptive' temperature or ameliorating the process and symptoms of infection may be detrimental to recovery. Children with chicken pox who were given paracetamol took on average about a day longer to recover than those who took placebo. Recovery from cold infections is slowed in those given aspirin as compared to those given a placebo, and the placebo group had a significantly higher antibody response.

The placebo—why would it have evolved?

'Placebo' is often used to pour scorn, but as a phenomenon it is quite remarkable. It is a word used by medical science and medicine to describe an awkward, puzzling and sometimes embarrassing phenomenon (for definitions and discussions of all the evidence see Chs 1–4). The placebo is consistently observed and is found when patients respond positively to an intervention that is known to be physiologically 'inactive' for the condition under scrutiny. However, as the reader will have already found in earlier chapters, it is also a consistent partner in 'active' treatments too. As a phenomenon, the placebo is unlikely to go away, and as a word it is frequently used in a derogatory and insulting way because it challenges the very foundations of medical intervention.

Even today, with the knowledge we have about the placebo, spontaneous recovery, regression to the mean and related phenomena, many doctors and Consultants regard physiotherapy as 'mere placebo'—something to keep the patient amused while they recover naturally, and something to prescribe to keep difficult patients out of their consulting rooms. In their view, the placebo is worthless and its presence provides evidence in support of an inorganic 'cause' of the patient's problem and that 'real' treatment is unnecessary and wasteful. Thankfully, such sentiments are being challenged seriously in favour of far more productive multidimensional models that embrace multidisciplinary co-operation and mutual respect (see earlier chapters and Gifford 2000).

As already argued by Pat Roche, Nigel Lawes, Mitch Noon and Richard Shortall (Chs 1–4), part of feeling comfortable with what we do as clinicians is feeling comfortable with the placebo. The word and the negative connotations that are associated with it are now wrong for clinical medicine and management, but the things that account for it are right. In particular I like the notion of the 'psychosocial' placebo (see Ch. 4) and the impact of the 'therapeutic alliance' (see Ch. 3) as better ways of taking this phenomenon on. It seems quite clear that the reassuring, activating, confidence-giving environment that good therapists can create has a very positive multidimensional impact. This includes positive biological responses. If positive interactions have consistent positive outcomes it is reasonable and useful to ask what their evolutionary underpinnings might be.

From an evolutionary perspective, it is proposed here that the observed placebo phenomena may be related to responses associated with:

1. The need to put healing on hold.
2. The need for help, safety, reassurance and satisfaction.
3. The need for pain variation.
4. The need for pain relief.

All four explanations will be discussed before tying the proposed reasoning together in a way that can be clinically useful.

The need to put healing on hold

Injury is a part of life; sometimes it causes death, but quite often the organism survives. All organisms have evolved some form of repair/healing physiology as well as a repair/healing reaction or behaviour. For the higher social mammals, this condition can be linked to altered moods and emotions, too (see Thayer 1996).

Healing/repair requires energy and nutrition and from an evolutionary/survival perspective has to be seen as a potentially expensive item. Organisms have evolved to conserve energy at all costs (recall the 'innate laziness' rule discussed earlier.) If an animal is in extreme environmental conditions, is in danger of losing its life for some reason, or perhaps has very meager energy stores—any available nutrients it does have need to be used in ways that are most likely to preserve its life. It makes sense for living things to have evolved very efficient systems that control the use of nutrients and energy efficiently, diverting resources to fuel only the most vital processes and actions. Putting lengthy and costly healing and repair processes 'on hold' while an animal escapes or is busy foraging for food makes sound 'evolutionary' survival sense.

In keeping with this line of reasoning, we know that stress inhibits vegetative (anabolic) functions (like growth and repair) powerfully, while at the same time promoting efficient nutrient delivery and energy provision for the appropriate threat/survival action response required.

In the evolutionary environment threat is commonplace; to stay alive requires hard work, and any energy or nutrient-preserving behaviour, reaction, or physiology is likely to be favourably selected from one generation to the next. From the perspective of the carer and the production of a placebo response (which promotes healing/recovery), turning this potent stress related energy conserving healing inhibitory mechanism off, by providing an environment that is safe and 'stress-less', may be an important governing feature for its occurrence.

The need for help, safety, reassurance and satisfaction

Humans, are societal; in a similar way to lions, hyenas, most monkeys, elephants, dolphins, termites and bees, we have evolved behaviours that in large part are community oriented. For us, and other social animals to survive requires co-operation in, for example, obtaining food, in nurturing, and in defence against predators and attackers. Such co-operation requires the exchange of information between individuals, and it is in social species that we find the most complex and sophisticated forms of animal communication. Think how capable and how necessary it is that we are expert at interpreting the mood states, friendliness and trustworthiness of others by vision alone.

In most successful communities there is the giving and taking of help. Issues involving social hierarchy and advantages were touched on earlier in this chapter, and the nature and evolution of altruism, an evolutionary paradox, can be investigated elsewhere (Wright 1994, Watson 1995). Clearly, for a community to maintain a successful working network individuals must help each other. Helping and needing help is part of our nature, a reason for our success, and logically must have biological underpinnings.

It makes sense that if we are injured, a requirement of the weakened injured tissues is some modification of behaviour that affords a degree of protection. If an injured tissue is vulnerable, so is the organism it belongs to. Why else would pain have evolved, but to provide a powerful background feeling that is so distressing it demands a change in attitude, thinking and behaviour? Surely this is the primary purpose of pain—to change behaviour?

One way of reasoning here is to consider the brain/CNS (the 'scrutinising' centre—see Gifford 1998) as receiving competing sensory inputs, each demanding some action or response. Thus, the brain/CNS might receive a massive sensory nociceptive barrage from injured tissues. Metaphorically the tissues are selfishly screaming, 'Me, me, me, look after me...forget all else, it's me you need to organise a response for, I'm the most important.' In this way, the first injury provision is for the tissues to selfishly try to get help—that is, to ask for, and selfishly try to get, a change in the behaviour of

135

'their' organism for their advantage. However, the brain/CNS may be busy elsewhere, tackling a marauding tribesman perhaps, or fleeing an attacking buffalo. The message back might be, 'Sorry bud, I might get back to you later, I'm busy right now, you'll just have to suffer. Tough. Bye.' (The pain gates, quite rightly, slam shut while the muffled nociception glumly continues). Later on, when life calms down a little, the tissue screaming may start to penetrate. The pain gate inhibitory currents gradually lift and our friend starts to suffer as the incoming messages reach consciousness. He feels pain in his badly twisted ankle, he starts limping, he orientates his attention towards the injured area, and he starts moaning and feeling very concerned (see Pat Wall's Introductory Essay in this volume). It doesn't look nice and it doesn't feel nice either. His instinctive reaction is to seek help or to find safety as soon as possible. He is weak, he hurts, he doesn't feel confident about looking after himself, he feels highly vulnerable, he is worried and he is only just coping. He is verging on feeling helpless (see Fig. 6.1). He needs help from others, or he needs to find a safe place to hide and rest up. Despite the intense pain he searches for help and safety. Pain now drives a very powerful 'help'/safety-seeking need state that, if satisfied, may enhance the chances of survival considerably.

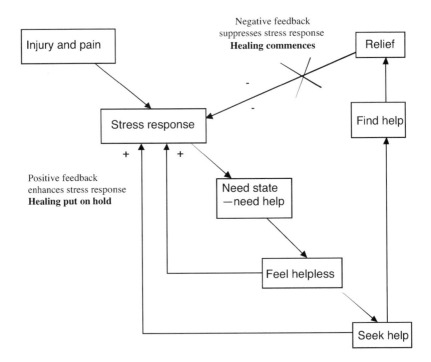

Fig. 6.1 Injury, pain and the stress response

Getting help and feeling safe reduces stress and consequently releases the powerful inhibitory controls on recovery/vegetative physiology. Recall that if we *perceive* that we are under threat (even though we may not be) our bodies mount a stress response that can instantly dampen down systems like those concerned with healing and repair. 'Maladaptive' perception of a situation may lead to unhelpful physiological responses. Feeling safe and feeling reassured may have powerful positive biological consequences in that it allows energy to be spent on the healing response.

The stress response has evolved so that it is switched on very rapidly— note the abruptness with which you become tense or your heart rate increases when you are uneasy or excited. Yet even though a *sense* of relief can be profound, it still can take a long time to fully calm-down afterwards. Clearly, evolution has preserved those who get worked up fastest and remain vigilant for a good while after. The doctor who frowns at a patient's X-ray and sighs at what he sees takes just a few seconds to wind up a prolonged stress response. Quelling the stress response, as all good therapists who deal with patients whom this has happened to know, can take a lot of words, a lot of reassurance, and a great deal of time. Careless talk can carry a high cost (see Ch. 5 this volume), but careful talk pays a good dividend.

The message here is that getting help, finding safety and feeling reassured on the one hand, allows the stress response to wind down and switch off, while on the other, the more vegetative functions like growth and repair to resume activity. Part of what happens when we get the help *we feel we need* might account for part of the placebo observation. Even if it is not, the arguments here provide some good reasons for providing actions and responses that help the patient feel reassured.

The need for pain variation

Pain varies all the time; it has to. Sadly, the inconsistent pain report and pain behaviour noted in many patients, especially in those with more chronic and difficult problems, is commonly/frequently used to challenge the authenticity of the pain and the patient. Sadly, too, if an observation doesn't fit with the pattern we perceive, rather than seek an explanation via thinking and research, we tend to blame the most obvious, though at times quite erroneous, factor we can think of. Time and again, the most obvious cause for an observation has been shown to be wrong (e.g. see Sagan 1997).

Pain needs to vary. As discussed in the previous section, the brain/CNS 'sorts and chooses' sensory information and prioritises its messages to best fit the needs of survival (see also the Introductory Essay to this volume). 'Disallowing' pain to reach consciousness, or dulling its intensity via gate control, is essential in times of need, like times of danger or when we perceive danger, or in times that require a great deal of attention and concentration. Hence, when under threat, or when busily occupied with 'important' tasks like gathering food, or having, or trying to have, sex, gate control may be at its most efficient. Since intense pain may inhibit actions that have survival (and health) benefits, it cannot always be permitted. Evolution clearly favoured those ancestors with the apparatus to vary the ability of nociception to produce pain and alter behaviour. Good pain can drive safety-seeking behaviour and recuperative actions at times of low threat, or low need, but can be powerfully dulled in times of important goal-seeking action. *Even in the acute situation, pain has evolved to be 'adaptively' inconsistent.* Pain is slippery.

Observe the inconsistency of a child's pain. One moment they are writhing and screaming in agony, the next minute they are running around as if nothing had happened. Call it naïve pain, or manipulating pain, but its major attribute is its *consistent* inconsistency through every culture. Pain can go when it suits just as easily as it can come when it suits. Pain at one level promotes behaviour that is beneficial to the tissues: it orientates us towards looking after the injured hurting part, it makes us go quiet, it promotes rest if rest is an option, it makes us move when the tissues crave movement, and it can make us feel concerned and want to seek help. At other less palatable levels, and let us not kid ourselves, it can also help provide advantages and rewards (remember survival advantages). Pain behaviour has a very smart but devious element. One difficulty is that providing rewards for pain and the accompanying pain behaviour further reinforces them and can amplify them. If crying and squealing very loudly when we hurt gets a sticky bun, then crying and squealing is very likely to be imprinted as a useful strategy in future. That the act is a conscious one can be challenged. Responses once reinforced quickly become learnt. If a pain and pain behaviour are subtly rewarded, their future activity may quickly become a conditioned habit that gets ever more permanently imprinted. Well-established habits require a great deal of effort to overcome.

Since a major part of the placebo effect relates to decreased pain, 'placebo analgesia', it is important to ask how the arguments above relate to this effect. There may be a slightly dangerous paradox, since relieving 'stress' and 'threat' via help and care during treatment may actually *allow* pain to feature more, rather than dull it. However, two forms of stress need to be considered: the first, associated with pure survival at and around the time of injury, which produces 'stress induced analgesia'; and the second, which relates to stress / distress associated with pain and the realisation of injury—which produces the feeling of vulnerability and the 'need for help' behaviour strategy. Our patients with acute pain are in this second category. Here, they are likely to be focused on the pain and the injury and anxious about it and its impact on their future. A good examination (in the patient's eyes), a clear explanation combined with a positive picture of management and the expected outcome are vital components during that first, and most important, therapist-patient session. As individuals, if we are concerned about an injury, or concerned about a pain, we dwell on it. If concern lessens, if the pain is 'normalised' in some way, our concern subsides and our attention and focus on the pain and injury can reduce significantly. Effective reassurance is a pain killer since it downgrades its importance. For reassurance to be effective, it requires patient belief in you and your examinations, your findings, and your explanations. Effective reassurance has little to do with the treatment offered and everything to do with you and your examination and explanation style.

In summary, on the one hand gate control can be initiated by fear and the need for survival activities, on the other it can be enhanced by changes in attention away from the pain. In the case of patients, shifting attention away from pain can occur with good quality reassurance in tandem with confidence building function and focused activity. Thus, a significant step in therapy occurs if attention can be directed away from the pain or the part that hurts and even further if it then includes some form of task fulfillment. If interactions with patients provide such things, then changes in pain, that may be termed a positive 'placebo' response in a trial setting, are likely to occur.

The need for pain relief

As argued so far, pain drives valuable safety-seeking behaviour. Pain orientates us to the site of damage and makes us investigate it and try to derive a meaning in order to formulate appropriate action. Since pain is so unpleasant, it also drives us towards behaviours that bring relief from it. If I get stung by a stinging nettle, I might immediately look around for a dock-leaf to press on the area (a dock-leaf feels very cool and distracts from the stinging). If I burn myself I look for the quickest way of cooling the part burnt. Pain drives behaviours to satisfy pain relief. Pain relief is what we all want. As Patrick Wall (Wall 1999 p. 155) has said, pain is 'best seen as a need state, like hunger and thirst, which is terminated by a consummatory act.' Part of the consummation for pain is the seeking and obtaining of a treatment. The importance of patient belief in relation to active and placebo treatments has already been discussed in earlier chapters.

Why would the need for pain relief have evolved? Surely that goes against the general purpose of pain? I would like to invite comments here, but would propose that while high pain early on is necessary to drive help-seeking behaviour, continued high levels are detrimental to best outcome. Once safe, it is paramount that pain is brought down to a manageable level so that life can go on and independence can return. Not only does high pain intensity stop you sleeping, make you moody and unpleasant and distressed, it may also prevent the restoration of normal movement and activity. Lack of normal activity and movement (and sleep too) quickly leads to a loss of fitness and deconditioning—which ultimately increases vulnerability and threatens survival capacity.

Activating the placebo response

Previous chapters in this section of the book show that placebo effects have two components: one that influences pain perception, and one that has measurable physiological effects. A clear message is that therapists should be looking to understand the placebo, appreciate its importance and integrate

139

aspects of therapy that relate to its effects. Problems have always arisen with the idea that if you use placebos you are deceiving the patient. Hopefully the chapters in this section of the book are helping to lay this perspective to rest. In fact, talking to your patients about the meaning of the placebo is an empowering thing for them. It is well worth reading what Norman Cousins said about the 'mysterious placebo' in his best-selling classic, *Anatomy of an Illness as Perceived by the Patient* (Cousins 1979).

In order to bring the material discussed together I would like to analyse some of the key components of a mother dealing with and comforting her young child who has just hurt himself. Although there is much subtle variability, most young children and their mothers react to injury and pain in stereotyped, and therefore arguably, in 'evolved' ways. Note that all the features discussed below occur very soon after the injuring incident and the onset of pain.

Seek help from someone trustworthy. When hurt in some way, most young children instinctively want their mother and their mother instinctively wants them. A mother is the one they trust and it takes a strong willed mother to let anyone else deal with their child. In hunter-gatherer times, and still in many regions and districts of the world, if you are hurt and vulnerable, it might be a very dangerous option to seek help from someone who is unknown. As a therapist, it helps if you are well known and have a good record in your local community. Successfully treated patients and positive referring doctors help here. Most people tend to stick with someone they trust and who has been effective in the past. People relax when they feel comfortable with someone trustworthy.

Attention and diagnosis. The mother attends to the area that is hurt— she shows concern, she finds out where it is, she looks and examines it, *she diagnoses the problem*. We all know how ineffective this part can be if the child feels the attention is inadequate—the mother who is too busy to be interested or take the time often gets an auditory savaging from the frustrated child. Therapists need to care, to show interest, to give adequate attention, and to take care to listen, question and do a high quality physical examination. Doctors would be advised to do the same. In the current culture, we all need more time.

Reassurance. The mother then reassures *herself* and then the *child* that the problem is not major. We need to do the same—the Red Flag guidelines that we now have are useful here (see Volume 2 of this series). As mentioned, the examination must be extensive enough to provide reassurance. This is an individual thing. Whether child or not, some people require a lot more time and a lot more reassurance than do others. If we do not give it, or it does not come across as convincing, it may not be sufficient. This involves listening, attention and the appropriate use of voice and touch.

Treatment. Thereafter, the mother's major concern is to quell the child's distress, attend to the pain, and get them active once more. She may rub the area, rub the child's back or 'kiss it better'; she may get a plaster or even give some medication. Throughout it all, touch is used very powerfully—the cuddles provide a feeling of protection, safety or distraction, the rubs and more precise touch may provide a comforting input and further reassurance. All combine to relieve anxiety and relieve the pain. Beneficial 'inputs' originate simultaneously from tissues as well as via the mind—'bottom-up' and 'top-down' inputs. Witness how social animals use touch when they care for their sick and vulnerable, elephants, many social monkeys, the whales and dolphins, for instance. Touch is a constant reminder to the nervous system and the organism that they are safe, that someone is there to protect. Early on and with high levels of disabling pain, this type of reasoning would predict that touch and closeness may need to be continuous and prolonged! Bedside vigils for the very sick—regular touch, gentle words, the application of soothing compresses may be fundamental to a recovery environment. Reactions like these seem instinctive with our children but as we mature they seem to be lost and forgotten. Is our current overly objective and cold mechanistic approach to illness with its 'no time for care' style, a problem to be addressed?

Distraction and reactivation. Once the tears and crying start to subside a mother might hold and play with a cuddly toy to further distract the infant's attention from the hurt. Reactivation and independent play soon follow. It seems likely that smiles and cuddles, laughter and fun (and the likely physiological effects) may represent many of the best attributes of good therapists and good therapy! Skilled parents can quickly turn terrible tears into chuckles and giggles. Pain gates slam shut and healing proceeds! Arguably, the goal of trying to get back to normal tasks and activities in a carefree way as soon as reasonably possible is paramount.

Having time to think about how we are going to perform our daily movements seems a ridiculous luxury when viewed from an evolutionary perspective. Re-education of *thoughtless, fearless movements* that are task and goal orientated needs to be taken more seriously by professions involved in treatment of pain conditions relating to musculoskeletal injury and dysfunction (Gifford 2001a, 2002). To teach a patient physical confidence and **not** to focus on their body during activity might be anathema to many, but to most normals it could be viewed as one of the most valued currencies of uncluttered survival!

Note that if help isn't immediately available, we have to cope. A child who is playing out of range of their mother may suffer scratches and blows that would normally elicit strong distress but in this instance do not. The child may self diagnose, they rub and squirm and shake the part, they try it and test it and find its OK, the more they move the better they feel and they're soon back playing in the game again. Lone sailors often report remarkable physical acts despite appalling injury and severe pain. When help is unavailable, we have to cope. There may be two extremes. At one end is not enough help—and we die! At the other end, is too much help—and we risk becoming disabled by it. The evidence is suggesting that we are giving and receiving far too much help for far too long for the majority of musculoskeletal problems.

Given the discussion here and that presented in earlier chapters, the overall stance is that specific environmental, psychological and physiological conditions exist that can promote more efficient recovery and normal function, and that there is a huge complex interplay between these conditions. Every individual and their condition is subtly different and therefore requires subtly different conditions. The clinician's role is to help the patient explore and gradually create the best recovery environment, the best psychological state and the best physiological activity. In the clinic I like to think that part of my role is to help set up the individual's system so that it responds best. It's a two way process (between patient and therapist) that attempts to adjust the 'gain' of the system to the most favourable setting for efficient recovery. This is definitely not 'soft' medicine, but powerful, biological and, due to lack of practical understanding, largely untapped. The word placebo, in a rather distorted 'proximal' or mechanistic way, is a poorly chosen word that is representative of some of the observations derived from the remarkable natural healing and recovery processes when they are given the opportunity to happen. Providing this opportunity is a skill that needs to be on offer and not one that is viewed with disdain because of some historical prejudices associated with a word.

Final comments

Evolutionary reasoning is all very well but dangers occur if concepts and reasoning so generated do not consider all possibilities and result in rigid approaches. For example, giving appropriate attention to the pain and injured part was discussed in the context of the child above, however, overindulging a child with attention or a patient with the passive component of therapy may be detrimental in the long run. For example, it can create dependency, passivity and lead to unnecessary physical incapacity. From earlier in the chapter, a therapist who tells all her patients that to be flexed and shifted is not a problem and as a result makes no attempt to improve or restore normal range or full physical potential is just as problematic as a therapist trying to correct the posture instantly.

Evolutionary reasoning in medicine and physiotherapy is a new way of thinking and viewing the situations and presentations of our patients. Pleasingly, its validity is being increasingly tested, while its utility at this stage, seems obvious and points towards interesting and exciting new management and research strategies.

REFERENCES

Adams MA, Hutton WC 1983 The effect of fatigue on the lumbar intervertebral disc. Journal of Bone and Joint Surgery British Volume 65B(2):199–203

Allison AC 1997 Protection afforded by sickle-cell trait against subterian malarial infection. In: Ridley M (ed) Evolution. Oxford University Press, Oxford 51–55

Charlton BG 1996 What is the ultimate cause of socio-economic inequalities in health? An explanation in terms of evolutionary psychology. Journal of the Royal Society of Medicine 89:3–8

Cousins N 1979 Anatomy of an Illness as Perceived by the Patient. Bantam Books, New York

Devor M 1990 Sources of variability in the sensation of pain. In: Dimitrijevic MR, Wall PD, Lindblom V (eds) Recent Advances in Restorative Neurology: 3 Altered Sensation and Pain. Karger, Basel 189–196

Devor M, Seltzer Z 1999 Pathophysiology of damaged nerves in relation to chronic pain. In: Wall PD, Melzack R (eds) Textbook of Pain 4th edn. Chruchill Livingstone, Edinburgh 129–164

Diamond J 1991 The Rise and Fall of the Third Chimpanzee. Vintage, London

Gifford LS 1997 Neurodynamics. In: Pitt-Brooke (ed) Rehabilitation of Movement: Theoretical bases of clinical practice. Saunders, London 159–195

Gifford LS 1998 Central mechanisms. In: Gifford LS (ed) Topical Issues in Pain 1. Whiplash—science and management. Fear-avoidance beliefs and behaviour. CNS Press, Falmouth 67–80

Gifford LS 1998 The mature organism model. In: Gifford LS (ed) Topical Issues in Pain 1. Whiplash—science and management. Fear-avoidance beliefs and behaviour. CNS Press, Falmouth 45–56

Gifford LS 2000 The patient in front of us: from genes to environment. In: Gifford LS (ed) Topical Issues in Pain 2. Biopsychosocial assessment. Relationships and pain CNS Press, Falmouth 1–11

Gifford LS 2001 Acute low cervical nerve root conditions—patient presentations and pathobiological reasoning. Manual Therapy 6(2):106–115

Gifford LS 2001a Perspectives on the biopsychosocial model Part 1: Some issues that need to be accepted? In Touch, The Journal of the Organisation of Chartered Physiotherapists in Private Practice Autumn issue No 97:3–9

Gifford LS 2002 Perspectives on the biopsychosocial model Part 2: The shopping basket approach. In Touch, The Journal of the Organisation of Chartered Physiotherapists in Private Practice Spring issue No 99:11-22

Groen GJ, Baljet B, Drukker J 1988 The innervation of the spinal dura mater: Anatomy and clinical implications. Acta Neurochirurgica 92:39–46

Lariviere WR, Wilson SG, Laughlin TM et al 2002 Heritability of nociception. III. Genetic relationships among commonly used assays of nociception and hypersensitivity. Pain 97:75–86

Linton SJ 1997 Overlooked and underrated? The role of acute pain intensity in the development of chronic back pain problems. Pain Forum 6(2):145–147

Main CJ, Spanswick CC 2000 Pain Management. An interdisciplinary approach. Churchill Livingstone, Edinburgh

Mogil JS 1999 The genetics of pain. Abstracts: 9th World Congress on Pain, Vienna, Austria IASP Press, Seattle 259

Mogil JS, Wilson SG, Bon K et al 1999 Heritability of nociception I. Responses of eleven inbred mouse strains on twelve measures of nociception. Pain 80:67–82

Mogil JS, Wilson SG, Bon K et al 1999a Heritability of nociception II. 'Types' of nociception revealed by genetic correlation analysis. Pain 80:83–93

Moore RJ, Latham JM, Vernon-Roberts B et al 1994 Does plate fixation prevent disc degeneration after a lateral annulus tear? Spine 19(24):2787–2790

Nesse RM, Williams GC 1994 Evolution and Healing. The new science of Darwinian medicine. Phoenix, London

Osti OL, Vernon-Roberts B, Fraser RD 1990 Annulus tears and intervertebral disc degeneration: An experimental study using an animal model. Spine 15(8):762–767

Roberts L 2000 Flagging the danger signs of low back pain. In: Gifford LS (ed) Topical Issues in Pain 2. Biopsychosocial assessment and management. Relationships and pain. CNS Press, Falmouth 69–84

Sagan C 1997 The Demon-Haunted World. Science as a candle in the dark. Hodder Headline, London

Thayer RE 1996 The Origin of Everyday Moods: Managing energy, tension and stress. Oxford University Press, New York

143

Waddell G 1998 The Back Pain Revolution. Churchill Livingstone, Edinburgh
Wall P 1999 Pain. The science of suffering. Weidenfeld & Nicolson, London
Watson L 1995 Dark Nature. A natural history of evil. Hodder & Stoughton, London
Watson P 2000 Psychosocial predictors of outcome from low back pain. In: Gifford LS (ed) Topical Issues in Pain 2. Biopsychosocial assessment and management. Relationships and pain. CNS Press, Falmouth 85–109
Wright R 1994 The Moral Animal: Why we are the way we are. Abacus, London

FURTHER READING—A SELECTION

As well as the literature cited above, many of the following books have impacted on and moulded my thinking on the topic of pain and health and some of the reasoning presented in the chapter. Some are from the 'pop' healing literature, several are written for the general public by respected academics, and some are more conventional science. Mostly, they provide easy and quite often amusing reading on a difficult topic.

Benson H 1996 Timeless Healing. The power and biology of belief. Simon & Schuster, Frome
Cassell EJ 1991 The Nature of Suffering and the Goals of Medicine. Oxford University Press, New York
Crick F 1994 The Astonishing Hypothesis. The scientific search for the soul. Touchstone books, London
Delvecchio Good M-J, Brodwin PE, Good BJ et al 1992 Pain as a Human Experience: An anthropological perspective. University of California Press, Berkeley
Dossey L 1993 Healing Words. The power of prayer and the practice of medicine. Harper, San Francisco
Edelman G 1992 Bright Air Brilliant Fire. On the matter of the mind. Penguin Books, London
Harrington A (ed) 1997 The Placebo Effect. An interdisciplinary exploration. Harvard University Press, London
LeDoux J 1998 The Emotional Brain. The mysterious underpinnings of emotional life. Weidenfeld & Nicolson, London
Martin P 1997 The Sickening Mind. Brain, behaviour, immunity and disease. Harper Collins, London
Montagu A 1986 Touching: The human significance of the skin 3rd edn. Harper & Row, New York
Morris DB 1991 The Culture of Pain. University of California Press, Berkeley
Pert CB 1997 Molecules of emotion. Why you feel the way you feel. Pocket Books, London
Plotkin H 1994 Darwin Machines and the Nature of Knowledge. Penguin, London
Price DD 1999 Psychological Mechanisms of Pain and Analgesia. Progress in Pain Research and Management Vol 15. IASP Press, Seattle
Robertson I 1999 Mind Sculpture. Your brain's untapped potential. Bantam Press, London
Rose S 1997 Lifelines:. biology, freedom, determinism. Penguin Books, London
Sapolsky RM 1997 Junk Food Monkeys and Other Essays on the Biology of the Human Predicament. Headline, London
Shapiro AK, Shapiro E 1997 The Powerful Placebo. From ancient priest to modern physician. John Hopkins University Press, Baltimore
Sutherland S 1992 Irrationality, The Enemy within. Penguin books, London
Whybrow PC 1997 A Mood Apart. A thinker's guide to emotion and its disorders. Picador, London
Williams GC 1996 Plan and Purpose in Nature. Weidenfeld & Nicolson, London
Wolpert L 1992 The Unnatural Nature of Science. Faber and Faber, London

2

Pain management

7

The biopsychosocial approach and low back pain

HEATHER MUNCEY

Physiotherapists working in an outpatient department today will expect the largest part of their caseload to be musculoskeletal pain and associated problems. Taking low back pain as a representative and frequently encountered condition, this chapter will consider evidence-based management, some models and approaches to care, and discuss the role of active rehabilitation in a physical therapy service.

In a busy department with high and often relentless caseloads it is sometimes difficult for therapists to keep their eyes on the ball of what the problem is and what is a desirable outcome from their treatment. The patient usually presents with pain as the main problem and will describe how this is affecting their daily life. Physiotherapy training encourages the analysis of the relationship between pain and tissue dysfunction. This leads seductively to a temptation to solve the problem by mobilising the stiff joint, strengthening the weak muscle, or correcting an imbalance. Of course, any of these may have a part to play in the overall treatment plan. However, a belief that 'clearing the pain' or 'altering the biomechanics' in itself will solve the patient's problem is, according to evidence, a faulty one.

So what exactly is the problem? The incidence and prevalence of low back pain have not changed over the past forty years. The natural history of non-specific low back pain is recurrent (CSAG 1994). However, statistics show that what has grown out of all proportion is pain associated disability (Waddell 1998).

Clearly, as well as relieving pain, physiotherapists must also consider the prevention of pain-associated incapacity as part of 'the problem.' Pain-associated incapacity or disability is multidimensional in nature; it may be biological, psychosocial, economic and work related.

Physiotherapists are familiar with the physical aspects of disability and how to tackle these. On the whole, however, they tend to be less confident about the psychosocial aspects, how to manage them and whether it is their role to do so. In addition, it is difficult from within the context of a healthcare system to affect the economic and work related aspects of ongoing pain.

Challenges to current models used in physical therapy

Over recent years an increasingly large body of evidence has shown that a purely biomedical approach to physical therapy in the management of low back pain is too reductionist. It often results in less than optimal outcomes for patients, therapists and purchasers. There is little evidence that symptomatic treatments for low back pain have a lasting effect (Koes et al 1991). In fact, in some cases these interventions may produce more harm than good (CSAG 1994a), especially if there have been delays whilst awaiting treatment.

Desirable outcomes are not simply reduced pain but improved function and ability to return to work as well as better health outcomes at a reasonable cost.

The biopsychosocial model relating to the assessment and management of pain takes into account aspects that affect the way individuals respond to pain. The model has been defined (Waddell 1993) and advocated for use by physiotherapists by many (Waddell 1993, CSAG 1994a, Kendall et al 1997, CSAG 2000, Watson & Kendall 2000).

How should this model be used in a physiotherapy department?

Integrating the biopsychosocial model

Changes to traditional physiotherapy approaches are needed to achieve desirable outcomes for low back pain sufferers. Changes are required:

1. To the information and advice given to patients.
2. In therapy aims and practice.
3. To shift resources to acute management of low back pain where this approach may reduce risk of poor outcomes (CSAG 1994a).

Information and advice to patients

Therapists usually advise patients with enthusiasm! This information and advice may be on the nature of the problems, on anatomy and biomechanics, ergonomics, or on how to avoid recurrences. It is important to consider two things when giving information and advice:

- **what** information/advice is being given, and the effect this will have on the patient (see Ch. 5)

- **how** the information/advice is being given and whether this is resulting in the desired change in behaviour.

Well chosen words linking the meaning with maintained or increased physical functioning are vital (Rose 1998). For example: 'There is nothing seriously wrong with your back although I appreciate that it hurts a lot. This is due to it being a bit out of condition and the best way to get it back into shape is to get it fitter again.' This analogy will make sense to many patients and sets the scene for a graded exercise programme and incremental return to usual activities.

Poorly chosen words, associating the problem with a desired behaviour of inactivity, may be damaging (Rose 1998; see also Ch. 5). For example: 'You have some wear and tear in your back and a nerve is being trapped.' To many patients this will mean that it is better not to move or do too much in case it makes the wear and tear worse. It also suggests a mechanistic 'techno-fix' cure such as a manipulation to provide a 'magic bullet', which will un-trap the nerve.

Information and advice is usually given in the hope of changing behaviour. Understanding how this happens is therefore important to physiotherapists. This is discussed further in the following chapter. Didactic methods of giving information and advice previously used by physiotherapists, such as some forms of Back School, should be considered carefully in the light of current knowledge on how behaviour is changed and treatment gains are maintained (Fordyce 1976).

Therapy aims and practice

The aim of therapy needs to shift from that of symptomatic treatment to an emphasis on education and rehabilitation to facilitate prevention and individual/personal responsibility and continued management (CSAG 1994a). Ostensibly this is an obvious shift. However, in practice it actually means a host of subtle changes in emphasis that are not immediately apparent. As in any change in practice, this will require education and training of therapists and time to implement (Muncey 2000).

The use of 'Active Rehabilitation' was strongly advocated by CSAG (1994a). This should be undertaken after biopsychosocial assessment. Active Rehabilitation aims to improve the patients' control over pain and how they cope with its consequences. Emphasis is placed on patient responsibility and continued self management. It focuses on restoring function and improving physical fitness despite residual or recurrent low back pain. This is done by way of a graded increase in activity rather than by symptom-focused and pain contingent exercise programmes which are 'prescribed' by the therapist. Guidance is given and it is the patient's responsibility to set the targets. Attitudes and beliefs towards physical activity and exercise and expectations of treatment and outcome need to be identified and considered as part of this process (Kendall et al 1997).

There is now considerable evidence to support Active Rehabilitation programmes as the best way of producing lasting relief of both pain and disability (Lindstrom et al 1992, Waddell 1993, Frost et al 1995). Ideally it is instituted early in management. Any pain relieving approaches should be used within the context of Active Rehabilitation in order to avoid harmful effects.

Clinical examination and assessment are the first steps that any physiotherapist will take towards deciding how best to advise the patient and manage their rehabilitation. Assessment of 'Red Flags' is vital (CSAG 1994a, Roberts 2000). However, it is equally as vital that assessment takes into account psychosocial factors as well as the physical ones. Some consideration must therefore be given to assessing psychosocial 'Yellow Flags.' How to do this is described in detail in Topical Issues in Pain Volumes 2 and 3 (see: Kendall et al 1997, Kendall & Watson 2000, Watson & Kendall 2000, Main & Watson 2002).

Broadly speaking the areas that should be assessed are:

- Attitudes and Beliefs
- Behaviours
- Compensation (including benefits)
- Diagnosis and Treatment
- Emotions
- Family
- Work

The treatment programme should be planned on the basis of *all* the relevant information. Missing a Yellow Flag can be as potentially harmful as missing a Red Flag, and care should be taken here.

Following thorough clinical examination and interview the treatment programme should be based on assessment of the findings. Patients with possible serious spinal pathology or requiring immediate medical opinion will be sifted out. The majority however will be those with non-specific back pain suitable for physical therapy. The evidence-based management of this group is to embark as early as possible on Active Rehabilitation in order to avoid risk of poor outcome (Watson & Main 1995, Kendall et al 1997).

Early management in particular should ensure that the patient keeps active, functioning and gains control over pain. Pain relieving techniques may be appropriate. However, it is important to deliver these within the framework of encouraging patients to take control over the pain themselves whilst at the same time acknowledging their difficulties. A belief that the technique alone was responsible for the improvement will work against active involvement in prevention of recurrences and self management.

Therapist/patient discussions should focus on changing function rather than on how the pain itself may be changing. The patients' active participation in their recovery should be sought. Patient responsibility should be nurtured whilst giving manageable chunks of information and guidance about how

150

to do this (see Ch. 8). Encouraging the patient to 'try it and see' will demonstrate to them how incremental changes can be made towards recovery. In this way, small successes assist with building confidence and making progress.

None of the above can be done successfully without first identifying *attitudes, beliefs and expectations* (Klaber-Moffett 2000). For example, fear avoidance *beliefs* around the pain and its relationship with physical activity must be dealt with before the patient is likely to engage in any active treatment programme (Muncey & Watson 1999, also, chapters in Volume 1 of this series). If the patient has *expectations* of the therapist to provide a passive 'cure' and then does not receive any 'treatment' it may create problems with the patient/therapist relationship. For example, the patient may be unwilling to engage in an active treatment programme when they think this is unlikely to help (Klaber Moffett 1995).

Barriers to change in the patient's environment should be identified. For instance, a spouse, family, friends or work colleagues who are either solicitous (see Volume 2 of this series) and unwilling to allow the patient to develop self responsibility, or punitive and demanding a quick-fix cure, will be a barrier to progress. Advice may be given to the patient on how to best overcome this and reassure others that an active approach is safe and the best way forward.

It is necessary to be clear on the difference between distress related to pain and the expression of pain severity, and distress that is not associated with pain, and to deal with each accordingly. Distress that is not pain related, for example the patient may have a mood disorder or be clinically depressed, is not for the physiotherapist to approach, and the patient should be advised to seek help for this elsewhere. However, it is for the physiotherapist to deal with worries and concerns related to the pain and how this affects function. Use of the approach and model of care being described is helpful in this respect. (The reader will find Chapter 8 in Volume 3 of this series very useful here (Main & Watson 2002)).

Treatment should avoid reinforcing pain contingent behaviour. For example, treatments that encourage the cessation of activity or exercise if the pain worsens strengthen fear-avoidance beliefs and behaviour (see Volume 1). This will militate against active participation in rehabilitation. It will also sanction inactivity and contribute to the development of the 'disuse syndrome' and all that accompanies this (Bortz 1984). It is not acceptable for physical therapy interventions to contribute to the development of pain associated incapacity and complex disability.

Although it is often difficult from within the healthcare system to be meaningfully involved in the patient's return to work, it will be helpful to have a clear idea of the issues around this (Kendall et al 1997). As well as giving the more traditional ergonomic advice, physiotherapists may also be helpful in advising both the patient and their employer on a graded return to their usual activities and how to plan and pace these.

151

Therapy resources

In the past, therapy services have been focused on dealing with what they have viewed as the main presenting problems. Treatments have been symptom-orientated, aimed at clearing the recurrent or chronic low back pain, and little attention has been paid to prevention of pain associated incapacity in the integrated way described above (Jette et al 1994). The evidence suggests that symptomatic treatments are either ineffective or sometimes positively harmful (CSAG 1994a, Spitzer et al 1995, van der Heijden et al 1995). Long delay whilst awaiting these treatments in itself contributes to chronic pain and disability, and also prevents the delivery of more effective treatments (CSAG 1994a, Kendall et al 1997, Waddell 1998, Watson 2000).

It is now known that suitable interventions in the early stages of low back pain can help prevent disability and this is reflected in the recommendations of several Clinical Guidelines to the management of low back pain (CSAG 1994a, RCGP 1996, Kendall et al 1997, CSAG 2000). All of these Guidelines recommend early access to physical therapy, usually within six weeks of onset if problems are not resolving. Although many GPs are now aware of this and are referring at this stage, it is common to find long waiting lists for therapy—which defeat this principle.

A shift in therapy aims and practice will help to direct resources where they are most effectively deployed. This should assist with reduction of waiting times so avoiding disabling delays. Accurate triage will also assist in the right management for the right patients in a timely way.

Clearly, what needs to occur is a shift away from long and sometimes repeated courses of symptom-focused treatments, which place the patient in a passive dependency role, and towards rehabilitation which enables the patient to be actively involved and to develop self responsibility for continued management. Some examples of physical therapy practice with these aims in mind are given below.

Two suggestions for improved practice

Integrating components of the cognitive-behavioural therapy (CBT) model

As a therapeutic model CBT lends itself well to the management of pain. The model generated within CBT hypothesises links between beliefs, adjustment and functioning. It aims to change views and coping (Phillips 1987) (see also Ch. 8).

Physiotherapists are not trained in the use of cognitive-behavioural therapy and should take care not to claim that they are using it. However, principles from the model applied to physical therapy have been described in the management of chronic pain (Harding & Williams 1995) and in the management of fear and avoidance relating to pain (Harding 1998).

Rehabilitation and exercise programmes delivered using the approach produce better long term outcomes (Fordyce et al 1986, Lindstrom et al 1992, Nicholas et al 1992).

Active rehabilitation: the fitness programme

Active rehabilitation may be done in a group or with the individual. The lead therapist must be trained in the use of cognitive-behavioural principles in physical therapy. A group approach is now often referred to as a Fitness Programme. This will use cognitive-behavioural principles (see Chs 8 & 9 this volume) and include:

- Stretch and circuit exercises to improve posture, mobility and fitness.
- Goal setting focused on return to usual daily activities.
- Relaxation skills to enhance the above and assist coping.
- Education and advice on self responsibility and continued management.

Outcomes of these programmes have been shown to be beneficial in several dimensions (Frost et al 1995). Further work is needed to show which particular sub-groups of low back pain sufferers benefit most from this approach and which may require a different approach (Muncey & Watson 1999).

Instigating a low back pain triage service

A delay for a second opinion may be harmful (Wells 1987, Kendall et al 1997). In particular, if this results in advice that conservative management is best then active rehabilitation has been delayed and appropriate early management missed (CSAG 1994a). Nevertheless, it is important for patients to feel that a thorough examination and appropriate investigations have been undertaken, and that accurate diagnosis has been made. A second opinion may be part of this reassurance. Thus, fast access to thorough and accurate diagnosis is a desirable feature in the management of low back pain (CSAG 1994a, RCGP 1996, Kendall et al 1997, CSAG 2000).

Physiotherapists are in a good position to facilitate or provide this. The role of physiotherapists working with an extended scope of practice within various outpatient medical specialties is now well established in the UK health service. It has been shown that their diagnosis is accurate and that patient satisfaction compares favourably with that found with medical practitioners (Croft & Joseph 1994, Dacr-White et al 1999).

In many instances this role is described as a triage role. That is, patients are allocated to the specialist physiotherapist for assessment and most non-surgical management. Any patients requiring a surgical opinion are referred on. The aims and detail of such services may differ but they are managed within secondary care and require a referral to whichever specialty or consultant is managing them.

Another model is that of an interface service between primary and secondary care. Here the specialist physiotherapist receives referrals direct

153

from GPs into the defined service. These follow certain criteria. In effect, the referrals are those that would usually go for an orthopaedic opinion where the GP is not certain of the diagnosis. If the diagnosis is more clear, e.g. inflammatory joint disease requiring referral to a rheumatologist, or nerve root pathology requiring surgical management, the referral will still go direct to the appropriate service.

When the specialist physiotherapist receives the referral, the patient will be seen within three weeks. Any investigations thought appropriate will support the specialist physiotherapist's opinion following examination of the patient. These investigations include CT and MRI scans, blood tests and plain X-rays. All are accessed directly by the specialist physiotherapist.

Patients requiring a surgical or medical opinion are referred on. However, the majority do not need further referral and are advised of the diagnosis and best management. Some are referred direct for the latter, i.e. to physiotherapy or to a pain management programme. The rest will be referred back with advice on management to their GP or advised by the specialist physiotherapist and discharged.

This type of triage requires medical supervision of the extended scope of practice of the specialist physiotherapist. It has been found to be successful in terms of reducing disabling delay for a second opinion, producing accurate diagnosis and being satisfactory to both patients and GPs and has been recommended accordingly (SW Regional Health Authority Good Practice Guide 1999, CSAG 2000). In addition, it may be viewed as a demand management strategy for services such as orthopaedics that have historically been inundated with referrals for low back pain which, in fact, do not require a surgical opinion.

Conclusion

This chapter has attempted to describe how physiotherapists using evidence-based management within an appropriate model of care can significantly improve the quality of outcome for low back pain sufferers.

Physiotherapists have the knowledge and skills to provide true rehabilitation rather than ineffective symptom-orientated treatments. This is crucial in the prevention of ongoing pain and chronic incapacity associated with low back pain.

This huge social, economic and individual problem has been poorly managed by medicine in the past. As rehabilitationists, physiotherapists should take the lead in instigating good quality and evidence based management of low back pain.

REFERENCES

Bortz WM 1984 The disuse syndrome. Western Newsletter of Medicine 141:691–694

Croft P, Joseph, S 1994 Low back pain in the community and in hospitals: A report to the clinical standards advisory group of the Department of Health. Arthritis and Rheumatism Council Epidemiological Research Unit, University of Manchester

CSAG 1994 Report of a clinical standards advisory group committee on the epidemiology of low back pain. Department of Health, HMSO London

CSAG 1994a Report of a clinical standards advisory group committee on back pain. Department of Health, HMSO, London

CSAG 2000 Report of a clinical standards advisory group on services for patients with pain. Department of Health, HMSO, London

Dacr-White G, Carr AJ, Harvey I, Woolhead G, Bannister G, Nelson I, Camerling M 1999 A randomised controlled trial: Shifting boundaries with doctors and physiotherapists in orthopaedic outpatient departments. Journal of Epidemiology and Community Health 53:1–7

Fordyce WE, 1976 Behavioural methods with chronic pain and illness. Mosby, St Louis

Fordyce WE, Brockway JA, Bergman JA, Spengler D 1986 Acute low back pain: A control group comparison of behavioural vs traditional management methods. Journal of Behavioural Medicine 9(2):127–141

Frost H, Kolaber Moffett JA, Moser JS, Fairbank JCT 1995 Evaluation of a fitness programme for patients with chronic LBP. British Medical Journal 310:151–154

Harding V 1998 Cognitive-behavioural approach to fear and avoidance. In: Gifford LS (ed) Topical Issues in Pain 1 Whiplash—science and management. Fear-avoidance beliefs and behaviour. CNS Press, Falmouth 173–191

Harding, V, Williams AC de C 1995 Extending physiotherapy skills using a psychological approach: Cognitive-behavioural management of chronic pain. Physiotherapy 81(11):681–688

Jette AM, Smith K, Haley SM, Davis KD 1994 Physical therapy episodes of care for patients with low back pain. Physical Therapy 74(2):101–115

Kendall NS, Linton SJ, Main CJ 1997 Guide to assessing psychosocial yellow flags in acute low back pain: Risk factors for long term disability and work loss. Accident and Compensation Commission of New Zealand and the National Health Committee, Wellington, New Zealand

Kendall N, Watson P 2000 Identifying psychosocial yellow flags and modifying management. In: Gifford LS (ed) Topical Issues in Pain 2. Biopsychosocial assessment and management. Relationships and pain. CNS Press, Falmouth 131–139

Klaber-Moffett J 1995 Influence of the physiotherapist patient relationship on pain and disability. Physiotherapy Theory and Practice 13:89–96

Klaber-Moffett J 2000 Pain: perception and attitudes. In: Gifford LS (ed) Topical Issues in Pain 2: Biopsychosocial assessment and management. Relationships and pain. CNS Press, Falmouth 141–151

Koes BW et al 1991 Physiotherapy exercises and back pain: A blinded review. British Medical Journal 303:1372–1376

Lindstrom I, Ohlund C, Eek C et al 1992 The effect of graded activity on patients with subacute low back pain: A randomized prospective clinical study with an operant-conditioning behavioral approach. Physical Therapy 72(4):279–290

Main C, Watson P 2002 The distressed and angry low back pain patient. In: Gifford LS (ed) Topical Issues in Pain 3. Sympathetic nervous system and pain. Pain management. Clinical effectiveness. CNS Press, Falmouth

Muncey H 2000 The challenge of change in practice. In: Gifford LS (ed) Topical Issues in Pain 2. Biopsychosocial assessment and management. Relationships and pain. CNS Press, Falmouth 37–54

Nicholas MK, Wilson PH, Goyen J 1992 Comparison of cognitive-behavioural group treatment and an alternative non psychological treatment for chronic low back pain. Pain 48:339–347

Phillips HC 1987 Avoidance behaviour and its role in sustaining chronic pain. Behaviour Research and Therapy 25(4):273–279

RCGP 1996 Clinical guidelines for the management of acute low back pain. Royal College of General Practice, London

Roberts L 2000 Flagging the danger signs of low back pain. In: Gifford LS (ed) Topical Issues in Pain 2. Biopsychosocial assessment and management. Relationships and pain. CNS Press, Falmouth 69–54

Rose MJ 1998 Iatrogenic disability and back pain rehabilitation. In: Gifford LS (ed) Topical Issues in Pain 1. Whiplash—science and management. Fear avoidance behaviour and beliefs. CNS Press, Falmouth 167–172

Rose MJ, Reilly JB, Pennie B, Slade PD, 1998 Chronic low back pain: A consequence of misinformation? Employee Counselling Today 5(1):12–15

South West Regional Health Authority 1999 Good Practice Guide. The Low Back Triage Service. Frenchay Healthcare NHS Trust

Spitzer XO, Skovron JL, Salmi IR et al 1995 Scientific monograph Quebec taskforce on whiplash associated disorders: Redefining whiplash and its management. Spine 28(suppl 1):2738–2745

Van der Heijden GJ, Beuerskins AJ, Icoes BW et al 1995 The efficacy of traction for back and neck pain: A systematic blinded review of randomised clinical trial methods. Physical Therapy 75(2):93–104

Waddell G 1993 A new clinical model for the treatment of low back pain. Spine 12:932–944

Waddell G 1998 The Back Pain Revolution. Churchill Livingstone, Edinburgh 1–8

Watson P 2000 Psychosocial predictors of outcome from low back pain. In: Gifford LS (ed) Topical Issues in Pain 2. Biopsychosocial assessment and management. Relationships and pain. CNS Press, Falmouth 85–109

Watson P, Main CJ 1995 Screening for patients at risk of developing chronic incapacity. Journal of Occupational Rehabilitation 5(4):207–217

Watson P, Kendall N 2000 Assessing psychosocial yellow flags. In: Gifford LS (ed) Topical Issues in Pain 2. Biopsychosocial assessment and management. Relationships and pain. CNS Press, Falmouth 111–129

Muncey H, Watson PJ 1999 Efficacy of a unidisciplinary outpatient fitness programme for patients with musculoskeletal pain. Abstract from proceedings of the 9th World Congress on Pain, International Association for the Study of Pain, Vienna.

Wells JCD 1987 The place of the pain clinic. Ballieres Clinical Rheumatology 1:123–153

8

Explaining pain to patients

HEATHER MUNCEY

Patients consulting a health professional regarding a pain problem will usually expect some explanation of their pain, even if it is not possible to provide a clear diagnosis. By the same token, most health professionals expect to provide information that may go some way to explaining why the pain is present. Physiotherapists may link this information with issues around movement, activity and function as a basis from which a change in exercise and activity behaviour leading to improved physical function may be encouraged.

There are two important points:

• When explaining pain to patients with this behaviour change in mind it is not enough to give information alone (Fordyce 1976);
• Studies show that many patients believe they are not told enough, often do not understand what they are told, or do not remember what is said (Ley & Llewellyn 1995).

So how do we explain pain to patients, their families, work colleagues and employers in a way which helps improve physical functioning?

The cognitive-behavioural therapy (CBT) approach to managing pain hypothesises links between beliefs, adjustment and functioning (Jensen et al 1994). Use of the approach aims to change patients' views and coping (Nicholas 1996). This may, therefore, provide a suitable framework for delivering explanations that promote and link with desirable behaviour changes.

Cognitive-behavioural theory has been applied to the management of pain for many years (Turk et al 1983). *Cognitive therapy* considers the attitudes and core beliefs of the individual, particularly those relating to pain. It argues that coping may be changed by developing alternative attitudes, beliefs and strategies. *Behavioural therapy* is based on the tenet that behaviour occurs as a result of controlling reinforcers which determine a range of reactions in response to these. The inter-relation of theory and therapy is presented as cognitive-behavioural therapy (CBT) (Beck 1989).

Physical therapists are not clinical psychologists and are not trained to use CBT. However, the therapeutic approach encompassed within this model may be used to enhance physical therapy (Harding & Williams 1995). Use of the approach will involve considering alternative attitudes to, and strategies for, improving physical function. It is important, however, to consider not only individuals but also the environment within which they exist. For example, if family and work colleagues do not support patients in the changes they are trying to make or even work against these, it will be difficult for a patient to make and maintain progress.

So instead of giving a well meant, straight forward explanation to the patient of what we think is going on to produce the pain, let us consider how a CBT approach might use information to link with what we want the patient to do.

Behavioural therapy methods

Behavioural therapy assists behaviour change to facilitate maintenance of treatment gains with:

- clear information
- goal setting
- operant learning through selective reinforcement
- pacing rather than overactivity/underactivity cycle
- training in strategies such as relaxation (also cognitive)
- use of cues, reminder plans and timetables

Behavioural therapy attempts to facilitate confidence building with physical activity via the use of a little information and a 'try it and see' approach. Incremental (gradually increasing) progress allowing the patient to plan and be in control provides the opportunity for the patient to test out the advice, achieve a predetermined goal and as a result feel rewarded for their achievements. Goal achievement necessarily reinforces their confidence and belief in the information given, and then leads to further progress.

Example

A female patient has ongoing low back pain. She has tried exercising, with painful consequences, and is fearful of trying again. She is not sure that the root of the trouble has been spotted and is worried that she may injure herself and make things worse.

Waddell et al (1989) described continuing pain behaviour despite accurate reassurance after thorough examination where fear-avoidance beliefs were present. An initial explanation of the pain might be couched in terms of the body being 'out of condition' thus implying the need for a planned and gradual return to fitness through paced activity and exercise.

As a first step the patient is advised how to calculate a starting point or 'baseline' for an agreed activity. There is no evidence to support the best way of doing this but a frequently used method is:

- Teach the activity, e.g. trunk curl stretches.
- Advise the patient to repeat this as much as they feel they can manage at the time.

Use of indicators such as pain increase should be avoided. Rather, concentrate on how well they are doing the activity despite pain whilst also encouraging them not to overdo the activity. An operant learning approach may be used at this stage (Harding & Williams 1995). For example, non-desirable behaviour such as excess pain behaviour whilst attempting the exercise, or even refusal to try, can be met with a lack of expression, no eye contact and a neutral level of interest in what they are doing. Desirable behaviour, such as tentatively trying the exercise, on the other hand, may be rewarded with smiles, praise for the achievement, and acknowledgement of how hard it is to achieve the exercise and how well they have done to make the effort. Care must be taken, however, not to appear patronising.

- Ask patients to use a diary to record the number of repetitions for that day.
- Repeat this process for three days asking patients to record the scores.
- Then average the scores and divide by 2 to calculate a conservative baseline. In this way the patient's baseline for the activity is considerably lower than the average. This may seem quite dramatic, but key to success with graded activity, improved confidence with function and return to fitness, is early success rather than failure which often follows from trying to do too much too early. Traditionally, pain management programmes have reduced the average by 20% (see chapters in Volumes 1 & 3 of this series and Ch. 9, this volume). The position here, from clinical experience, is that halving the average, rather than reducing by only 20%, leads to better compliance and outcomes for the majority of patients.
- An important aim is for the baseline exercise to be achieved every day despite the pain. Halving the 'average' as discussed above, is one way of helping ensure that this is possible.

Once a routine of doing this every day is established, and the patient has actually experienced that it does not provoke unmanageable, new, exercise-related aches and pains or result in further damage, their confidence will grow, not only in the exercise itself, but also in their ability to work out what is safe to do. This skill, the first step in goal setting, can then be transferred into all other activity planning.

A sensible programme of pacing up the activity can then be agreed by negotiation using the patient's new found knowledge and experience of how well she can do if her planning and pacing is right. For example, she might determine that the trunk-curl exercise could be increased to two sessions a day, or that every third day one more repetition could be added.

Prioritising activities through the day and considering overall planning and pacing using goal setting is a practical behavioural method very applicable to physical therapy (Cott & Finch 1991). If applied to activity cycling (where patients 'cycle' from overactivity to prolonged periods of inactivity) it can assist in smoothing this out so that the patient has better control over the pain and activity levels and is able to plan their life more satisfactorily.

This practical application may assist with shifting patient beliefs and attitudes to physical activity to support the use of the cognitive approach.

Cognitive methods

Cognitive methods and approaches help patients to:

- recognise, challenge and re-structure unhelpful thoughts, beliefs and emotions regarding pain
- aim to reduce the frequency of maladaptive and catastrophising cognitions and make the shift towards more realistic thinking
- use coping strategies such as coping self statements
- establish habits of self reinforcing 'well' behaviour
- improve self efficacy.

An important component in the this part of management is for the therapist to help patients re-conceptualise the problem as being due more to the consequences of the pain and appreciate that they can have considerable impact on their own well-being and recovery. It is then possible to focus on challenging unhelpful cognitions in a much more useful way (Nicholas 1996).

Example

A good way of doing this is to work through a hypothetical patient example with the patient. Give a short case history of a chronic pain sufferer such as:

John is 37 and is an engineer in a large firm in the city. He is married with three children under 10 and the family have recently moved to a new house. John is a keen rugby player and belongs to the local club. He is also involved with the school Parents' Association.

John was putting up some curtains when he fell off a stepladder. He injured his back and sprained some ligaments in his wrist. This was three months ago and the wrist has healed but he still has back pain although the X-ray was normal.

Now ask the patient to work through the scenarios for John and his family at 6 months after the accident, one year afterwards and, finally, two years afterwards. Encourage them to consider all the dimensions of his life that might be affected. The three pictures produced will usually display increasing physical, psychological and social consequences of the ongoing pain. Brief discussion on the progress of the pain itself usually reveals that it is more or less the same albeit with good times and bad times. This can be represented pictorially as a graph drawing the pain line as undulating but travelling at a similar level over the period. However, the effects/consequences line rises steadily over the period.

It can then be seen that these two things, although related, are not directly linked in terms of their complexity or impact upon quality of life. So, if the consequences can rise whilst the pain remains more or less the same, then they can also reduce despite a 'no change' situation with the pain. It can then be possible to work with the patient on changing the consequences in an active way.

Maladaptive cognitions such as praying and hoping or catastrophising need to be identified. A start can be made on shifting these with recognition of achievements as a result of better planned and paced activity patterns as above. Encourage the use of alternative coping strategies such as coping self statements or distraction techniques as frequency of maladaptive cognitions decreases. A link with behavioural methods will help improve self efficacy.

Example

The female patient with low back pain in the first example has successfully maintained her trunk-curl programme and further goals have been tackled in similar ways. She has achieved a modest walking goal after determining an agreed baseline distance and gradually pacing it up as described. At this stage discussions with her might be considering her worries and fears as to the nature of the pain and what it means regarding activity. She has already achieved some progress and this can be used to develop positive self reinforcement and encourage coping self statements such as 'I can do it!'

This will assist in reducing maladaptive and catastrophising cognitions such as 'There must be something seriously wrong that they've missed' or 'I'll probably end up in a wheelchair.' Reassurance that clinical examination and possibly investigations have revealed no signs of anything seriously wrong is now more meaningful as she is starting to see a little improvement in her function.

Patients believing that their pain is a mystery may benefit initially from sound objective information on the nature of their pain and what coping skills have worked well for others (Williams & Keefe 1991). In the majority of cases of low back pain, a precise diagnosis cannot be made. However, a description of 'non-specific back pain' may be made much less worrying and more reassuring if the fact that 'there is no evidence of anything seriously wrong' can be fostered by facilitating use of more effective coping skills and confidence in physical ability. Careful use of descriptive language such as 'Your back is a bit out of condition' rather than 'Your joints are degenerating' may result in the patient wanting to 're-condition' her back with some exercise rather than wanting to protect it from further wear and tear by resting it!

More positive cognitions can then be used to facilitate maintenance of treatment gains. This way of explaining pain to patients, helping them to work through what is happening and how this relates to their coping, is more likely to result in useful rehabilitation than simply telling the patient what you think and hoping they believe you!

Stress management techniques, such as training in relaxation and the use of distraction techniques, will reduce anxiety and increase self control. The ability to relax is a helpful skill to develop. It will help to reduce muscle tension and the anxiety that may contribute to this. This assists in physical performance as well as in flare-up management and improved sleep (Keefe & Gill 1986).

In practice, behavioural and cognitive methods are integrated. This helps patients recognise that they can improve their function and quality of life despite pain. The ideas incorporated in the CBT approach are, therefore, central to therapy where pain problems recur or persist. They are also of great value in the early stages of a pain presentation where the physiotherapist is key in preventing ongoing pain and the development of chronic incapacity.

As we have seen, identifying beliefs and coping strategies is an important aspect of the CBT approach and some more discussion on this may be helpful.

Pain beliefs

Pain beliefs are defined as a sub-set of the belief system that represents a personal understanding of the pain experience as a whole (Williams & Thorn 1989). Beliefs may lead to maladaptive coping and cause ones own efforts to be viewed as ineffective. Understanding beliefs may:

- help modify coping strategies
- facilitate the therapeutic relationship
- help engagement with treatment
- influence outcome.

When explaining pain to patients, family or work colleagues it is important not to make assumptions but first of all to identify *their* present understanding of what is going on, attributions of the cause, what it means for them and what they are doing in response to the problem and what is likely to help. That is, what they think, feel and do (cognitions, emotions and behaviour). This will help individuals to feel they have been listened to and to build up trust in order to engage them with treatment.

What beliefs and attitudes might be relevant to physical therapy? Some common beliefs and attitudes found in chronic pain sufferers are:

Beliefs

Perception of pain as mysterious, long lasting, the patient's 'fault', or uncontrollable. Fear-avoidance beliefs such as that pain will increase with activity, or that activity may cause injury.

Attitudes and expectations

There may be a passive attitude to rehabilitation, expectation of a 'cure', or decreased self efficacy where the individual has poor expectations to use coping strategies successfully (Bandura 1977).

Pain coping strategies

As well as identifying beliefs, attitudes and expectations it is also important to identify pain coping strategies (Rosensteil & Keefe 1983). Cognitive and behavioural coping strategies are present in the non pain population but those which are of interest in pain sufferers are defined as: 'Thoughts and behaviours people use to manage pain or emotional reactions to it to reduce distress' (Turner & Clancy 1986).

Cognitive coping strategies

The patient may use catastrophising, diverting attention from the pain, re-interpreting pain sensations, generating coping self statements, ignoring pain sensations, or simply praying and hoping.

Behavioural coping strategies

The patient may exhibit increasing or decreasing activity levels.

Research supports the idea that identifying beliefs and coping strategies has important clinical implications (Schwartz et al 1985, Williams & Thorn 1989, Williams & Keefe 1991). It has been found that there is likely to be lower engagement with physical therapy in chronic pain sufferers who have beliefs that pain is never-ending and is mysterious. In addition, when these beliefs are present patients are less likely to use adaptive cognitive coping strategies, as they do not see them as likely to help control or decrease pain. Patients with these beliefs are more likely to catastrophise (Williams and Keefe 1991).

In this situation the therapy plan may need to focus on encouraging the patient that even if they do not fully understand their pain it may still be influenced positively by improved activity levels. It will then be helpful to use behavioural approaches such as diaries or graded return to activity to support them in making these changes. This will help them to link their change of behaviour with better coping in their daily tasks.

Many patients who understand their pain and believe it is of short duration engage well with CBT as a whole. Therefore agreeing an effective treatment plan will be relatively easy.

Fear-avoidance beliefs and behaviour are key for the therapist to identify and acknowledge in treatment strategies (see Harding 1998 in Volume 1 of this series and Main & Watson 2002 in Volume 3). Here activity is avoided because there is a belief that this will cause more pain and/or further harm or damage.

Use of a multidimensional model will help to describe the development of chronic low back pain. It helps us to understand the biological, psychological and social influences in this process. Fear avoidance beliefs and behaviour may be viewed in context in this way and hence more clearly appreciated (Hill 1998 in Volume 1 of this series).

Fear-avoidance behaviour was initially thought to be a direct result or consequence of pain. Later, Phillips (1987) put forward a model that recognised the important role of cognitions in influencing avoidance behaviour. It was considered that the avoidance of stimuli played an active part in reducing sense of control over pain and an increasing *expectation* that exposure to stimuli would increase pain. These cognitive changes, i.e. in expectations and sense of control, clearly encourage further withdrawal from usual activities and growing intolerance of stimulation.

An example of this would be reduced activity resulting from a belief that there is a structural cause for pain experienced on movement. For instance, the belief that a 'slipped disc' has resulted from a forward bend may lead to future avoidance of forward bending with an increasing intolerance of it over time. Behaviour such as this contributes to disability (Zusman 1998). Beliefs such as these, which have generated avoidance behaviour, may easily be compounded iatrogenically (Rose 1998, see also Ch. 5). This kind of behaviour leads to physical de-conditioning and the setting up of a 'vicious circle' which may further add to the problems.

The influence of others

The cognitive-behavioural approach helps to explain pain to patients in a way that engages them in physical therapy. But what about the influence of their family, friends, work colleagues and employers? Others may be solicitous (over protective) and/or punitive in their approach to the patient. This will not support the desired behaviour change (Newton-John 2000).

If others are *over protective* this will emphasise fear-avoidance beliefs and encourage catastrophising. So if a spouse encourages the patient to remain lying on the sofa this will contribute to physical de-conditioning, more pain or discomfort on movement, and the cognitive changes described above. The patient may then begin to think that things will never get better, that they will end up in a wheelchair, etc.

Punitive behaviour, on the other hand, such as the spouse who chastises the patient when they are not eliciting a diagnosis and cure from their doctor, will encourage anxiety, a decrease in self confidence, and negative cognitions.

Appropriate *support* from others assists return to usual activities, e.g. for pacing of activities, for maintenance of other pain management strategies, or for graded return to work. Thus, a change in beliefs, attitudes and behaviour of others may also be required. How may this be achieved?

Handouts, and documentation such as diary sheets, may be worked through with significant others by the patient. It will be necessary to encourage this. Communication skills may be taught to the patient to help them to reassure others. It may be possible to have the family in during treatment in order to expose them to the approach being used.

Ideally work visits take place to advise on the ergonomic aspects of work as well as how attitudes and behaviour of work colleagues may hinder or help. In the absence of this opportunity, it may be necessary to work on problem solving and assertiveness skills with the patient. This helps them to challenge the worries of others, to problem solve and to continue with their self management plan including an appropriate return to work strategy (Nicholas 1996).

Conclusion

One of the most important messages is that *giving information alone is not enough to change behaviour*. The therapist must consider all the dimensions of a biopsychosocial model (Waddell 1992). The cognitive-behavioural approach hypothesises a link between beliefs, adjustment and function and aims to change views and coping. As such, it is an ideal therapeutic framework from within which to deliver physical rehabilitation.

This is important in all stages of the pain experience. The way in which pain is explained to patients and to those around them should be considered carefully. Explanation should be provided within an evidence-based therapeutic framework that ensures clinical effectiveness in its fullest sense (see Ch. 7). The aim is that, as well as having a positive effect, no further harm is done.

REFERENCES

Bandura A 1977 Self efficacy: towards a unifying theory of behaviour. Psychological Review 84(2):191–215

Beck AT 1989 Cognitive Behavioural Therapy and Emotion Disorders. Penguin, Harmondsworth

Cott C, Finch E 1991 Goal setting in physical therapy practice. Physiotherapy Canada 43(1):19–22

Fordyce WE 1976 Behavioural Methods for Chronic Pain and Illness. Mosby, St Louis

Harding V 1998 Application of the cognitive-behavioural approach. In: Pitt-Brooke J, Reid H, Lockwood J et al (eds) Rehabilitation of Movement: Theoretical bases of clinical practice W B Saunders, London

Harding VR, Williams AC de C 1995 Extending physiotherapy skills using a psychological approach: Cognitive behavioural management of chronic pain. Physiotherapy 81(11):681–688

Hill P 1998 Fear-avoidance theories. In: Gifford LS (ed) Topical Issues in Pain 1. Whiplash—science and management. Fear-avoidance beliefs and behaviour. CNS Press, Falmouth 159–166

Jensen MP, Turner JA, Romano JM, Lawler BK 1994 Relationship of pain specific beliefs to chronic pain adjustment. Pain 5(7):301–309

Keefe FJ, Gill KM 1986 Behavioural concepts in the analysis of chronic pain syndromes. Journal of Consulting and Clinical Psychology 54(6):776–783

Ley B, Llewellyn S 1995 Improving patients understanding, recall, satisfaction and compliance. In: Broome A, Llewellyn S (eds) Health Psychology: Process and applications Chapman & Hall, London 75–98

Main CJ, Watson PJ 2002 The distressed and angry low back pain patient. In: Gifford LS (ed) Topical Issues in Pain 3. Sympathetic nervous system and pain. Pain management. Clinical effectiveness. CNS Press, Falmouth 177–204

Newton-John T 2000 When helping does not help: Responding to pain behaviours. In: Gifford LS (ed) Topical Issues in Pain 2. Biopsychosocial assessment and management. Relationships and pain. CNS Press, Falmouth 165–175

Nicholas MK 1996 Theory and practice of cognitive behavioural programmes. In: Campbell JM (ed) Pain 1996—An Updated Review. IASP Press, Seattle 287–293

Phillips HC 1987 Fear avoidance behaviour and its role in sustaining chronic pain. Behaviour Research and Therapy 25(4):273–279

Rose MJ 1998 Iatrogenic disability and back pain rehabilitation. In: Gifford LS (ed) Topical Issues in Pain 1. Whiplash—science and management. Fear-avoidance behaviour and beliefs. CNS Press, Falmouth 167–172

Rosensteil AK, Keefe FJ 1983 Use of coping strategies in chronic low back pain patients: Relationship to patient characteristics and current adjustment. Pain 17:33–44

Schwartz DP, de Good DE, Shutty MS 1985 Direct assessment of beliefs and attitudes of chronic pain patients. Archives of Physical Medicine and Rehabilitation 676:806–809

Turk D, Michenbaum D, Genest M 1983 Pain and Behavioural Medicine: A cognitive behavioural perspective. Guildford Press, New York

Turner JA, Clancy S 1986 Strategies for coping with chronic low back pain: Relationship to pain and disability. Pain 24:355–364

Waddell G 1992 Biopsychosocial analysis of low back pain. Clinics in Rheumatology 6:523–557

Waddell G, Pilowsky I, Bond M 1989 Clinical assessment and interpretation of abnormal illness behaviour in low back pain. Pain 39: 41–53

Williams DA, Thorn BE 1989 An empirical assessment of pain beliefs. Pain 36:351–358

Williams DA, Keefe FJ 1991 Pain beliefs and the use of cognitive behavioural coping strategies. Pain 46(2):185–190

Zusman M 1998 Structure-oriented beliefs and disability due to back pain. In: Gifford LS (ed) Topical Issues in Pain 1: Whiplash—science and management. Fear avoidance behaviour and beliefs. CNS Press, Falmouth 199–213

9

Improving physical function in chronic pain syndrome patients

BABS HARPER

Introduction

There is much evidence (reviewed in Waddell 1998, Main & Spanswick 2000) that the prevalence of chronic pain *disability* is increasing. There is also evidence (also reviewed in Waddell 1998, Main & Spanswick 2000) to support the idea that the medical system and societal factors reinforce chronicity albeit often unwittingly (see Ch. 5).

Many people with chronic pain are able to get on with their lives and do not experience the same degree of disability as those who eventually end up attending a pain management programme. A major aim of these programmes is to decrease the level of disability, help patients cope better, and ultimately to become physically fitter. The programmes utilise a cognitive-behavioural (CB) approach and as such require a multidisciplinary team. Physiotherapy is one of the core elements and requires patients to take part in and build up, exercises. In so doing patients learn to improve their physical confidence and physical fitness, and increase levels of activity generally. The emphasis is on a self management approach where the goal is to work *with* the pain, not on it.

The following account focuses on the physiotherapy component dealing with improvement in physical functioning through the exercise component of the programme. It will become obvious that the physical aspect of the intervention cannot be executed in isolation from other aspects of the programme. The multidimensional impact of ongoing pain is respected and attended to by pain management programmes.

All the physiotherapy sessions take place in a group setting.

The chronic pain sufferer

The patients seen on a CB pain management programme have chronic pain syndrome. In pain management, what we are dealing with is the impact of pain on the sufferer's life. Many people with chronic pain have adequate coping strategies and skills to deal with their pain and get on with their lives. Others do not and can become physically and emotionally disabled. Pain has the potential to impact all the areas illustrated in Figure 9.1.

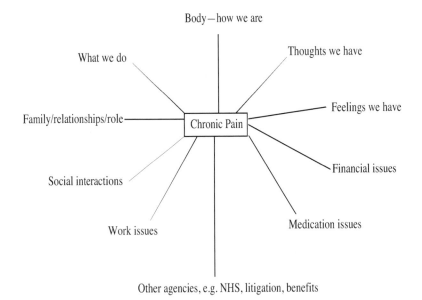

Fig. 9.1 Diagram built up with patients to illustrate the impact of chronic pain syndrome on the sufferer. It also illustrates the multidimensional nature of chronic pain.

Setting the scene: recognising the problems

In the first group session the physiotherapist invites patients to build-up a diagram like that in Figure 9.1. This is done by asking them to relate how their body has been affected. They may reply with, 'The whole of my body is in pain' or, 'The pain is spreading and affecting most of my body'. The physiotherapist can then ask, 'So how has this affected your body? For example, do you feel that you are as strong as before?' Patients often then report that they feel generally weaker; their muscles feel weaker and they may have lost muscle bulk, or put on weight. Each of the factors illustrated

168

in Figure 9.1 can be brought to the attention of the patients by asking appropriate questions. For example, 'So how does that make you feel?' or, 'Has that affected your social life?' By doing this, patients can draw their own picture/illustration of how chronic pain has impacted their lives and that of others around them. This starts the process of reconceptualising the problem for the sufferer. It is the identification, not of the chronic pain, but of chronic pain *syndrome*. The aim is to highlight the fact that the distress experienced and the broad impact on the sufferer is much greater than the chronic pain itself and that many areas need to be addressed and worked on.

Patients with chronic pain syndrome often feel disbelieved and frightened, and have a sense of loss of control over their lives. Often a great many areas of their life are affected. This may come out in the discussion and can be discussed helpfully and shared in the group. Specific situations provide useful examples of the impact of pain. For instance, a patient may mention having become stuck in a distressing place and as a result become avoidant of many issues and activities thereafter. Patients frequently experience, or exhibit, maladaptive cognitions and behaviours. While these and other maladaptive strategies may be the only way they know how to deal and manage their life, they may be the very things that keep them locked into the problem. In part pain management programmes using a CB approach help patients recognise and deal with maladaptive cognitions and behaviour. Physiotherapy is very much a part of the process.

The role of the physiotherapist

What follows is a list that illustrates the broad approach and skills required by physiotherapists working with chronic pain syndrome patients. Physiotherapists need to:

- Acknowledge the pain is real and believed but that no attempts will be made to alleviate or eliminate it as this is no longer helpful or appropriate.
- Listen to and work with the patient.
- Provide space, time and support.
- Address the issues of avoidance.
- *Not* take over control.
- Introduce the idea that the pain may be 'here to stay'.
- Educate the patient about chronic pain mechanisms and to emphasise that ongoing pain does not equate to ongoing damage.
- Engage the patient in a process of living life with pain where the emphasis is not on fighting the pain but one of accepting that pain is now a part of life and finding ways to move on despite the pain.
- Enable the patient to reconceptualise the chronic pain syndrome. With these patients their focus is mostly on the pain and any associated distress and disability they have is usually all attributed to the pain. By reconceptualising the syndrome for the patient the need to find other ways of dealing with the situation becomes more apparent.

169

- Change unhelpful patterns of activity and behaviour to more normal acceptable ones despite ongoing pain.
- Normalise the ongoing pain and help patients understand that there is no ongoing serious pathology.
- Reassure the patient that the emphasis now needs to be on regaining an improved level of fitness and not on a need to treat the pain as this is no longer helpful.
- Introduce the idea that they are normal well people with chronic pain who can have full and meaningful lives.
- Be able to offer training to improve quality of life with persistent pain.
- Facilitate the sufferer to discover appropriate ways of dealing with life in an active yet non-striving manner that enables the person to have a better quality of life despite the ongoing pain.
- Help the sufferer to regain and retain control over their lives.

The cognitive behavioural therapy approach to exercise/activity

A very simple way of viewing the process is shown in Box 9.1.

Box 9.1 The cognitive-behavioural therapy approach to exercise/activity

- **The problem**: fear and therefore avoidance of exercise. Fear of 'If I do exercise, then what? Exercise has increased my pain in the past and made me worse.'
- **The plan**: graded exposure to the barrier/fear. In this case exercise.
- **The process**: desensitisation.

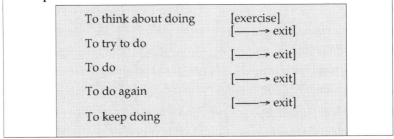

The patient can exit the process at any stage shown above. However, the task for the physiotherapist is to enable the patient to re-engage and to continue with the process successfully. This means identifying the thing they fear, facing it and challenging it using a process of rationalisation. This means weighing up the pros and cons, and what the likely outcome might be. Questions like, 'What is the worst thing that can happen? What is the likelihood of this? Is there a way to approach this that reduces the likelihood of this happening?' are often useful and also help the patient to learn problem solving skills that may be used in other situations.

Getting started—setting the scene for exercise and activity

Engage the patients. Allow each patient briefly to review past interventions and outcomes and the effectiveness of these. The physiotherapist has to bring the patients into the present and appreciate the reality of the current situation. This is highly skilled. Chronic pain sufferers often reflect repeatedly on how things were prior to the pain problem, on the events that brought them to their present state, and on what is wished for. By relating events like these and outlining the various treatments they have had the patient is undergoing a process of review. Once done, the physiotherapist can then invite patients to comment on the effectiveness of their treatments. It is important that the physiotherapist avoids judging the patient or any other professionals who have been involved. Rather than 'colleague bash,' if the patient expresses anger over past treatments it is far more productive for the physiotherapist to suggest that past treatments were offered with the very best of intention.

This type of discussion sets the scene for introducing a new approach to the management of the current situation—one that will encourage the patients to take control of their own management even though they may be reluctant to do this at first. The physiotherapist needs to keep handing control back to the patient while offering an appropriate level of support.

The physiotherapist can invite each patient to look at current patterns of activity and levels of fitness and what influences these. Discussion/debate may then take place on whether they need to change. The aim is for the intervention to be patient-driven with the physiotherapist playing a role in providing research and educational material to validate/support the need for change. It is important for patients to know that they have control and the decision for change is theirs. Maintenance will only be achieved with these circumstances in place.

All these discussions take place within the context of the chronic pain syndrome scenario. It is part of a reconceptualisation process whereby the pain is seen in a different way, and one where something positive can be done about life with pain. It is part of the process of acceptance.

Normalisation is part of this process too and the importance of achieving an improved level of fitness is explored. The physiotherapist plays an important facilitator role in the sufferer seeing himself/herself as a well person with pain who can still become fitter with no risk of further damage. That a life that has pain in it can be a meaningful life and have quality despite the pain is an important concept for patients to understand. In order to achieve this a major focus is on improved levels of fitness and not on one where activity is governed by pain and fear of what effect the activity may have on the pain.

As part of this normalisation the physiotherapist needs to share with the sufferer that when anyone embarks on a fitness programme there is an expectation that some muscle soreness will occur. This is not a sign of damage but the way that the muscles let their owner know that they have been worked hard! It needs to be added that the best way to deal with this normal soreness is to do the same exercise again but more gently. This is the most effective way to embark on a fitness programme. Examples can be quoted from well known athletes and from personal experience, and better still from the patient's past pre-pain experience! It is useful to ask if the sufferer is currently engaging in any form of exercise. Establishing their thoughts on exercise can also be useful.

The exercise programme

I consider a total body exercise programme incorporating varied and functional starting positions to be more favourable than an individual, problem area focused programme. There are several reasons for choosing such a programme.

- *First* it broadens the focus from one attending to the problem area alone to one of a total body fitness programme. The goal is to move away from the concept of treating an area that needs fixing. Thus, a total body programme minimises the risk of the patient focusing on the 'problem' area with the hoped for outcome being one of pain reduction i.e. that by moving the part that had previously been kept still an answer to the pain problem will be found.
- *Secondly* it allows sufferers to self assess. They find out information about themselves. For example, patients might report with surprise, 'I can move more on my bad side than on my good side!' At times like this there is a good opportunity to reinforce the fact that they can move what they perceive to be their bad side. Questions can be asked like, 'Does that surprise you?' 'Does it please you?' It also highlights the unpredictable nature of chronic pain and provides an opportunity to work within this context.
- *Thirdly* a total body programme may actually help patients find out about their fear and avoidance and be helped to address it (see Ch.8, and also Volume 1 of this series). All total body programmes obviously include individual components that move and stress the perceived problem area(s). As a result the patient may well come to focus on the area and exhibit fear-avoidant behaviour. The patient may even discover new activities that s/he is avoidant of but of which s/he was previously unaware. This 'flooding' can occur even at very low levels of exposure in a person who has been avoidant for many years. By being vigilant for this the physiotherapist can help the patient address the problem. This often requires carefully establishing an exercise quota to work to for all the exercises as well as a more discrete desensitisation programme where issues of avoidance can be addressed in a more subtle way. Once patients become aware that they are actually addressing avoidance a more overt desensitisation process can be executed and progressed.
- *Fourthly* it provides a means by which sufferers may come to identify and discover things they can do and do well. This discovery and increased confidence may then provide the encouragement to go on to address other challenges and fears. The notion that 'I can try to do it' rather than 'There's no way I'm doing it' is often engendered.

Doing it!

Getting feedback from the patients about the exercise programme helps identify any misconceptions and fears that they may have. It also provides an opportunity to start challenging these by gently questioning and asking for clarification.

An example of this: 'I did the exercises as I was told to do them but it made me much worse and I'm not doing exercise again.' The therapist can ask the sufferer for help in gaining a better understanding of what *worse* means. 'The exercise made you worse? Tell me how it made you worse.' Allowing the person to describe how it was for them and letting him/her know that you are listening helps to build up a trust that will enable the person to work with you. The conversation can continue with, 'So tell me what happened then.' The patient may relate that they were incapacitated for a while. The therapist might then ask the patient if this had frightened them and the response is usually 'Yes.' The therapist can then support the idea that being fearful is quite understandable and proceed with, 'So what happened next?' The patient will eventually describe how their activity eventually increased. The physiotherapist can highlight the point that activity levels did increase. 'So let me get this right. You did the exercises. You experienced an increase in pain that stopped you doing things. This was very frightening for you. Eventually you did manage to get going again.' The therapist might then ask, 'What do you think helped you get going again?' and if the time is right the therapist can refer back to previous discussions of how activity levels have diminished and what the possible benefits of exercise are for someone with persistent pain. This has to be done in a gentle manner that is non-coercive, non-judgmental, non-blaming and also non-patronising. The therapist can continue with, 'So what do you think will enable you do the exercises again? A different approach maybe? Doing them as gently as possible with virtually no effort—doing effortless exercise. How does that sound to you? Does that seem more possible?' By doing this you are letting the sufferer know that you believe they can do exercise again in a relaxed, slow, controlled, effortless way. Note that there is no opportunity to reinforce avoidant behaviour, only the opportunity to problem solve and find alternative ways of proceeding. The therapist can now help guide, talk and come up with a modified plan of action, for example, what their new starting point might be. Importantly, there is always something that a patient can manage to do.

A common response encountered is one of activity cycling. Here patients can lurch into an overdoing phase when embarking on an exercise regime, despite fear of the consequence of exercise. This may be due to their desire to let the physiotherapist know that they will do their very best or that they are determined to 'get better'. For some it may be an indication of their sense of frustration and even helplessness. There may even be an element of self punishment. The outcome of this over-active approach is that the sufferer experiences increased pain, is concerned about the possibility of further damage and becomes even more fear avoidant with a more pronounced sense

173

of failure. If this occurs the physiotherapist needs to engage the patient in a process of reasoning, discussion and review so that they are able understand and solve their 'failure.' In this difficult process the physiotherapist has to facilitate the patient by gently challenging any unhelpful thoughts and fears that they may be experiencing.

Some details of the physical process

Establishing baselines

Setting and readjusting goals. Having set the scene for relaxed slow controlled exercise (effortless exercise) the patients are invited to participate. They are encouraged to set an exercise baseline below what they perceive to be their maximum number (see Ch. 8, and also chapters by Shorland in Volume 1 and Brook in Volume 3 of this series). They proceed with this through all the exercise programmes (stretches, water exercise, and circuit sessions) at the identified times.

Acknowledging that *overestimating* one's ability when identifying goals is part of the human condition, the next stage in the physical process is to readjust goals downwards or to keep them the same for the next session.

Planned exercise not pain-contingent exercise

Sticking to goals and reviewing patterns. For the next stage the patients are advised to continue with relaxed 'effortless' exercise and to stick to their set goals. They are then encouraged to set a goal (the same number or a slightly higher number) for subsequent session after completing each exercise. This process continues for several sessions.

In the event of a patient having a 'good day' they are reminded of the approach to the exercise, and of sticking to set targets. There is an opportunity here to discuss with the patient the temptation of putting maximum effort in on this good day and the possible outcomes. If the patient does happen to overdo their exercises and suffer the consequences, it can be useful as it will provide an opportunity to review the effectiveness of the approach taken and to problem solve a more effective one—for example, being more relaxed or going more slowly.

If the patient is experiencing a 'bad day' an opportunity is provided to challenge avoidance and to perform the gentlest possible exercise and still stick to set goals. On such occasions, it is common for patients experiencing a bad day to actually gain some relief by performing gentle exercise and often even manage to stick to the goals set for that session. Importantly the patient will have gained a positive experience from managing to complete their exercise programme—a powerful factor in challenging avoidance.

The patients continue with the above process for several sessions to identify their own pattern. This involves carrying out the goals set and then setting the same or a slightly higher goal for the following session. Occasionally the patterns exhibit activity cycling and / or avoidance of certain exercises. This provides the opportunity for the therapist to review with the patient what has taken place and why. Discussion may involve such things as challenging underlying fears about exercise or the consequence of erratic exercise patterns. A better quota system can be identified and negotiated. Ideally, the aim is for the patient to use their own reasoning to adjust their exercise pattern. This helps establish a sense of responsibility, control, ownership and achievement.

Maintenance

How to keep it going and progress with quotas. At some stage it is important to discuss obstacles that might get in the way of continuing with the exercises. This takes place in a group setting and patients are encouraged to share with others their particular barriers to maintenance of the programme. This session can be very helpful. The group often offer suggestions of how to deal with perceived barriers and offer encouragement to fellow group members.

Each patient needs to have time with the therapist to discuss a long term plan with identified timescales. The patient is invited to nominate their own plan of when and how they will increase the number of exercises performed, e.g. to perform an exercise 3 times for the next 2 sessions and then to increase it to 4 for the following 2 sessions and so on. A date for the patients to review their own programme is also set. Discussion can take place on how to progress the programme further for the future.

Patients need the opportunity to discuss options with the therapist but the ultimate control should always remain in the patient's domain. In this way the therapist takes on a facilitatory role, for example, by inviting the patients to challenge and make sense of their own decisions. Questions like, 'So how have you come to that decision?' or, 'What do you expect to happen?' may be appropriate stem questions.

Re-engagement

How to deal with setbacks. 'Setbacks' need to be reviewed as they are common and will happen to most patients. Sessions need to discuss the sorts of things that might precipitate a setback and then how the patient can go on to deal with them and get started again. For example, it is important for patients to know how to work out the number of exercises to do when restarting—or at what level to re-engage. The patient should be encouraged to look at all the options and to explore each in turn and what the outcomes might be. Here again, the therapist takes the role of facilitator and requests clarification from the patient of the thoughts behind any decisions made. This can help the patient to challenge underlying fears and to identify other options that may prove more helpful. Each patient is invited to write their own setback plan. The setback can be viewed as an unpleasant but nevertheless useful event in that patients find out that they can get through it and can come to re-engage in activity once more. It can be an empowering experience.

175

Dealing with obstacles

During any exercise or activating process many obstacles are encountered. One frequently met in the early stages is the response to the invitation to engage in exercise that involves the patient getting on to the floor. The response often encountered is 'I can't get on to the floor.' Rather than accept this, it is important to keep working with the patient. 'So you are unable to get right down on to the floor. What do you think will happen if you do try to get on to the floor?' Or, 'Help me by explaining to me how you used to do this' and then, 'So let's see which bit of this is still possible' and so on. In this way it is possible to slowly establish how much of the activity the patient can still do. Patients often see a task in an 'all or nothing way' and therapists may be guilty of accepting the patient's position too easily. There is always at least a part of a movement, exercise or activity that the patient can comfortably do or try and then build from. It is important not to give the patient the opportunity to avoid something they fear. Identifying a feared activity needs to be seen as providing an empowering opportunity. Establishing, trying and achieving the bit that can be done for the patient who is resistant to getting down on the floor nicely identifies a baseline for eventually going on to achieving it. As therapists we need to be careful in our assumptions of what the patient might actually want to try and achieve. In the getting onto the floor example it might be useful to ask, 'Is this something you would like to be able to do—maybe to play with children (or grandchildren)?' In this way the activity of getting on to the floor can become more relevant to the patient since it means being able to play with young family members and goes towards lessening a sense of isolation.

This is just one example of the many physical obstacles that can occur with chronic pain syndrome patients. It also illustrates the distress a patient may have and the complex work of the physiotherapist in this area. While difficult it is often very rewarding.

Final comments

All the processes described have used a general exercise programme in a group setting as an example. The same principles can be generalised for tackling any physical/functional activity difficulties.

These principles of a CB approach for exercise and activity can also be utilised with modification in an outpatient setting and on an individual basis for chronic pain sufferers. In order to avoid things like conflicting information, different forms of advice, different approaches and the dangers of creating confusion, there is a great need to liaise and discuss management with other involved parties—physiotherapists, general practitioners, consultants, psychologists, family members, employers, and any others as appropriate. Ideally, a consistent team approach that reinforces the same messages to the patient is in place to manage this complex problem.

It must be recognised that patients who have a chronic pain **syndrome** will need input from experienced professionals and a referral to a specialist unit is the best course of action.

The principles of cognitive behavioural therapy can be generalised to many chronic illnesses, for example, coronary heart disease, rheumatoid arthritis and diabetes. Many of the intervention strategies discussed are also relevant to acute conditions and to conditions with active ongoing pathology. The importance of CBT is that it can have a major impact in reducing and minimising unnecessary physical disability and the negative psychosocial consequences that accompany it.

NOTE

For further information and Workshops on the approach please contact Babs Harper, Training Consultant, on: 0117 9860494 or 0776 1224814

SUGGESTED READING

Crombez G, Vlaeyen, JWS, Heuts PHTG, Lysens R 1999 Pain-related fear is more disabling than pain itself: Evidence on the role of pain-related fear in chronic back pain disability, Pain 80:329–339

Gifford LS (ed) 1998 Topical Issues in Pain 1. Whiplash—science and management. Fear-avoidance beliefs and behaviour. CNS Press, Falmouth

Gifford LS (ed) 2000 Topical Issues in Pain 2. Biopsychosocial assessment. Relationships and pain. CNS Press, Falmouth

Gifford LS (ed) 2002 Topical Issues in Pain 3. Sympathetic Nervous System and Pain. Pain Management. Clinical Effectiveness. CNS Press, Falmouth

Main CJ, Spanswick CC 2000 Pain Management. An interdisciplinary approach. Churchill Livingstone, Edinburgh

McCracken LM, Spertus IL, Janeck AS, Sinclair D, Wetzel FT 1999 Behavioral dimensions of adjustment in persons with chronic pain: Pain-related anxiety and acceptance. Pain, 80:283–289

Kabat-Zinn J 1990 Full Catastrophe Living. Delta, New York

Waddell G 1998 The Back Pain Revolution. Churchill Livingstone, Edinburgh

Muscles and pain

10

Psychophysiological models of pain

PAUL J WATSON

Physiotherapy is increasingly viewing musculoskeletal pain from a biopsychosocial perspective (Watson 1999, Watson 2000, Watson & Kendall 2000), which represents an advance in the way we manage such problems. We no longer see these problems as being either pathological or psychological but recognise that both are inextricably linked. Very few therapists would deny today that a person's reaction to a disease influences what they do about it and that this has more influence on the ultimate level of disability than biomechanical dysfunction alone. Research over many years in the area of psychophysiology has demonstrated that stress, disease conviction and coping not only influence the development of disability but also the development and perpetuation of abnormal physiological states which can lead to physiological dysfunction and even disease. Once labelled as 'psychosomatic' disease or hypochondriasis, and therefore largely dismissed as untreatable by physiotherapy, we are now starting to investigate the powerful physiological effects these states can have. How physiotherapists manage psychosocial dysfunction challenges the traditional way painful conditions have been viewed in physiotherapy practise.

The purpose of this chapter is to give a brief overview of some research that has been conducted into the possible role of muscle/mind interaction and the development of abnormal muscle activity which could contribute to chronic pain states. Examples from the author's own research and some previously unpublished data will be presented. It will offer an alternative model based on a more dynamic view of the interaction between beliefs about pain and injury, the stress that accompanies disability, and changes in muscle responses and perception of stressful or threatening stimuli.

The spasm–pain–spasm model

Initial models of myogenic pain tried to explain the perseverance of pain following injury according to a model which suggested that, following injury, muscle activity increases around the affected area to protect it. The underlying mechanisms of this theory have not been demonstrated clearly, but it is often assumed that pain increases γ-motor neurone activity which in turn leads to an increase in α-motor neurone activity which goes on to precipitate hyper-reactivity and spasm. This then results in local ischaemia as increased muscular pressure produces forces that exceed the local tissue perfusion pressure causing capillaries and arterioles to become compressed. The net result of this is the release of algogenic (pain producing) substances (Christensen 1986, 1986a). These enhance the transmission of nociceptive impulses by reducing the threshold for stimulation of nociceptive specific neurones and reduce the sensitivity of wide dynamic range neurones causing previously non-nociceptive stimuli (e.g. pressure) to become painful (Coderre et al 1993, Mense 1997, Gifford 1998, 1998a). This model might serve in the acute state or in short-term acute flare-up in recurrent or chronic pain states where increased muscle activity can be demonstrated in some muscle groups in particular over injured joints. However, inhibition of other muscle groups also occurs and the relationship between the muscle activity and the report of pain is unclear (Simons & Mense 1998). Research into identifying elevated muscle activity in chronic pain states without obvious spasm has not substantiated a role for consistently elevated levels of muscle tension (Ahern et al 1988, Arena et al 1991, Letchuman & Deusinger 1993, Watson et al 1997).

When chronic pain patients are compared to pain free controls using electromyography most research has failed to demonstrate any difference in muscle activity at rest. Researchers who have been able to demonstrate elevated muscle activity in subjects with chronic pain report levels that would be insufficient to cause the increase in intramuscular pressure required to reduce muscle circulatory perfusion (Cram & Steger 1983, Cram 1990).

If those who report pain do not have elevated levels of muscle tension, why do we frequently hear patients complain that they feel tense in painful muscle groups, for example in the neck? Research conducted in occupational settings has helped to throw some light on this area. Through a sequence of experiments in industrial settings a Norwegian group has looked at the relationship between neck and shoulder pain, muscle activity, and the perception of tension (Vasseljen & Westgaard 1995, Westgaard 1999). This is discussed further below.

Muscle hyper-reactivity

In order to overcome the objections to the spasm–pain–spasm model because of the insubstantial nature of the evidence, many researchers suggested that the increase in muscle activity may not be permanent but may occur with sufficient frequency to perpetuate the painful condition. In this model both physiological and psychological stress can increase muscle activity.

Westgaard and colleagues (see Westgaard 1999 for a summary) recorded the muscle activity during a typical working day in a group of office workers and another group working on a production line. Subjects were asked to rate their neck and shoulder pain and the perception of muscle tension. As might be expected, those working on the production line had more muscle activity than those working in the office because of the nature of the work; furthermore, their perception of muscle tension through the day correlated with the EMG measures. It has often been suggested that the pain reported by office workers is due to increased muscle tension that develops during prolonged sitting in a biomechanically ineffective position; this was not demonstrated in this study.

The best predictor of the development of pain in the *production line* workers was indeed the actual level of muscle activity. However, in the *office workers*, who demonstrated much less muscle activity, the best predictor of the development of pain was the *perception* of muscle tension even though there was no relationship between self-report of muscle tension and measured EMG. This further appears to have been closely related the *psychological status* of the worker at the time. This calls into question the presumed linearity of the relationship between pain and muscle activity in the office workers:

- The postures that they maintained during their work did not lead to high levels of muscle tension.
- Their beliefs and perception of muscle tension appeared to be most influential in reporting pain.

However, when looking at the effect of 'cognitive demand' on trapezius muscle tension during VDU operation, the team found that muscle tension *increased* proportionately with the *complexity* of the task to a point where pain was reported. This was found in healthy controls (Waersted & Westgaard 1996).

These findings suggest that the biomechanical demands of the task (sitting at a VDU) alone, are insufficient to cause increases in muscle tension sufficient to cause pain; but increasing the complexity of the task, and the attention required to perform it, are of greater importance in the development of myogenic neck/shoulder pain. Furthermore, when the same experiments were conducted on pain sufferers the responses were repeated but there was a more marked development of pain than in the healthy controls (Bansevicius et al 1999).

The diathesis stress model

An individual can be placed under stress—for example by being asked to do more complicated tasks and this may eventually lead to increased muscle tension as described earlier. But, this may be a general stress to which we all might be expected to respond. *Diathesis*, in this model, refers to an individual's susceptibility to a stressor, in this case it is specific and results from a previous experience. Re-exposing the individual to the specific stressor, or a similar experience, will result in psychological stress that can be seen as a physiological response.

The findings discussed in the previous section relate to a non-specific stressor and relate only to the trapezius muscle. Other authors believe that for patients to develop a stereotypical muscular response to stressful situations; the stressor should be personally relevant. This may be an experience that evokes memory of the original painful episode, for example driving a car after whiplash, performing an occupational task that provoked pain, or it can be the result of other such stressors.

Flor et al (1991a) proposed a *diathesis-stress model* to explain pain. In this the chronic pain sufferer exhibits stereotypical increased muscle activity in response to stressful experiences. These increases in muscle tension are seen only in personally relevant situations, occur only in the painful muscles, and do not generalise to other muscle groups.

Chronic low back pain (CLBP) patients and healthy controls were asked to relate a personally relevant stressful situation while muscle activity was monitored in the low back and control site muscles. An arithmetical task served as a non-personally-relevant control stressor. The back pain group demonstrated increased lumbar paraspinal muscle activity during the personally relevant stressor. This increase was not seen in the healthy controls and did not generalise to other muscle groups. This indicated to the authors that muscle tension may contribute to the pain state through a stereotypical response in a stressful situation. They further suggested that pain itself may be able to trigger this response (although this was not tested).

It should be noted that the back pain patients did not report pain during the personally relevant stressor. This may be because the increase in muscle activity was not maintained for long enough to cause pain or that the increases observed were remarkably small and therefore unlikely to lead to significant enough ischaemia to cause pain. The role of the perception of muscle tension may be an important factor here (see previous section).

Interestingly, even though the response was only small, there was a clear demonstration that the muscles of the CLBP patients responded differently to different stressors.

These investigators went on to compare the responses in tempero-mandibular joint (TMJ) dysfunction subjects and CLBP subjects. As predicted by the model, the CLBP group responded to the personally relevant stressors in the muscles of the low back and the TMJ subjects responded in the jaw muscles (Flor et al 1991, 1992).

A group in the UK has investigated stereotypical responses to *painful stimuli*. It is an anecdotal observation that chronic pain patients sometimes report that pain in other areas 'sets off' or leads to an increase in their usual pain.

Watson et al (1998) investigated the role of a non-specific pain stressor in 14 subjects with chronic low back pain and 12 healthy pain free age and sex matched controls. The two groups were subjected to a cold pressor test (Lavallo 1975), which involves the subject placing their hand in water at near freezing point. This results in a cramping type pain after typically 15–20 seconds. The subjects are instructed to keep their hand in the water until they can no longer tolerate the pain or until a pre-determined time (usually 4 minutes). The pain ratings, and the muscular responses of the lumbar paraspinal and trapezius muscles were recorded using sEMG (surface electromyography). The method involved: after baseline readings the right hand was immersed in cool water at 15°C, the 'cool water phase'. This was followed by quiet sitting and then the 'cold pressor phase'. Here, the hand was placed in water at 1°C as described above. This was followed by a final baseline reading. The patients' pain responses were recorded throughout using the method described by Chen et al (1989).

In the analysis of the results it was found that:

- Throughout the experiment there were no significant differences between the groups for pain report or pain tolerance. This demonstrated that back pain individuals *do not have* a lower lowered pain tolerance in general as has sometimes been asserted (Cohen et al 1986, Peters & Schmidt 1991).
- CLBP patients demonstrated *much higher levels* of activity in the lumbar paraspinal muscles during both the 'cool water' and 'cold pressor' phases and these reached statistical significance during the cold pressor (pain challenge) phase (see Fig. 10.1). Surprisingly, back pain subjects demonstrated lower levels of activity than controls in the trapezius muscles (see Fig. 10.2).

This experiment suggests that those with back pain demonstrated a stereotypical response of increased guarding of the painful area (the low back) in the presence a painful stimulus elsewhere. This must be a learnt response as a result of the chronic pain problem. The relationship between this and the development of pain cannot be clarified because the subjects were required to report only the pain felt in their hand and not in the back.

The role of muscle learning in response to pain has been investigated by pairing auditory tones with electric shocks administered to the fingers. The investigation used a group of pain free students who were conditioned to anticipate the administration of pain (Flor & Birbaumer 1994). As expected, increases in muscle activity accompanied painful shocks. After a conditioning period the auditory tone alone was sufficient to cause an increase in muscle activity in the subjects. Pictures with negative emotional connotations (e.g. angry faces) were then paired with the tones and shocks and a further increase in the muscle responses was observed. The researchers also found that those students who reported that they suffered from neck and shoulder complaints when studying became conditioned sooner and that their responses were more resistant to extinction.

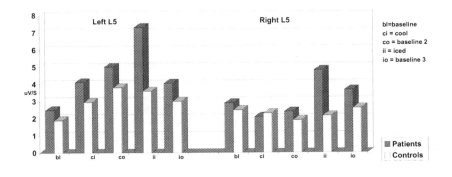

Fig. 10.1 Cold pressor test sEMG responses for lumbar paraspinal muscles to the right and left of L5 in patients with chronic low back pain and controls. (From Watson et al 1998)

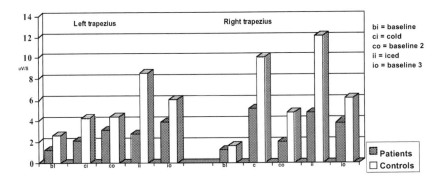

Fig. 10.2 Cold pressor test sEMG responses for trapezius muscles in patients with chronic low back pain and controls. (From Watson et al 1997)

Changes in dynamic movement patterns

These results of the experiments discussed in the previous section demonstrate that the muscles underlying the area of pain in chronic pain patients respond differently to painful and stressful stimuli when compared to healthy controls. However, these experiments involved only static and relatively relaxed postures (sitting, fully supported).

In recent years there has been much interest in differences in muscle activity during movement. The fact that muscle recruitment patterns in CLBP patients is different from that in normal controls is far from new and was first identified on EMG in the 1950s. Recently it has been suggested that these abnormalities of recruitment are a possible cause of the back pain, and treatment strategies aimed at correcting this have developed. This is in advance of clearly convincing evidence for specificity of effect.

It is important to remember that although the paraspinal muscles perform skilled integrated activities automatically and unconsciously, they are still under a great degree of cortical, conscious control and subject to learning like any other skeletal muscle. Also, the action of such muscle is a measure of physical *performance* and as such it is influenced not only by physiological factors but also psychological ones (Watson 1999a).

One of the best known and researched abnormalities of muscle action in back pain is loss of the 'flexion relaxation phenomenon' (FRP). When moving from standing into full lumbopelvic flexion the paraspinal muscles demonstrate a characteristic and highly reproducible pattern of activity (Floyd & Silver 1955). At the completion of the lumbar flexion component the paraspinal muscles demonstrate electrical silence; i.e., the flexion relaxation phenomenon or FRP. During this silent phase the weight of the body is supported through the thoracolumbar fascia and the rest of the motion is performed through rotation of the pelvis on the hips. On rising back to upright the paraspinal muscles demonstrate a sudden increase in activity to bring the lumbar spine into extension. This has been repeatedly demonstrated to be abnormal in back pain patients and has been demonstrated to return to normal on the resolution of symptoms (Haig et al 1993).

A group of us (Watson et al 1997) developed an algorithm for measuring the FRP, the 'flexion relaxation ratio' (FRR). This was demonstrated to be highly reproducible over time and discriminated back pain patients from healthy controls with a remarkable degree of accuracy (Watson et al 1997). This work also showed that the FRR changed significantly towards the normal following a pain management programme in a group of 36 CLBP subjects (Watson et al 1998). In the research we predicted that if there was a straightforward biomechanical or myogenic cause to the patients' pain, then a normalisation of the muscle pattern should lead to a reduction in pain.

We were surprised to find that the normalisation of the muscle function was most closely related to changes in fear-avoidance beliefs and an increase in the patients' confidence that they could move despite the pain. This demonstrated a powerful role for beliefs about pain, injury and movement in the maintenance of abnormal muscle activity.

It may be the case that when clinicians spend time:

- giving a relatively benign attribution which supports self management
- reassuring that it is safe to move
- explaining that movement will be beneficial
- giving patients the opportunity for regular guidance and practise of movement

that it will result in the reduction in fear and an increase in self-confidence (self efficacy) in controlling their pain.

187

The particular *type* of exercise performed may be relatively unimportant. Separating the changes in fear and self-confidence about movement and the effect of specific exercises on muscle activity would be an interesting area of further investigation.

Experimental pain and psychological influences

Our group (Watson et al 1996) has also addressed the issue of the relationship between fear of injury and muscle sensitivity as measured by pressure algometry.

It has been well established that those who report chronically painful muscles demonstrate increased pain sensitivity evidenced by reduced thresholds for pressure-induced pain *over the painful muscles*. This has been reported widely in fibromyalgia, low back pain and whiplash associated disorders (Wolfe et al 1990, Fischer 1987, Olivegren et al 1999). In an acute state this might be closely associated with the underlying pathology, particularly the inflammation processes and its accompanying protective secondary sensitisation. In the chronic pain state there is rarely, if ever, any observable, *significant* muscle pathology.

In our research (Watson et al 1996) we investigated two series of patients, one with chronic low back pain and one with a diagnosis of fibromyalgia. The pressure pain thresholds for the lumbar and lower thoracic spine, and the 18 'American College of Rheumatology fibromyalgia tender points' (Wolfe et al 1990) in 21 patients with chronic low back pain, and 21 age and sex matched controls were studied.

Chronic low back pain (CLBP) subjects were taken from the waiting list at a local pain management clinic. Only those reporting pain in the low back and/or both legs were included in the study. Those reporting widespread pain (i.e. pain in the upper body and upper limbs) were excluded. Subjects were aged between18 and 60, there was no history of chronic pelvic pain, no other significant medical condition, and no inflammatory or neoplastic disease. Patients continued to take medication as routine.

Healthy control subjects were drawn from University and health care communities. They were aged between 18 and 60 years, had no history of consulting for low back pain, no back ache in the previous year, no history of chronic pain, and were not under going any current medical treatment.

In the first experiment the low back was divided into 48 points based on defined anatomical landmarks. The American College of Rheumatology fibromyalgia points were also tested (Wolfe et al 1990). Prior to testing, the patient group completed the Modified Somatic Perception Questionnaire (MSPQ) (Main 1983), the physical component of the Fear Avoidance Beliefs questionnaire (FABQ) (Waddell et al 1993) and a visual analogue scale of 'current pain status'.

Pressure pain thresholds (PPT) were assessed using a Somedic bridge amplifier pressure algometer with a rubber tipped 1cm probe to each of the points in a random order leaving at least 10 seconds between point testing to prevent the cumulative effect of repeated local stimulation. The rate of increase of progression was 100 kPa (kilopascals) per second, assessed by visual feedback. The subject was required to press a button indicating the pressure pain threshold at the point where 'the pressure ceases to be pressure alone and begins to feel painful'. The pressure was stopped and the next point then tested.

Scores for the pressure pain threshold for each of the sites were derived using analysis of variance (ANOVA) based on group (patient or control) membership (see Table 10.1).

Table 10.1 Pearson product moment correlations between pressure pain threshold scores, pain report and somatic anxiety in CLBP patients (n=21)

	Mean Score Low Back PPT (kPa)	Mean Score ACR points PPT (kPa)
Fear Avoidance Beliefs (FABQ Physical activity)	-.58 p=.007	-.67 p=.001
Current Pain (VAS)	-.48 p=.03	-.47 p=.03
Somatic Anxiety (MSPQ)	-.44 p=.05	-.44 p=.05

Results for the CLBP group

- The patient group had significantly lower pressure pain thresholds than the control group for each of the 48 points ($p<.05$–$.001$). The mean score for low back pressure pain thresholds was significantly lower in the CLBP pain group (F=16.6, $p<.0001$).

- The CLBP group also demonstrated significantly lower pressure pain thresholds for 14 of the 18 ACR (Wolfe et al 1990) fibromyalgia points. The mean score for all the fibromyalgia points was significantly lower in the CLBP group than in the control group (F=17.2, $p<.0001$). Simply, the CLBP patients reported the onset of 'pain' with the pressure algometer earlier than did the control groups.

- The 'Current pain status' scores demonstrated significant correlation with the mean of the scores for low back tenderness (the higher the pain reported, the lower the threshold for pain on PPT) ($p<.03$). Current pain status scores demonstrated a significant correlation with the mean of the ACR fibromyalgia points, too ($p<.03$).

189

- Highly significant correlations were identified between the mean of the PPT scores for the back and the FABQ (physical)(p<.007).
- Highly significant correlations were identified between mean of the PPT for the ACR FM points and the FABQ (physical) (p<.001). For both sets of these results the more fearful the patient was, the lower the pain threshold.
- Weak but significant correlations were observed between the PPT scores and the modified somatic perception questionnaire. The more anxious or aware the patient was about bodily sensations, the lower the threshold for pain.

The results for the low back PPT were subjected to multiple regression analysis. Mean back tenderness was entered as the dependant variable and the FABQ (physical) and current pain status were entered as independent variables in a stepwise regression model.

- FABQ (physical) accounted for 29% of the variance (adj. R^2) (sig =.007).[1]
- FABQ (physical) and current day pain combined accounted for 39% of the variance (adj. R^2) (sig =.05).

This demonstrates that in this group the current level of pain, although closely related to the report of tenderness in the back, was *less important than the fear of injury*.

Results for the fibromyalgia group

The same experiment was repeated in a group of 44 fibromyalgia patients who were compared to 33 healthy, pain-free controls. In this study the FABQ physical score was substituted by the Tampa Scale of Kinesiophobia (TSK) (Kori et al 1990). This broader questionnaire does not include questions on work and is specifically designed to assess fear of movement and re-injury. Patients also completed the Short-form McGill Pain Questionnaire (SF-MPQ). The SF-MPQ has three compartments that assess respectively: the affective, sensory, and intensity components of pain (see Table 10.2 and results discussion below). Only the results for the ACR FM pressure points will be described here for brevity.

In the CLBP experiment it was noted not only that the patients had a reduced pressure pain threshold (PPT) but also that the pain sensation they experienced at the 'threshold' was much stronger than in the normal control subjects.

As a result of this a measure was developed called the Pressure Pain Threshold Intensity (PPTI). This measure requires subjects to report the point at which pain starts and at the same time to rate the intensity of the pain on a scale of 1–10. The PPTI was recorded for all the points tested and used to assess whether in fibromyalgic patients:

- there was a lower PPT
- there was any influence of pain and fear on the magnitude of the pain reported to the experimental pressure stimulus.

In a previous study (Georgoudis 1996), the PPTI was demonstrated to be highly reliable and much better at discriminating patients from controls than the ACR point score alone. The scores for the PPT and the PPTI were calculated and these were compared with the results from the SF-MPQ and the TSK. Independent t-tests were used to assess group differences.

- As expected the fibromyalgia patients had much lower PPTs for the ACR points (controls mean 469.3 kPa, SD 109; patients mean 214.3 kPa, SD 84; p<.001).
- The PPTIs for the patient group were much higher than the controls (controls mean 2.7, SD .75; patients mean 6.5, SD 1.6; p<.001).

The relationships between pain report, tenderness, experimental pain response and the TSK are given in Table 10.2. The following points are relevant:

- The relationship between the report of pain and tenderness (PPT) demonstrated a significant but relatively weak correlation in the patient group.
- The relationship with the sensory component was not significant.
- The strongest relationship was with the affective dimension of the (SF-MPQ).
- The same pattern is seen for the report of intensity of experimental pain (PPTI).
- The correlation between the TSK and the mean score for muscle tenderness (PPT) was significant but weak.
- The TSK was highly correlated with the report of mean pain intensity (PPTI) during the experiment. In other words, those patients who were high on fear, rated the pain at threshold, as being more intense.

Table 10.2 Pearson product moment correlations between fear/avoidance beliefs, muscle tenderness and report of experimental pain in fibromyalgic patients (n=44)

	PPT mean score	PPTI mean score	TSK
Fear avoidance beliefs (TSK)	-.32 p=< .03	.42 p=<.007	–
SF-MPQ Affective	-.33 p=<.03	.38 p=.01	.53 p=<.001
SF-MPQ Sensory	-.25 ns	.2815 ns	.39 p=<.01
SF-MPQ VAS	-.31 p=<.05	.30 p=<.05	.38 p=<.01

MPQ = Short-form McGill Pain questionnaire
PPT = Pressure Pain Threshold
PPTI = Intensity of Pain at PPT

- The relationship between the current pain report (SF-MPQ VAS) and the scores for the TSK is significant.
- The relationship with the tenderness scores was less so.

The above evidence lends some support to the model suggested by Lathem et al (1983), which is one of a fear-avoidance model of exaggerated pain perception. Vlaeyen and Linton (2000) have postulated that fear leads to the development of hypervigilance to symptoms which may be reflected in an increased report of pain.

Clearly the results in this series of experiments are only cross-sectional and so we cannot draw conclusions about the process of increased sensitivity to pain. However, what has been found does support the idea that heightened fear is closely associated with increased pain report and increased responses to experimentally induced pain. The results from the chronic low back pain experiments, discussed earlier, also demonstrate a role for heightened somatic awareness which is analogous to the hypervigilance in the Vlaeyen and Linton (2000) model.

Some clinical implications

What relevance does all this experimental work have for physiotherapy practice? Pressure algometry is a good analogy for palpation used in patient examination. Just as with palpation, pressure algometry exerts pressure over an area until the patient reports pain. In the case of palpation the patient's response is often used to guide treatment. The good news for therapists is that the response to pressure over tissues is different in patients and healthy controls and is related to the current report of pain in the patients. However, in both the low back pain group and the fibromyalgics the pain reported in relation to pressure or palpation is influenced more by *the patient's fear of being hurt or injured* than by the current pain state.

Physiotherapists must understand that when making clinical decisions based on how a patient responds to palpation that it involves a *combination* of:

- local tenderness as a result of local changes,
- secondary sensitisation, and
- the patient's fear of injury.

The latter may be the most important factor in determining tenderness in those with chronic pain conditions.

How can we bring all this material together into a whole? In Figure 10.3 I have tried to illustrate how different strands of the data presented here might be incorporated into a working model. Many of these factors have been addressed in other volumes of Topical Issues in Pain. Readers may be interested to overview the model proposed by Gifford (1998b) in Volume 1 of this series, as well as the model suggested by Waddell (1998 p. 233) which has many of the features in Figure 10.3.

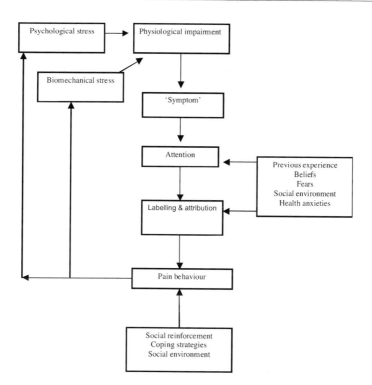

Fig. 10.3 An integrated model of symptom, attention and stress in musculoskeletal pain.

At the centre of the model proposed in Figure 10.3 there is a physiological stimulus or symptom that I believe is the focus of the problem. This may be nociceptive; it may be noxious (unpleasant) but non-nociceptive; or it may be non-nociceptive and benign. Our beliefs about the nature of the sensation lead us to label it (Cioffi 1991). We then try to assign meaning to it. This is influenced by our knowledge and beliefs about the nature of damage and harm and the social environment at the time. All are vitally important in influencing our subsequent reaction to the pain—our 'pain behaviour'. For example, whether we report pain or behave as though we are in pain (e.g., develop abnormal movement, or muscular guarding). If uncorrected, inappropriate or 'maladaptive' pain-related behaviours can lead to avoidance of exercise, secondary deconditioning, the development of guarded movement and abnormal patterns of movement. Patients may also demonstrate abnormal responses to aversive stimuli or to any stimuli that they perceive as potentially damaging or that may have been associated with previous pain and injury. These contribute to changes in biomechanical stresses in the affected area and beyond.

The secondary effects of continued pain and physical incapacity will have psychological consequences. These factors are discussed at length in this and previous volumes in this series. It is important to note however, that depression and anxiety are common sequelae in painful conditions (Magni 1994) and are well known to affect the perception of pain, attention to symptoms and treatment seeking (Croft et al 1994). Anxiety, in particular, increases autonomic nervous system activity that can result in increased muscle activity/tension (the autonomic nervous system is reviewed in Volume 3 of this series, but also see Wall's Introductory Essay and Ch. 2 in this volume in relation to anxiety, attention, fear and depression).

Pain and its psychological consequences have an effect on the quantity and quality of sleep and it has been clearly demonstrated that lack of sleep is associated with the development of muscle pain (Moldofsky & Scarisbrick 1976). Interestingly, lack of sleep results in a reduction in the normal levels of growth hormone secreted during sleep. It is thought that this may be responsible for a failure of muscle to repair resulting in observable muscle micro-damage and the development of pain (Bennett et al 1992).

Altered patterns of muscle activity in the affected area eventually become automatic responses to the presentation of stimuli that are painful or may be associated with pain. Altered muscle activity can be seen as an unconscious 'preparation' by the brain, which has become conditioned by experience and learning, and may serve to maintain abnormal input into the system.

Heightened attention to the painful area may lead to misinterpretation of various physical stimuli as well as normal body sensations. For example if we really give attention to our body we often easily feel pins and needles and modest discomfort that we hadn't noticed. Heightened attention to stimuli and other sensations may reinforce the perception of an abnormal stimulus (pain) arising from the tissues. Simply, increased attention can amplify a sensation or lead to its misinterpretation so that it may be processed by the nervous system in terms of pain (see Gifford 1998a p. 73).

Note that in this model (Fig. 10.3) there is no attempt to separate nociceptive and non-nociceptive stimuli; it encompasses both. The pain cannot be ascribed clearly to a single pathological event, although one may have begun the process, or to a psychological cause. Consequently, the problem is unlikely to respond to a single modality approach:

- Psychologists cannot effectively correct guarded movement and deconditioning using solely psychological techniques, and physiotherapists cannot overcome the misattribution of sensations or aberrant beliefs by adopting a single exercise approach or by manipulating tissues.
- It is my opinion that a clinician unacquainted with the complexity of the pain experience will regard painful conditions as either psychological or pathological; a more informed clinician will unconsciously ascribe a percentage to each area; but an enlightened clinician will see pain as a dynamic interaction between a multitude of influences and manage it accordingly and appropriately.

194

Conclusions

Hopefully this chapter has achieved its aims—to demonstrate the considerable interaction between muscle activity, pain, the nervous system and a patient's psychological status. In essence, all pains are psychophysiological phenomena and need to be considered as such in the clinic. It seems that muscles in particular are influenced heavily by what we may be thinking and how we are feeling. The following points are worth reiterating:

- Beliefs (fears) about injury and ability to cope with pain change muscle action in CLBP patients, these are unconscious but objectively observable.
- In CLBP the resolution of abnormal dynamic muscle activity is mediated by changes in fear of movement and patients' confidence in their ability to manage the pain.
- Chronic pain patients demonstrate abnormal muscle responses to stressful situations including pain.
- Response to palpation are highly influenced by fear of re-injury in chronic pain patients.
- Perceptions about increases in muscle tension may be more important in the development of pain than objectively measured increases in some situations.
- Stereotypical responses to pain can be conditioned in normal subjects. Once conditioned, an associated stimulus is sufficient to elicit the muscular response independently from pain.
- The combined effect of psychological stress and physical stressors on the development and maintenance of chronic pain is under-researched.

ENDNOTE

1   Regression techniques try to explain how variables in research relate to each other. The statistic used is not important here but the concept is. For example, in a population tall people are generally heavier than short people. This is by no means true for all. Increase in height explains 50% of the variance for increase in weight; the rest is explained by increased muscle (10%), increased fat (10%), and other factors (water content, bone density). Eventually you might explain 100% of the variation in weight. This is rare in multiply-determined things like disability.

REFERENCES

Ahern DK, Follick MJ, Council JR, Laser-Wolston N, Litchman H 1988 Comparison of lumber paravertebral EMG patterns in chronic low back pain patients and non-pain controls. Pain 34:153–160

Arena JG, Sherman RA, Bruno G, Young TR 1991 Electromyographic recordings of low back pain subjects and non-pain controls in six different positions: Effect of pain levels. Pain 45:23–28

Bansevicius D, Westgaard RH, Sjaastad OM 1999 Tension-type headache: Pain, fatigue, tension, and EMG responses to mental activation. Headache 39(6):417–25

195

Bennett RM, Clark SR, Campbell SM, Burkhardt CS 1992 Low levels of somatomedin C in patients with fibromyalgia syndrome. A possible link between sleep and muscle pain. Arthritis and Rheumatism 35:1113–1116

Chen ACN, Dworkin SF, Haug J, Gehrig L 1989 Human pain responsivity in a tonic pain model: Psychological determinants. Pain 37:143–160

Christensen LV 1986 Physiology and pathology of skeletal muscle contraction: Part 1 Dynamic activity. Journal of Oral Rehabilitation 13:451–456

Christensen LV 1986a Physiology and pathology of skeletal muscle contraction: Part 2 Static activity. Journal of Oral Rehabilitation 13:463–477

Cioffi D 1991 Beyond attentional strategies: A cognitive-perceptual model of somatic interpretation. Psychological Bulletin 109:25–41

Coderre TJ, Katz J, Vaccarino AL, Melzack R 1993 Contribution of central neuroplasticity to pathological pain: Review of clinical and experimental evidence. Pain 52:259–285

Cohen MJ, Swanson GA, Nabiloff BD, Schandler SL, McArthur DL 1986 Comparison of electromyographic response patterns during posture and stress tasks in chronic low back patients and normal controls. Journal of Psychosomatic Research 30:135–141

Cram JR 1990 Clinical Electromyography Vol 2. Clinical Resources, Nevada City

Cram JR, Steger JC 1983 EMG scanning in the diagnosis of chronic pain. Biofeedback and Self-Regulation 8(2):101–108

Croft P, Schollum J, Silman A 1994 Population study of tender point counts and pain as evidence of fibromyalgia. British Medical Journal. 309:696–699

Fischer AA 1987 Pressure threshold measurement for the diagnosis of myofascial pain and evaluation of treatment results. Clinical Journal of Pain 2:207–214

Flor H, Turk DC, Birbaumer N 1985 Assessment of stress-related psychophysiological reactions in chronic back pain patients. Journal of Consulting and Clinical Psychology 53:354–364

Flor H, Birbaumer N, Schulte W, Roos R 1991 Stress related EMG responses in patients with chronic tempero-mandibular pain. Pain 46:145–152

Flor H, Birbaumer N, Turk DC 1991a The psychobiology of chronic pain. Advances in Behavioural Research and Therapy 12:47–84

Flor H, Birbaumer N, Schugens MM, Lutzenburger W 1992 Symptom specific responding in chronic pain patients and healthy controls. Psychophysiology 29:452–460

Flor H, Birbaumer N 1994 Basic issues in the psychobiology of pain. In: Gebhart GF, Hammond DL, Jensen TS (eds) Proceedings of the 7th World Congress on Pain. Progress in pain research and management Vol 2. IASP Press, Seattle

Floyd WF, Silver PHS 1955 The function of the erector spinae muscles in certain movements and postures in man. Journal of Physiology 129:184–203

Georgoudis G 1996 Pressure pain threshold and intensity of pain responsiveness in fibromyalgia and normal healthy controls. M.Sc dissertation, University of Manchester

Gifford LS 1998 Tissue and input related mechanisms. In: Gifford LS (ed) Topical Issues in Pain 1. Whiplash—science and management. Fear-avoidance beliefs and behaviour. CNS Press, Falmouth 57–65

Gifford LS 1998a Central mechanisms. In: Gifford LS (ed) Topical Issues in Pain 1. Whiplash—science and management. Fear-avoidance beliefs and behaviour. CNS Press, Falmouth 67–80

Gifford LS 1998b The mature organism model. In: Gifford LS (ed) Topical Issues in Pain 1. Whiplash—science and management. Fear-avoidance beliefs and behaviour. CNS Press, Falmouth 45–56

Haig AJ, Weisman G, Haugh LD, Pope M, Grobler LJ 1993 Prospective evidence for change in paraspinal muscle activity after herniated nucleus pulposus. Spine 18(7):926–930

Kori SH, Miller RP, Todd DD 1990 Kinesiophobia: A new view of chronic pain behavior. Pain Management Jan/Feb:35–43

Letchuman R, Deusinger RH 1993 Comparison of sacrospinalis myoelectric activity and pain levels in patients undergoing static and intermittent lumbar traction. Spine 18:1361–1365

Lethem J, Slade PD, Troup JDG, Bentley G 1983 Outline of a fear-avoidance model of exaggerated pain perception. Behavioural Research and Therapy. 21:401–408

Lovallo W 1975 The cold pressor test and autonomic function: A review and integration. Psychophysiology 12(3):268–282

Magni G 1994 Prospective study on the relationship between depressive symptoms and chronic musculoskeletal pain. Pain 56:289–297

Main CJ 1983 The modified somatic perception questionnaire. Journal of Psychosomatic Research 27:503–514

Mense S 1997 Pathophysiologic basis of muscle pain syndromes. An update. Physical Medicine and Rehabilitation Clinics of North America 8:23–53

Moldofsky H, Scarisbrick P 1976 Induction of neuraesthenic musculoskeletal pain by selective sleep deprivation. Psychosomatic Medicine 38:35–44

Olivegren H, Jerkvall N, Hagstrom Y, Carlsson J 1999 The long-term prognosis of whiplash-associated disorders (WAD). European Spine Journal 8(5):366–370

Peters ML, Schmidt AL 1991 Psychophysiological responses to repeated stimulation in chronic low back pain patients. Journal of Psychosomatic Research 35:59–74

Simons DG, Mense S 1998 Understanding and measurement of muscle tone as related to clinical muscle pain. Pain 75:1–17

Vasseljen O, Westgaard RH 1995 A case-control study of trapezius muscle activity in office and manual workers with shoulder and neck pain and symptom-free controls. International Archives of Occupational and Environmental Health. 67(1):11–18

Vlaeyen JWS, Linton SJ 2000 Fear-avoidance and its consequences in chronic musculoskeletal pain: a state of the art. Pain 85:317–332

Waddell G 1998 The Back Pain Revolution. Churchill Livingstone, Edinburgh

Waddell G, Newton M, Henderson I, Henderson D, Main CJ 1993 A fear-avoidance beliefs questionnaire (FABQ) and the role of fear-avoidance beliefs in chronic low back pain and disability. Pain 52:157–168

Waersted M, Westgaard RH 1996 Attention-related muscle activity in different body regions during VDU work with minimal physical activity. Ergonomics. 39(4):66–176

Watson PJ 1999 Psychosocial assessment: The emergence of a new fashion, or new tool in physiotherapy for musculoskeletal pain. Physiotherapy 85(10):530–535

Watson PJ 1999a Non-physiological determinants of physical performance in musculoskelatal pain. In: Max M (ed) Pain 1999—An Updated Review. IASP Press, Seattle 153–158

Watson PJ 2000 Psychosocial predictors of outcome from low back pain. In: Gifford LS (ed) Topical Issues in Pain 2. Biopsychosocial assessment and management. Relationships and pain CNS Press, Falmouth 85–109

Watson PJ, Johnson TW, Main CJ 1996 Low back tenderness in CLBP: The influence of pain report and psychological factors. In: Abstracts of the 8th International Association for the Study of Pain, World Congress. Vancouver, Canada

Watson PJ, Booker CK, Main CJ, Chen ACN 1997 Surface electromyography in the identification of chronic low back pain patients: The development of a flexion relaxation ratio. Clinical Biomechanics 12(3):165–171

Watson PJ, Booker CK, Main CJ 1997a Evidence for the role of psychological factors in abnormal paraspinal activity in patients with chronic low back pain. Journal of Musculoskeletal Pain 5(4):41–56

Watson PJ, Chen ACN, Booker CK, Main CJ, Jones AKP 1998 Differential electromyographic response to experimental cold pressor test in chronic low back pain patients and normal controls. Journal of Musculoskeletal Pain 6(2):51–64

197

Watson P, Kendall N 2000 Assessing psychosocial yellow flags. In: Gifford LS (ed) Topical Issues in Pain 2. Biopsychosocial assessment and management. Relationships and pain CNS Press, Falmouth 111–129

Westgaard RH 1999 Effects of physical and mental stressors on muscle pain. Scandinavian Journal of Work, Environment and Health 25 Suppl 4:19–24

Wolfe F, Smith HA, Yunus MB et al 1990 The American College of Rheumatology 1990 criteria for the classification of fibromyalgia. Report of the multicenter criteria committee. Arthritis and Rheumatism 33:160–172

11

Back muscle function and low back pain

PATRICIA DOLAN

Introduction

Low back pain has replaced the common cold as the most frequent medical cause of absence from work in the UK, with approximately 90 million working days lost each year (CSAG 1994). Associated financial costs are escalating, and recent studies suggest that this is largely due to the small percentage of sufferers who go on to develop chronic pain and disability (Waddell 1998, Watson et al 1998).

The reasons some people become chronically disabled by back pain remain obscure. Psychological factors are undoubtedly important because they influence how people cope with persistent pain (Williams & Keefe 1991, Jensen et al 1994), how they respond to treatment (Waddell 1992), and whether they return to work (Hildebrandt et al 1997, Symonds et al 1996). Evidently, psychosocial factors play an important role in determining levels of disability experienced by patients in response to back pain. However, they do not appear to be important *causes* of this pain (Adams et al 1999, Mannion et al 1996) suggesting that, in the majority of cases, back pain has a physical basis, at least at the outset.

In recent years, attention has become more focused on preventing the disability that accompanies low back pain, and whilst much effort has been concentrated on cognitive approaches that address people's beliefs and attitudes about back pain, there is still considerable evidence that exercise and functional restoration programmes have an important part to play in this respect too.

The purpose of this chapter is to review the role of the back muscles in low back pain. The first section describes the normal mechanical function of the back muscles and considers how changes in back muscle activity can influence spinal loading. The next section discusses associations between muscle function and low back pain, and the final part of the chapter considers whether poor muscle function can be improved by exercise and what effect this has on clinical outcome in patients with low back pain.

The mechanical role of the back muscles and their influence on spinal loading

The back muscles are largely responsible for determining the magnitude and distribution of loads acting on the spine. As well as providing the forces and moments required to produce trunk movements, they also act to stabilise the spine and protect it from excessive bending which might otherwise sprain the intervertebral ligaments (Adams et al 1980) or cause intervertebral disc prolapse (Adams & Hutton 1982, 1985). However, the back muscles, when they contract, can also apply high compressive forces to the spine (Dolan & Adams 1993, Dolan et al 1994, 1999) and these may damage the vertebral bodies especially if they are applied on a repetitive basis (Adams & Hutton 1985, Brinckmann et al 1988). One of the main roles of the back muscles, therefore, is to optimise spinal loading to ensure that neither the bending nor compressive stresses rise to damaging levels. Normally, the back muscles perform this role effectively. However, under some circumstances the back muscles may act inappropriately and this can cause spinal loading to increase to potentially damaging levels.

One factor which can compromise the action of the back muscles is their susceptibility to fatigue. Prolonged or repetitive activity can cause the force and speed of contraction of the back muscles to decrease making them less able to protect the underlying spine from excessive flexion. Repetitive loading studies have shown that muscle fatigue is associated with increased lumbar flexion during lifting (Dolan & Adams 1998, Potvin & Norman 1993) and consequently, increased bending stresses acting on the lumbar spine (Dolan & Adams 1998). In some subjects, muscle fatigue caused the bending moment during lifting to rise above 50% of the value at the elastic limit of the ligaments (Dolan & Adams 1998, Dolan & Adams 2000). Although this level of bending moment would not cause injury in a single loading cycle, it may cause fatigue damage to accumulate in the intervertebral discs and ligaments if applied on a repetitive basis (Green et al 1993).

A further consequence of sustained or repeated bending is that it causes creep in spinal tissues, and this can also compromise the protective action of the back muscles. Reflex contractions normally occur during forward bending movements in response to signals from stretch receptors in ligaments, tendons and muscles, and in this way the back muscles act to limit lumbar flexion. However, experiments on anaesthetised cats have shown that repeated stretching of the supraspinous ligament over a 10 minute period (to simulate repetitive spinal flexion) almost eliminates this protective reflex (Solomonow et al 1999), as does just 3 minutes of sustained stretching (Williams et al 2000). In recent unpublished experiments on living people, we examined the effect of both repeated and sustained lumbar flexion on reflex activation of the back muscles by measuring the onset of electromyographic (EMG) activity during a standardised forward bending task. We found that 100 toe touches resulted in a significant delay in the reflex response.

- The toe touching caused lumbar flexion to increase by 4.2°, on average, before the onset of back muscle activity.
- This effect was even more marked after sitting in a low chair for one hour when lumbar flexion was increased by approximately 7.5° before reflex activation of the back muscles was elicited during the forward bending task.

These results suggest that physiological levels of creep *in vivo* may influence reflex activation of the back muscles, and *in vitro* experiments suggest that under these circumstances the intervertebral discs would then have to resist proportionately more of the applied bending moment (Adams & Dolan 1996).

While the above studies have highlighted circumstances where the activation of the back muscles is impaired, in some circumstances the opposite effect is observed and the back muscles tend to over-react. For example, several studies have shown that sudden or unexpected perturbations of the trunk, such as might occur during a stumble or fall, cause large increases in the EMG activity of the back muscles (van Dieen et al 1998, Magnusson et al 1996, Wilder et al 1996), and it is likely that such increases in muscle activation will lead to increased spinal compression. We investigated this possibility in a series of experiments in which loads of unknown mass were dropped into a box held in the subjects' hands.

- We found that the compensatory increase in back muscle EMG caused peak spinal compression to increase by between 30% and 70% above that required simply to decelerate the falling load (Mannion et al 2000).
- We also found that the increase in spinal compression was similar regardless of whether subjects could see the weight being dropped, and therefore anticipate it, or were blindfolded.

These findings suggest that the increase in spinal loading was largely due to reflex contractions of the trunk muscles caused by stimulation of muscle spindles and Golgi tendon organs.

Other factors that influence how the muscles distribute loads between the tissues of the underlying spine include asymmetries or imbalances in muscle activity. These can result in small changes in posture and spinal movements which may lead to high concentrations of compressive stress in the apophyseal joints (Dunlop et al 1984) and the annulus of the intervertebral discs (Adams et al 1994, 2000) (Fig. 11.1). The apophyseal joint capsule and outer annulus are both highly innervated (Bogduk 1997), and so concentrations of stress at these sites could conceivably give rise to pain. The size of such stress concentrations is influenced by the water content, height, and degenerative state of the disc (Adams et al 1996), and is likely to be greater in middle-aged than in young discs, and in dehydrated compared to hydrated discs. This may explain why back pain is more common in middle-aged people and why it often worsens over the course of the day.

201

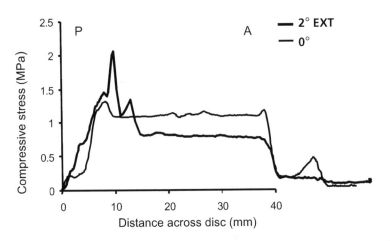

Fig. 11.1 Profiles of vertical compressive stress along the mid-sagittal diameter of a cadaveric lumbar intervertebral disc (L4–5 level, male 61 years) subjected to a compressive load of 2kN. Profiles were obtained with the specimen in the neutral position (0°), and also in 2° of extension to simulate the angle in erect standing. Evidently, just 2° of extension is sufficient to reduce the pressure in the nucleus and generate large stress peaks in the posterior annulus. P=posterior; A=anterior.

Associations between back muscle function and low back pain

Recent investigations indicate both structural and functional abnormalities of back muscles in patients with low back pain. Their back muscles are:

- smaller (Cooper et al 1992, Hides et al 1994, Parkkola et al, 1993)
- weaker (Cassisi et al 1993, Mayer et al, 1989), and
- fatigue more easily (Biering-Sorensen 1984)

when compared to healthy subjects, and their spinal movements are often:

- restricted (Burton et al 1989)
- slower (Szpalski et al 1992) and
- associated with abnormal 'accessory' movements (Stokes et al 1981).

These findings are interesting but do not enable us to distinguish between cause and effect when considering the relationship pain and muscle function.

In order to identify whether certain aspects of back muscle function are important in determining the risk of first time low back pain, we carried out a large-scale prospective study on 403 nurses and other healthcare workers who had no history of serious low back pain that required medical attention or time off work. On entering the study, subjects underwent a full assessment of spinal function, after which they were followed-up for three years by postal questionnaires. The spinal function assessment included measurements of posture, hip and spinal mobility, spinal loading during lifting, and back muscle strength and fatiguability. The latter was assessed from changes in the median frequency of the EMG power spectrum evaluated during the Biering-Sorensen test (Biering-Sorensen 1984, Mannion & Dolan 1994) and during a high level contraction at 80% of maximum voluntary contraction (Dolan et al 1995). The questionnaires, which were completed at 6-month intervals throughout the study, were used to identify those subjects who had suffered 'any' or 'serious' low back pain in the preceding 6-month period, where *serious* referred to pain that required medical attention or time off work. They also included a number of psychometric evaluations that were used to determine whether psychological factors influenced the risk of developing first-time low back pain. These included the *ZUNG* to assess depression (Zung 1965), the *Modified Somatic Perception Questionnaire (MSPQ)* to assess heightened somatic awareness (Main 1983), and the *Health Locus of Control* to evaluate beliefs and attitudes about pain (Wallston et al 1976).

A preliminary analysis of the fatigue data for the first 200 subjects at 12 months showed that people who had more fatiguable back muscles (indicated by a higher rate of decline in median frequency during the Biering-Sorensen fatigue test) were at greater risk of developing serious first-time low back pain (Mannion et al 1997). However, subsequent analysis of the data for all subjects over the 36 month follow-up period suggested that muscle fatiguability was an inconsistent predictor of future low back pain. The reason for this discrepancy between the early and later results was not clear so a more detailed analysis of this data is currently being undertaken.

Other factors which were found to be significant and consistent predictors of serious low back pain included: a reduced range of lumbar lateral flexion, a reduced lumbar lordosis, a long back, increased psychological distress, and a history of previous non-serious low back pain (Adams et al 1999). We also found that those nurses who applied lower peak bending moments to their spine during lifting also had a lower risk of developing low back pain (Mannion et al 1998).

The incidence of *serious* or *any* low back pain during the three year follow-up was greatest in the first 12 months when values reached 11.6% and 39.4% respectively. At three years, the corresponding percentages of new cases had fallen to 6.5% and 21.7% (Fig. 11.2). One factor which contributed to the increased risk of back pain during the first year was the higher incidence of low back pain in student nurses who represented 32% of the total study population. This group had just begun working on the wards at their time of entry into the study, and during the first 12 months of such work their incidence of *serious* or *any* low back pain was approximately 25% higher than that of more experienced workers. Furthermore, during the first 12 months of follow-up, physical factors such as poor lumbar mobility and a long back carried an even greater risk of low back pain in this group when compared to more experienced nurses (Adams et al 1999). Similar results have been reported previously in a prospective study of student nurses which found that their risk of low back pain was highest during the first nine months of working on the wards (Klaber-Moffet et al 1993).

203

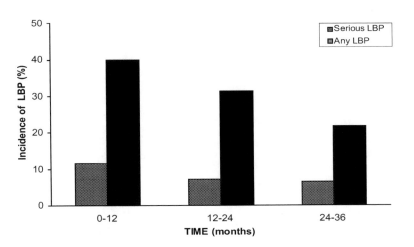

Fig. 11.2 Incidence of new episodes of 'serious' or 'any' low back pain (LBP) in 403 nurses and other healthcare workers over a 3-year follow-up period. At the time of entering the study, subjects had never suffered from serious low back pain. Incidence is expressed as a percentage of those subjects who, at the beginning of that time period, had not suffered 'serious' or 'any' low back pain respectively since the start of the study.

These findings highlight an important issue with regard to occupational loading: *sudden increases in loading may greatly increase the risk of low back pain, and this may be due to the different adaptive capability of spinal tissues.*

When people move from a sedentary to a more arduous occupation, the muscles and bones strengthen quickly, but intervertebral discs and ligaments are much slower to respond and this may leave them more vulnerable to injury during the first months of starting such a job (Adams & Dolan 1997). With time, the musculoskeletal system may become fully adapted to the new job, and improvements in skill and co-ordination may also act to reduce loading of the musculoskeletal system. Together, these factors may act to protect the spine and this could explain the reduced incidence of back pain that we observed with increased time in nursing (Adams et al 1999). This suggestion is further supported by the fact that nurses who had a poor lifting technique when they entered the study and applied high bending moments to their spines, also had an increased risk of developing future low back pain (Mannion et al 1998).

The results of our study and those of other prospective studies suggest that there is a link between poor muscle function, high levels of spinal loading and the risk of developing low back pain, especially when the magnitude of loading is increased suddenly. Consequently, improvements in function and / or reductions in spinal loading might be expected to reduce the risk of future back pain. We are currently examining this possibility in a further prospective study of subjects with acute low back pain. Sixty-three subjects have been recruited into the study, 17 of whom were assessed in our earlier study at a time when they had never suffered from low back pain. Subjects were assessed 6–12 weeks after the onset of their pain, and at 6 month intervals thereafter to determine whether a recovery of normal function was associated with improvements in pain and disability. The follow-up of these subjects is currently continuing; however, a preliminary analysis of the short-term results has revealed some interesting findings.

At the time of their first assessment following back pain, those subjects who had been measured in our earlier study showed reduced mobility in the lumbar spine and a reduced lumbar lordosis when compared to their pre-back pain values, and some of these changes were significant (Fig. 11.3). These subjects also showed evidence of *reduced* fatiguability of the back muscles following back pain when assessed during the isometric fatigue tests described earlier. This was indicated by a *slower* rate of decline in the median frequency of the EMG power spectrum (Fig. 11.4), suggesting a slower rate of muscle fatigue (Mannion & Dolan 1994, Dolan et al 1995). This may reflect hypertrophy of type I fibres which are more fatigue-resistant than type II fibres, in which case it might be construed as a beneficial adaptation that would act to improve the endurance capacity of the muscles. However, it could equally reflect atrophy of type II fibres so that a greater proportion of the force (and EMG signal) is generated by the more endurant type I fibres. In this case, the improved fatigue properties would be gained at the expense of reduced strength and this may not be beneficial. At this point in time we have no evidence to support either of these suggestions since both strength and endurance capacity were not significantly altered following back pain.

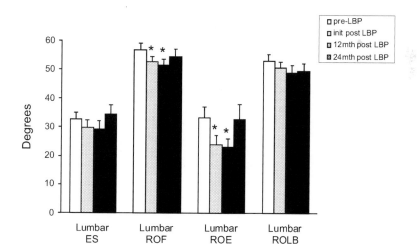

Fig. 11.3 Changes in spinal posture and mobility following a first attack of low back pain (LBP). ES=lumbar lordosis in erect standing; ROF=range of lumbar flexion; ROE=range of lumbar extension; ROLB=range of lumbar lateral bending. *Pre-LBP* before low back pain; *init post-LBP* initial test after onset of low back pain; *12m and 24m post-LBP* 12 months and 24 months after initial post-back pain test. (Bars indicate standard error of the mean; * indicates a significant difference from pre-back pain values at p<.05.)

Subsequent assessments on these same subjects showed that changes in spinal function persisted, on average, for 18–24 months (Figs 11.3 & 11.4) indicating that recovery of function was naturally slow. A comparison of those subjects who reported further pain at 6 months with those who did not, indicated that the former had higher levels of pain, disability and functional impairment on entering the study. These findings suggest that there may be a correlation between pain, disability and spinal function, and that recovery of certain aspects of spinal function may help to protect against future episodes of back pain.

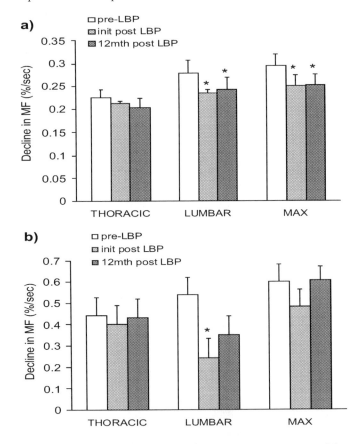

Fig. 11.4 Decline in median frequency (MF) of the EMG power spectrum of the erector spinae during a) the Biering-Sorensen test, and b) a fatigue test at 80% MVC. A high percentage decline in MF indicates a high rate of muscle fatigue. Thoracic and lumbar values of MF decline refer to recordings made at T10 and L3 respectively; max indicates the maximum rate of decline at either site. *Pre-LBP* before low back pain; *init post-LBP* initial test after onset of low back pain; *12m post-LBP* 12m follow-up after initial post-back pain test. (Bars indicate standard error of the mean; * indicates a significant difference from pre-back pain values at p<.05.)

Can aspects of muscle function be altered by exercise?

Our most recent work has turned to the problem of how best to improve or recover back muscle function. A training study was carried out in 56 healthy volunteers, 27 of whom took part in a 4-month training programme, while the remaining 29 acted as controls. The training programme involved some aerobic exercises but concentrated on specific exercises for the back and abdominal muscles including abdominal curls, straight-leg raises, back extension and side flexion exercises, all performed in a variety of different ways. The training programme brought about highly significant improvements in lumbar and hip mobility, and in back muscle endurance time during the performance of two different fatigue tests, the Biering-Sorensen test and a test at 60% of maximum voluntary contraction (MVC) of the back muscles (Wood et al 1997). Improvements were substantial even though these subjects had no initial functional impairment. Patients with impaired back function may therefore benefit to a similar or even greater extent from a similar type of programme.

This possibility was investigated in a pilot study carried out on 20 patients with sciatica of less than 12 months duration who were undergoing microdiscectomy for disc prolapse (Dolan et al 2000). These patients were blindly randomised into a control group who received normal post-operative care and an exercise group who received a 4-week post-operative exercise programme six weeks after surgery. The programme consisted of a mixture of aerobic exercises as well as specific exercises for the back and abdominal muscles. Patients were assessed in the week before surgery and at 6 weeks, 10 weeks, 6 months and 12 months afterward. At each time point, pain, disability and psychological distress were assessed, and patients underwent a full functional assessment that included measures of posture, hip and lumbar ranges of motion, and back muscle fatiguability. The latter was assessed from changes in the EMG median frequency during the performance of the Biering-Sorensen fatigue test, as described elsewhere (Mannion & Dolan 1994).

At the first assessment, prior to surgery, these patients had greater levels of pain, disability and functional impairment than patients with acute back pain, and also demonstrated a slight increase in the combined MSPQ+ZUNG score when compared to healthy controls. Six weeks after surgery, both the control and exercise groups showed significant reductions in pain, disability and MSPQ+ZUNG scores compared to pre-operative values. These improvements in pain and disability were accompanied by significant increases in hip and lumbar ranges of flexion. However, no changes in the EMG measures of muscle fatiguability were observed in either group as a result of surgery.

Ten weeks after surgery, the exercise group showed further improvements in pain and disability but these did not reach significance. However, this group also demonstrated a significant increase in hip range of flexion, as

207

well as a significant improvement in muscle fatiguability indicated by an increase in endurance time and a reduction in the median frequency gradient in the Biering-Sorensen fatigue test. These subjects also showed an increase in initial median frequency, at the start of the fatigue test, indicating a relative increase in high frequency EMG signal that may reflect fibre hypertrophy. By way of contrast, the control group showed no further improvement in any outcome measure at 10 weeks compared to 6 weeks after surgery.

At the later follow-up assessments, at 6 and 12 months after surgery, further reductions in pain and disability were observed in the exercise group, such that values at 12 months were significantly improved compared to 6 weeks after surgery. Furthermore, all of the functional measures also continued to improve significantly. The control group, however, showed no further significant improvements in any of the measures except for the endurance time in the Biering-Sorensen test.

The results of this study are encouraging, and suggest that improvements in pain and disability may be related to recovery in back muscle function, and that such recovery, although naturally slow, can be enhanced by appropriate exercise. However, other studies have raised doubts about the effectiveness of exercise therapy in the treatment of low back pain. Negative results may be attributable to small numbers of patients, or the use of poor, non-objective outcome measures, or they may reflect the fact that differences in exercise regimes or the types of patients undertaking them can result in different outcomes. Several reviews have attempted to account for these influences in order to provide recommendations regarding the efficacy of exercise treatments (Faas 1996, Koes et al 1991). Well-controlled studies suggest that the benefits of *specific* back exercises are doubtful in acute low back pain (Faas et al 1993, Malmivaara et al 1995), although 'McKenzie' exercises can produce some short-term symptomatic improvement (Koes et al 1991). In subacute back pain, data is very limited, but graded exercise appears to improve function and reduce sickness absence compared to usual care (Lindstrom et al 1992). In non-specific chronic low back pain, the case for exercise therapy is stronger. Intensive dynamic trunk exercises have been reported to improve outcome compared to more general exercise (Hansen et al 1993, Manniche et al 1991) or placebo therapy (Hansen et al 1993, Spratt et al 1993), and supervised fitness programmes were found to enhance the beneficial effects of home-based exercises (Frost et al 1995). More recently, a study which compared several different types of exercise including group aerobic/stretching classes, that provided by physiotherapy, and muscle strengthening/co-ordination exercises using training devices found that all were equally effective in reducing pain and disability in patients with chronic low back pain (Mannion et al 1999).

Post-surgical rehabilitation programmes have received relatively little attention despite the fact that many patients undergoing spinal surgery report a poor outcome. Even with pathology as well-defined as disc prolapse, approximately 20–30% of patients report residual back and/or leg pain and reduced work capabilities (Dvorak et al 1988). Part of the problem may lie in the long delay between the onset of symptoms and eventual surgery. During this time, patients are relatively inactive and may adapt their posture and movement patterns in order to accommodate their pain. Furthermore, prolonged inactivity may lead to muscle atrophy and weakness, and such changes are unlikely to be corrected by surgery. A number of randomised trials have reported improvements in pain, disability and various aspects of spinal function as a result of an early post-operative exercise programme following lumbar discectomy (Kjellby-Wendt & Styf 1998, Manniche et al 1993) supporting the preliminary findings of our own study.

The current consensus of opinion seems to suggest that specific exercise programmes can benefit patients with chronic low back pain, including those having surgery for disc prolapse. However, there is still little information available to indicate whether improvements in muscle function or more central beneficial effects of exercise are responsible for the improvements in clinical outcome observed.

Conclusions

The back muscles play an important role in the mechanical function of the spine. They effect movements, provide stability, and normally prevent excessive loading of underlying spinal structures. Under some circumstances the action of the back muscles can become compromised or abnormal and this can lead to increased spinal loading and an increased risk of developing low back pain. Changes in back muscle function can also occur as a result of low back pain, and preliminary results suggests that subjects showing the greatest changes may be more likely to suffer future back pain. Under normal circumstances, full recovery of muscle function is naturally slow. However, there is some evidence that recovery can be speeded up by appropriate exercise therapy aimed at strengthening and mobilising the back muscles.

Further work is still needed to demonstrate the long-term effectiveness of exercise therapy in larger and more diverse groups of patients. However, if causal relationships between improvements in function and improvements in pain and disability can be identified in well-controlled prospective studies, then this will provide a basis for devising improved treatment protocols in the future that can be tailored to meet the needs of various patient groups.

ACKNOWLEDGEMENTS

Patricia Dolan is partly supported by a Research Fellowship from the Arthritis Research Campaign. The author would like to acknowledge the following people who have collaborated on the work from our laboratory which is reviewed in this paper: Michael Adams, Anne Mannion, Keith Greenfield, Ian Nelson, Richard Nelson, Ian Wootton, Kherrin Wood, John Kirwan and Iain Hine. Chris Standell and Nicola Latham are also thanked for providing technical support.

REFERENCES

Adams MA, Dolan P 1996 Time-dependent changes in the lumbar spine's resistance to bending. Clinical Biomechanics 11:194–200

Adams MA, Dolan P 1997 Could sudden increases in physical activity cause intervertebral disc degeneration? Lancet 350:734–735

Adams MA, Hutton WC 1982 Prolapsed intervertebral disc. A hyperflexion injury. Spine 7:184–191

Adams MA, Hutton WC 1985 Gradual disc prolapse. Spine 10: 524–531

Adams MA, Hutton WC, Stott JRR 1980 The resistance to flexion of the lumbar intervertebral joint. Spine 5:245–253

Adams MA, McNally DS, Chinn H, Dolan P 1994 Posture and the compressive strength of the lumbar spine. Clinical Biomechanics 9:5–14

Adams MA, McNally DS, Dolan P 1996 Stress distributions inside intervertebral discs: the effects of age and degeneration. Journal of Bone and Joint Surgery 78B:965–972

Adams MA, Mannion AF, Dolan P 1999 Personal risk factors for first-time low back pain. Spine 24:2497–2500

Adams MA, May S, Freeman BJC, Morrison HP, Dolan P 2000 Effects of backward bending on lumbar intervertebral discs. Relevance to physical therapy treatments for low back pain. Spine 25:431–437, discussion 438

Biering-Sorensen F 1984 Physical measurements as risk indicators for low back trouble over a one-year period. Spine 9:106–118

Bogduk N 1997 Clinical Anatomy of the Lumbar Spine 3rd edn. Churchill Livingstone, Edinburgh

Brinckmann P, Biggemann M, Hilweg D 1988 Fatigue fracture of human lumbar vertebrae. Clinical Biomechanics 3 (Supplement 1)

Burton AK, Tillotson KM, Troup JDG 1989 Variation in lumbar sagittal mobility with low back trouble. Spine 14:584–590

Cassisi JE, Robinson ME, O'Connor P, MacMillan M 1993 Trunk strength and lumbar paraspinal muscle activity during isometric exercise in chronic low-back pain patients and controls. Spine 18:245–251

Clinical Standards Advisory Group 1994 Back Pain. London, HMSO

Cooper RG, Forbes WSTC, Jayson MIV 1992 Radiographic demonstration of paraspinal muscle wasting in patients with chronic low back pain. British Journal of Rheumatology 31:389–394

Dolan P, Adams MA 1993 The relationship between EMG activity and extensor moment generation in the erector spinae muscles during bending and lifting activities. Journal of Biomechanics 26:513–522

Dolan P, Adams MA 1998 Repetitive lifting tasks fatigue the back muscles and increase the bending moment acting on the lumbar spine. Journal of Biomechanics 31:713–721

Dolan P, Adams MA 2000 Biomechanical factors affecting the intervertebral disc. Journal of Orthopaedic Medicine 22:3–9

Dolan P, Earley M, Adams MA 1994 Bending and compressive stresses acting on the lumbar spine during lifting activities. Journal of Biomechanics 27:1237–1248

Dolan P, Mannion AF, Adams MA 1995 Fatigue of the erector spinae muscles: A quantitative assessment using 'frequency banding' of the surface EMG signal. Spine 20:149–159

Dolan P, Kingma I, van Dieen JH, de Looze MP, Toussaint HM, Baten CTM, Adams MA 1999 Dynamic forces acting on the lumbar spine during manual handling: can they be estimated using EMG techniques alone? Spine 24:698–703

Dolan P, Greenfield K, Nelson RJ, Nelson IW 2000 Can exercise therapy improve the outcome of microdiscectomy? Spine 25:1523–1532

Dunlop RB, Adams MA, Hutton WC 1984 Disc space narrowing and the lumbar facet joints. Journal of Bone and Joint Surgery 66-B:706–710

Dvorak J, Gauchat M-H, Valach L 1988 The outcome of surgery for lumbar disc herniation. Spine 13:1418–1422

Faas A 1996 Exercises: which ones are worth trying, for which patients, and when? Spine 21:2874–2879

Faas A, Chavannes AW, van Eijk JThM, Gubbels JW 1993 A randomized, placebo-controlled trial of exercise therapy in patients with acute low back pain. Spine 18:1388–1395

Frost H, Klaber-Moffett JA, Moser JS, Fairbank JCT 1995 Randomised controlled trial for evaluation of fitness programme for patients with chronic low back pain. British Medical Journal 310:151–154

Green TP, Adams MA, Dolan P 1993 Tensile properties of the annulus fibrosus. Part II Ultimate tensile strength and fatigue life. European Spine Journal 2:209–214

Hansen FR, Bendix T, Skov P et al 1993 Intensive, dynamic back-muscle exercises, conventional physiotherapy, or placebo-control treatment of low back pain. Spine 18:98–107

Hides JA, Stokes MJ, Saide M, Jull GA, Cooper DH 1994 Evidence of lumbar multifidus muscle wasting ipsilateral to symptoms in patients with acute/subacute low back pain. Spine 19:165–172

Hildebrandt J, Pfingsten M, Saur P, Jansen J 1997 Prediction of success from a multidisciplinary treatment program for chronic low back pain. Spine 22:990–1001

Jensen MP, Turner JA, Romano JM, Lawler BK 1994 Relationship of pain-specific beliefs to chronic pain adjustment. Pain 57:301–309

Kjellby-Wendt G, Styf J 1998 Early active training after lumbar discectomy. A prospective, randomized, and controlled study. Spine 23:2345–2351

Klaber-Moffett JA, Hughes GI, Griffiths P 1993 A longitudinal study of low back pain in student nurses. International Journal of Nursing Studies 30:197–212

Koes BW, Bouter LM, Beckerman H, van der Heijden CJMG, Knipschild PG 1991 Physiotherapy exercises and back pain: A blinded review. British Medical Journal 302:1572–1576

Lindstrom I, Ohlund C, Eek C, Wallin L, Peterson L, Nachemson A 1992 Mobility, strength, and fitness after a graded activity program for patients with sub-acute low back pain. Spine 17:641–652

Magnusson ML, Aleksiev A, Wilder DG et al 1996 Unexpected load and asymmetric posture as etiologic factors in low back pain. European Spine Journal 5:23–35

Main CJ 1983 The modified somatic perception questionnaire (MSPQ). Journal of Psychosomatic Research 27:503–514

Malmivaara A, Hakkinen U, Aro T, et al 1995 The treatment of acute low back pain: Bedrest, exercises or ordinary activity? New England Journal of Medicine 332:351–355

Manniche C, Lundberg E, Christensen I, Bentzen L, Hesselsoe G 1991 Intensive dynamic back exercises for chronic low back pain: A clinical trial. Pain 47:53–63

Manniche C, Skall HF, Braendholt L et al 1993 Clinical trial of postoperative dynamic back exercises after first lumbar discectomy. Spine 18:92–97

Mannion AF, Dolan P, 1994 EMG median frequency changes during isometric contraction of the back extensors to fatigue. Spine 19:1223–1229

Mannion AF, Dolan P, Adams MA 1996 Psychological questionnaires: Do 'abnormal' scores precede or follow first-time low back pain? Spine 21:2603–2611

Mannion AF, Connolly B, Wood K, Dolan P 1997 The use of surface EMG power spectral analysis in the evaluation of back muscle function. Journal of Rehabilitation Research and Development 34:427–439

Mannion AF, Adams MA, Dolan P 1998 People who load their spines heavily during standard lifting tasks are more likely to develop low back pain. Proceedings of the International Society for the Study of the Lumbar Spine, Brussels, June 1998

Mannion AF, Muntener M, Taimela S et al 1999 A randomized clinical trial of three active therapies for chronic low back pain. Spine 24:2435–2448

211

Mannion AF, Adams MA, Dolan P 2000 Sudden and unexpected loading generates high forces on the lumbar spine. Spine 25:842–852

Mayer TG, Vanharanta H, Gatchel RJ, Mooney V et al 1989 Comparison of CT scan muscle measurements and isokinetic trunk strength in postoperative patients. Spine 14:33–36

Parkkola R, Rytokoski U, Kormano M 1993 Magnetic resonance imaging of the discs and trunk muscles in patients with chronic low back pain and healthy control subjects. Spine 18:830–836

Potvin JR, Norman RW 1993 Quantification of erector spinae muscle fatigue during prolonged, dynamic lifting tasks. European Journal of Applied Physiology 67:554–562

Solomonow M, Zhou BH, Baratta RV et al 1999 Biomechanics of increased exposure to lumbar injury caused by cyclic loading: Part 1. Loss of reflexive muscular stabilization. Spine 24:2426–2434

Spratt KF, Weinstein JN, Lehmann TR, Woody J, Sayre H 1993 Efficacy of flexion and extension treatments incorporating braces for low-back pain patients with retrodisplacements, spondylolisthesis, or normal sagittal translation. Spine 18:1839–1849

Stokes IAF, Wilder DG, Frymoyer JW, Pope MH 1981 Assessment of patients with low-back pain by biplanar radiographic measurement of intervertebral motion. Spine 6:233–240

Symonds TL, Burton AK, Tillotson KM, Main CJ 1996 Do attitudes and beliefs influence work loss due to low back pain? Occupational Medicine 48:3–10

Szpalski M, Spengler D, Keller T et al 1992 Trunk function in asymptomatic subjects with normal and abnormal X-ray findings compared with low back pain patients. Proceedings of the Society for Back Pain Research, Spring Meeting, Bristol UK

van Dieen JH, van der Burg P, Raaijmakers TAJ et al 1998 Effects of repetitive lifting on kinematics: inadequate anticipatory control or adaptive changes? Journal of Motor Behaviour 30:20–32

Waddell G 1992 Biopsychosocial analysis of low back pain. Clinical Rheumatology 6: 523–557

Waddell G 1998 The Back Pain Revolution. Churchill Livingstone, Edinburgh

Wallston BS, Wallston KA et al 1976 Development and validation of the health Locus of Control scale. Journal of Consulting and Clinical Psychology 44:580–585

Watson PJ, Main CJ, Waddell G, Gales TF, Purcell-Jones G 1998 Medically certified work loss, recurrence and costs of wage compensation for back pain: A follow-up study of the working population of Jersey. British Journal of Rheumatology 37:82–86

Wilder DG, Aleksiev AR, Magnusson ML et al 1996 Muscular response to sudden load. A tool to evaluate fatigue and rehabilitation. Spine 21:2628–2639

Williams DA, Keefe FJ 1991 Pain beliefs and the use of cognitive-behavioural coping strategies. Pain 46:185–190

Williams M, Solomonow M, Zhou BH et al 2000 Multifidus spasms elicited by prolonged lumbar flexion. Spine 25:2916–2924

Wood KA, Standell C, Adams MA, Dolan P, Mannion AF 1997 Exercise training to improve spinal mobility and back muscle fatigability: A possible prophylaxis for low back pain? Presented at the Physical Medicine Research Foundation Symposium 'Clinical approaches to spinal disorders', Prague 1997

Zung WWK 1965 A self-rating depression scale. Archives of General Psychiatry 12:63–70

12

Fibromyalgia–a single case study

LORRAINE L MOORES

Introduction

A single case study was carried out to assess the efficacy of a multidisciplinary pain management programme in the treatment of a patient with fibromyalgia.

Fibromyalgia is a non-articular chronic pain disorder of uncertain aetiology affecting the musculoskeletal system. Specific areas of localised tenderness referred to as 'tender points' distinguish fibromyalgia from other soft tissue rheumatoid disorders. Onset of symptoms occurs most commonly between the ages of 20–40 years mainly in women (McDermid et al 1996, Wolfe et al 1990).

Fibromyalgia sufferers often report severe widespread pain, fatigue and difficulty performing daily activities (Wolfe et al 1995). Although there is no known cure for fibromyalgia, treatments aimed at symptomatic relief, pain management and physical conditioning, frequently include pharmacological treatment, psychological intervention and physiotherapy (Mason et al 1998).

Recent research has made recommendations for a multidimensional cognitive-behavioural approach to the management of fibromyalgia (Rossy et al 1999, Consensus document on fibromyalgia 1992). Multidisciplinary group treatment programmes are especially suited to such techniques. In fibromyalgia, as for other chronic pain syndromes, multidisciplinary treatment programmes have been recommended (Bennett 1996, Rossy et al 1999).

This chapter reports on the effects of a multidisciplinary pain management programme for a 42 year old female patient with a 6-year history of fibromyalgia. A re-assessment of the study subject's performance is reported 6 months following the intervention phase in order to assess the long-term efficacy of treatment. This is particularly important, as fibromyalgia is a chronic disorder.

Literature review

Presentation and definition

Fibromyalgia syndrome is a common rheumatological condition characterised by widespread musculoskeletal pain. It is a chronic condition rarely ending in total remission of symptoms (Ledingham et al 1993). Although fibromyalgia patients suffer primarily muscular pain, they may also report localised articular pain, subjective swelling of joints ,and numbness or coldness of the extremities (Boissevain & McCain 1991). Patients also frequently experience fatigue, non-restorative sleep, stiffness, disturbance of mood, headache, temporomandibular joint dysfunction, dysmenorrhea, irritable bladder, and irritable bowel syndrome (Henriksson & Mense 1994, Consensus report on fibromyalgia 1996).

In 1990, a multicentre study established the criteria for the diagnosis of fibromyalgia (Wolfe et al 1990). The American College of Rheumatology (ACR) adopted these criteria. The definition as stated by the ACR includes:

- At least a three-month history of widespread pain defined as pain in the axial skeleton and two contra-lateral quadrants of the body above and below the waist.
- There must also be the presence of hyperalgesia or allodynia in 11 or more of 18 specific anatomical points when 4kg of digital pressure is applied.

This definition has been criticised for being too inclusive and failing to reflect the idea of truly diffuse and widespread pain (Hunt et al 1999). It is possible to satisfy the ACR criteria for chronic widespread pain with, for example, pain restricted to the lumbar area, left wrist and right ankle. Also if all other criteria are present but the patient has only 10 out of the 18 tender points (rather than 11 of the 18) what is the appropriate diagnosis? The diagnostic criteria do not include the multitude of other symptoms often associated with fibromyalgia (Wolfe et al 1995). A consensus document on fibromyalgia accepted the ACR definition as a basis for diagnosis, and added other symptoms to that definition including persistent fatigue, generalised morning stiffness and non-restorative sleep (Consensus document on fibromyalgia 1992).

MacFarlane et al (1996) suggested a refinement of the ACR definition. This still required the presence of axial pain and contra-lateral limb pain; however, each limb is divided into four anatomical areas. Pain must be present in at least two areas before the limb is considered to be painful. The modified criteria require pain to be more generally widespread and have been found to be more closely related to associated symptoms such as psychological distress and fatigue (Chaitow 2000, Hunt et al 1999).

Aetiology

The precise aetiology of fibromyalgia is incompletely understood. Routine testing such as haematological or imaging have not proved to be diagnostically useful except to exclude potential disorders that may mimic fibromyalgia (Consensus report on fibromyalgia 1996, Pellegrino 2000). Research into the aetiology has lead to a number of theories focusing on the following main areas:

- muscular changes
- alteration in serotonin metabolism
- other neuroendocrinological changes
- sleep disturbance
- environmental factors
- changes in the function of the autonomic nervous system and psychological aberrations (Henriksson 1994 Chaitow, 2000).

In some cases the patient may report precipitating events such as trauma, infection, surgery, physical and emotional stress. Studies suggest that there is no single explanation encompassing all the clinical findings in patients with fibromyalgia and it is likely that the aetiological mechanisms involve a complex interaction of multiple factors (Yunus 1992).

Prevalence

Epidemiological statistics suggest that fibromyalgia is a common syndrome. Croft et al (1993) reported a prevalence of 11.2% in the UK using the ACR criteria. Hunt et al (1999) in an epidemiological study in the UK reported a prevalence of 4.7% using the Macfarlane et al (1996) more specific definition of chronic widespread pain, compared to a 12.9% prevalence rate using the ACR criteria. These studies demonstrated that fibromyalgia occurs more commonly in women.

Treatment

Currently there is no intervention that eradicates the symptoms of fibromylagia. As for many chronic conditions the absence of an obvious ongoing inflammatory or nociceptive process renders the traditional medical/disease model inappropriate and ineffective. Medical treatments have been reported as relatively ineffective (White & Harth 1996, Consensus report on fibromyalgia 1996, Rossy et al 1999). Nevertheless, various interventions may help some individuals even if the condition cannot be cured (Pellegrino 2000). Medications such as the tricyclic antidepressant amitriptyline have been moderately successful in reducing the pain and sensitivity of the characteristic tender points (Carette et al 1994).

There are a number of research trials, which lend support to exercise, self-management, stress-management and education in the treatment of fibromyalgia.

Burckhardt et al (1994) compared a 6-week group self-management education programme, with the programme plus physical training, and a control group in fibromyalgia patients. They found improvement in quality of life and self-efficacy in both treatment groups. Wigers et al (1996) compared an aerobic exercise group, a stress management training group, and a control group receiving treatment as usual, in 60 fibromyalgia patients. The

215

experimental groups reported improvements in global subjective variables. The aerobic exercise group reported an improved work capacity when compared to the stress management group. Vlaeyen et al (1996) compared a group education programme with cognitive-behavioural treatment, a group education programme with discussion group, and a no treatment control group. The study demonstrated improvements in both the cognitive-behavioural and the discussion group but no significant difference was found between groups except for 'fear,' which was significantly reduced in the discussion group. It was suggested that poor compliance, and difficulty with homework assignments, might have limited the effectiveness of the cognitive-behavioural treatment group.

Bailey et al (1999) reported the benefits of a multidisciplinary rehabilitation programme consisting of 36 sessions delivered over a 12-week period. The programme included exercise and self-management skills such as management of fatigue and sleep, coping skills, goal setting and education.

In a review of studies using self-management training skills for fibromyalgia, Sandstrom and Keefe (1998) suggest that formal self-management programmes have an important role in the treatment of fibromyalgia patients. White and Nielson (1995) reported favourable results in a follow-up study of 22 fibromyalgia patients who had attended a 3-week cognitive-behavioural programme.

A recent meta-analysis of fibromyalgia treatment interventions has provided a review of the efficacy of non-pharmacological and pharmacological treatment interventions for fibromyalgia (Rossy et al 1999). Forty-nine outcome studies met the criteria to be included in the analysis, assessing outcome across four main domains including, daily function, physical status, self-report of symptoms and psychological status.

- Treatment with antidepressants gave rise to an improvement in the self-report symptoms of fibromyalgia and physical status.
- All non-pharmacological interventions resulted in significant improvements in all four categories of outcome measurements. The exceptions to this were physically based (primarily exercise) treatments, which did not yield a significant improvement in daily functioning.
- Non-pharmacological treatments were particularly more beneficial in the management of self-reported symptoms of fibromyalgia (such as pain and fatigue) and daily function, than pharmacological treatment alone.

The analysis concluded that optimum intervention for fibromyalgia includes a non-pharmacological approach, specifically exercise and cognitive-behavioural therapy, in addition to appropriate medication use as necessary to manage sleep and pain symptoms.

It would seem likely that as fibromyalgia is a multidimensional syndrome the most effective treatment approach should include multiple strategies (Burckhardt et al 1994).

A multidisciplinary pain management programme is particularly suited to such an approach. Pain management programmes are founded on the principles of cognitive-behavioural therapy. They are psychologically based rehabilitative treatment programmes for people with chronic pain which remains unresolved by other treatments (Pain Society 1997). A major treatment aim is restoration of functional activities and providing patients with the necessary skills to control pain and disability (Rosen 1994, Bennett 1996). The Pain Society (1997) outlines the overall aim of a pain management programme as, 'to reduce the disability and distress caused by chronic pain, by teaching sufferers physical, psychological and practical techniques to improve quality of life.' A recent review and meta-analysis (Morley et al 1999) concluded that there is strong evidence for the efficacy of cognitive-behavioural therapy in the restoration of adaptive function, improved mood and the reduction of disability in adults with chronic pain. Cognitive-behavioural therapy attempts to redress maladaptive thoughts and behaviours. Intervention includes relaxation, exercise, provision of information and education, cognitive pain coping strategies and self-management techniques (Harding 1998, Harding & Williams 1995).

Much of the research literature evaluating treatment outcome in fibromyalgia is open to criticism. For example, limitations in study design such as incomplete blinding of outcome assessors and inadequate randomisation are noted. Typically patients included in studies were recruited from rheumatology clinics and may not be a representative sample of fibromyalgia sufferers in the general population.

In evaluating literature on treatment outcome:

- There are obvious differences in length of follow-up evaluation and treatment delivery.
- Frequently the contents of treatment programmes are not clearly defined.
- There is often a reliance on self-report data in research studies, which may not be an accurate representation of performance.
- A diversity of outcome measurements is evident; no two trials used the exact same outcome measurements.
- Also, important clinical outcomes such as functional and psychological status are often omitted in data collection.

Failure to cover such important outcome domains may produce a misleading picture of treatment outcome and long-term gains that does not relate closely to the aims of a pain management programme. This was also noted in a recent survey evaluating follow-up procedure for pain management programmes (Peat et al 2001). Variation in the length of follow-up, and outcome measurements demonstrate that there is no clear agreement on when patients should be followed up and exactly how they ought to be evaluated (Peat et al 2001, Rossy et al 1999).

Use of a common set of outcome measures would facilitate comparisons amongst studies.

Literature review summary

- Although some controversy may exist as to the precise diagnostic criteria there seems to be general agreement that fibromyalgia patients exhibit unique symptoms and signs, which readily distinguish them from individuals with other chronic pain syndromes (Boissevain & McCain 1991).

- Fibromyalgia is a challenging disorder to treat, partly due to the incomplete understanding of aetiology, as well as the multitude of symptoms characteristic of fibromyalgia (Rossy et al 1999).
- Despite limitations in the research studies there is extensive literature that indicates treatment of fibromyalgia can achieve good results.
- Research supports the multidimensional treatment of fibromyalgia and has made recommendations for a cognitive-behavioural approach.

The single case study

Single case studies involve the application of an intervention and careful evaluation of its effects. They are a cost-effective method of determining whether improvement is due to specific intervention or the passage of time (Barlow & Hersen, 1988). The single case study documents the course of progress over time as well as outcome, examines the course of variability and gives an indication of when most improvement takes place. They may also be useful as pilot studies (Kazdin 1982).

In carrying out this study an ABA single case design was utilised. This method examines the effect of the intervention by alternating the baseline condition (phase A1), when no intervention is taking place, with the intervention condition (phase B). The follow-up phase A2 (when no intervention is taking place) completes the third stage of the study.

Continuous assessment during phase A1 allows the investigator to examine the pattern and stability of performance before the intervention is instigated. When the treatment is eventually initiated the subject's performance is continuously observed while the intervention is in effect. The observations are continued and the investigator is able to examine whether behaviour changes coincide with the treatment (Kazdin 1982).

The effects of the intervention are clear if performance improves during the intervention phase (phase B), and reverts to or approaches original baseline levels when treatment is withdrawn during phase A2. Such a reversal is required to demonstrate an effect of the intervention (Barlow & Hersen, 1988). However, it must be said that the investigator has an explicit hope that performance will be maintained after treatment is withdrawn.

The ability to demonstrate long-term benefits in patients with chronic pain is a key factor in evaluating the effectiveness of multidisciplinary pain management programmes (Melzack & Wall 1996). Indeed, the intended aim of most interventions is to achieve a permanent change even after the intervention is withdrawn (Kazdin 1982, Hicks 1999).

The study subject

The subject was a 42-year old female recruited from the list of patients waiting to attend the multidisciplinary pain management programme at Manchester and Salford Pain Centre. As is normal procedure at the centre, the subject was assessed carefully by a medical practitioner, senior physiotherapist and clinical psychologist before being offered a place on the pain management programme. The purpose of the study was explained to her and an outline of her commitment to attend repeated assessments during each stage of the study was explained fully. Her participation was on a voluntary basis and prior to commencement of the study she gave her written consent to attend.

The subject had a 6-year history of fibromyalgia syndrome ascertained by medical examination. The condition was precipitated by a viral illness in 1993 from which she did not fully recover. Associated symptoms included fatigue, premenstrual syndrome, depressed mood, and irritable bowel syndrome.

She had in the past had a series of appointments following a conventional physiotherapy approach directed at the cervical spine and shoulders, which produced short-term benefit only. Reflexology did not give her long-term benefit. Aromatherapy and massage was stopped due to an immediate increase in her pain.

Study design

The ABA design was used in this study, the total investigation lasted 9 weeks. The 3 phases were as follows:

A1 Weeks 1–3, baseline measurements carried out twice each week at equally spaced intervals.
B   Weeks 4–6, multidisciplinary pain management programme and measurements carried out twice each week at equally spaced intervals.
A2 Weeks 7–9, follow-up measurements carried out twice each week at equally spaced intervals.

Measurements

In order to ensure the main outcome domains of a pain management programme (as described by the Pain Society, 1997) were addressed, measurements were selected on the basis that they are standardised tests used widely in studies of chronic pain patients.

Self-report measures

- **The Kirwan and Reeback Health Assessment Questionnaire** (Kirwan & Reeback 1986). This questionnaire has been shown to reliably assess disability in patients with rheumatological conditions.
- **The Modified Somatic Perception Questionnaire (MSPQ)** (Main 1984)
- **The Modified Zung Questionnaire (MZ)** (Main 1984) The MSPQ and MZ were developed by Main (1984) and examine the two constructs of heightened somatic awareness and depressive symptomatology respectively. Depressive symptoms and somatic anxiety/hypervigilance

219

to bodily symptoms are characteristic of fibromyalgia and chronic pain sufferers.

- **The Tampa Scale of Kinesiophobia (TSK)** (Kori et al 1990). A measure of fear of re-injury, movement and avoidance of activity.
- **The Short Form McGill Pain Questionnaire** (Melzack 1987). The questionnaire includes a visual analogue scale for current pain intensity, and a list of 11 sensory and 4 affective pain description words which patients select to give a self-reported description of their pain.

Physical function measures

The following physical function tests were included. (As already stated, self-report measures may not be an accurate representation of performance). The reliability and validity of these tests are documented by Harding et al (1994) and Sweet (1995).

- **Step-up test.** The number of completed step-ups achieved in a 30 secondtime period using a 20cm step-up block (adapted from Harding et al 1994).
- **Psychophysical lifting test.** The maximum load lifted and transferred from a plinth onto a chair and back up onto the plinth (Sweet 1995).
- **5 minute walking distance.** The number of 20 metre laps covered in a 5 minute time period (Harding et al 1994).
- **Timed 20 metre speed walk.** The time taken to walk 20 metres measured in seconds (Harding et al 1994).

These physical measures form part of the standardised pre and post programme assessment for all patients attending the pain management programme at Manchester and Salford Pain Centre.

To minimise bias and contamination of results, throughout the investigation measurements were carried out by a senior physiotherapist not involved in the subject's treatment.

During phase B the MSPQ, MZ, and TSK were not repeated as it was felt the subject would remember the individual questions and this would bias the answers.

In order to assess long-term outcome, all the measures were repeated 6 months after the intervention phase. At this point the subject attended the routine 6-month review at the centre.

Method

The subject attended the 3-week multidisciplinary pain management programme at the Manchester and Salford Pain Centre on an outpatient basis. The programme ran from Monday to Friday each week from 9.00 a.m. to 5.00 p.m. and was based on a cognitive-behavioural approach to chronic pain. It combined active rehabilitation with educational sessions and psychological approaches to coping with chronic pain. The group size in this case was 10 patients all suffering chronic pain but not necessarily all with a diagnosis of fibromyalgia.

The time was split into sessions led by a senior physiotherapist, clinical psychologist and medical consultant. Physiotherapy sessions involved the teaching and daily practise of a stretching routine for the whole body, and a strengthening programme. Aerobic exercise was carried out once each week and exercise in water carried out twice during the programme. The amount of exercise planned and achieved daily was recorded by each patient. The physiotherapy sessions lasted 3 hours with a half-hour break.

Exercise sessions usually lasted 1.5 hours per day. The physiotherapist also taught patients about the effects of inactivity, benefits of exercise on the body, posture, anatomy, body mechanics, lifting, pacing and goal setting.

Cognitive-behavioural principles were applied during these sessions to encourage progress (see Chs 7–9).

Psychology-led sessions also lasted 3 hours with a half-hour break and included daily practical relaxation techniques, teaching and discussion on the psychophysiology of pain and stress, problem-solving techniques, automatic thinking errors, communication skills and assertiveness training.

Medical input included one-hour teaching sessions on pain physiology, use of medication, appropriate use of the health care system and flare-up management.

Practice of these self-management skills was expected between sessions. Patients set their own goals at the end of the programme and adherence to a self-management home programme was encouraged strongly.

Procedure

The measurements taken were carried out by a senior physiotherapist not involved in the pain management programme that the study subject attended. The assessments took place at equal intervals during the working week, e.g. Monday and Wednesday, or Tuesday and Thursday. Measurements were carried out at various times during phase A1 and phase A2, at a mutually convenient time for both physiotherapist and subject. During Phase B measurements were carried out at lunch time (12.45 p.m.). A quiet room was available for the subject to complete questionnaires. The physical tests were carried out in a standardised way (see Appendix for full description).

Analysis of data

The results of the study are presented in the form of graphs. Statistical procedures may be used in single case studies as they may reveal a change that is of importance, even though it is not obvious from visual inspection.

In this investigation the 'Two Standard Deviation Method' was employed. The level of significance for the statistical test was set at $p<0.05$. This is identified by calculating the mean value +/- 2 standard deviations of the baseline measurements (for each variable), and then, by comparing the scores from phase B and phase A2 to see if they fall outside the 95% confidence interval band. Two successive data points must fall outside the 2 standard deviation band for a statistically significant change to have occurred (Barlow & Hersen 1988).

Results

The raw data collected during all phases of the study are presented in the form of tables and graphs in the Appendix. On the graphs the 'long dash–dot–dot' line represents the mean score for phase A1 and the dashed horizontal line indicates +/- 2 standard deviations from the mean of the baseline phase A1. For the purpose of this study the baseline phase A1 was considered stable if the measurements during this phase fell inside the 2 standard deviation band.

Each phase of 3 weeks duration produced 6 observations for each variable except for the TSK, MSPQ and MZ. For these variables only one measurement was taken during phase B; this coincided with the routine post programme assessment carried out on the last day of the pain management programme.

Data collected at the 6-month follow-up session of the pain management programme is also presented in order to determine the longer-term benefit of the programme.

During the 8th week of the investigation the subject took a holiday, consequently one set of data during that week is missing.

Discussion

The purpose of this investigation was to examine the effect of a multidisciplinary pain management programme on the treatment of a fibromyalgia patient. Observation of raw data is the primary means of evaluation in single case studies, as they do not lend themselves to formal statistical techniques. However, statistical analyses performed with caution provide objective evidence in support of trends or differences observed in the raw data. With the exception of the step-up test, a generally improving trend can be observed for all physical function tests (see Graphs 1–4). An improving trend can also be seen in Graphs 5–8 evaluating changes in self-reported disability, fear of movement/re-injury, depressive symptomatology and somatic anxiety. Graphs 9–11 clearly indicate the highly variable nature of pain intensity levels; no clear trend or change can be observed.

Using the Two Standard Deviation Band Method to evaluate the results, *statistically* significant improvements in: the physical function tests; time taken to walk 20 metres; distance walked in 5 minutes; and lifting test can be seen (Graphs 1–3 respectively). Using the same method, self-reported disability levels, fear of movement/re-injury, and depressive symptomatology all reveal *statistically* significant improvement (Graphs 5–7 respectively). Furthermore, these *statistically* significant improvements in physical function tests and self-report measures are maintained at 6-month re-assessment.

222

Although two successive data points fall outside the 2 standard deviation band for the MSPQ scores in phase A2 (Graphs 8), a rather variable picture can be observed. In view of this, it is difficult to confirm a statistically significant improvement.

Spanswick and Peat (2000) suggest that a *clinically* significant improvement in outcome data for pain management programmes may be defined as an improvement of more than 2 standard deviations from the pre-treatment scores for each self-report measure, and that this should be maintained at 6 months. Following these recent guidelines it can be seen that a *clinically* significant improvement has also been achieved in the self-report measures for disability, fear of movement/re-injury and depressive symptomatology.

For physical function measures Spanswick and Peat (2000) suggest a *clinically* significant improvement may be reported if, following treatment, there is an improvement of greater than 50% from pre-treatment measures. Following these guidelines, a *clinically* significant improvement cannot be recorded for any of the physical function measures.

The step-up test did not reveal a clinically or statistically significant improvement. This is likely to be a result of the ceiling effect. Results reveal that the study subject scored highly with this test, achieving an average score of 10 step-ups in 30 seconds during phase A1. In a recent investigation of functional limitation in chronic pain patients prior to rehabilitation, Peat (1998) reports an average number of 8 step-ups achieved in 30 seconds. It is unlikely that the study subject could improve upon an already high score.

It must be said that the physical function tests may be subject to practice effects. Self-report measures of pain intensity were very variable throughout the study (Graphs 9–11). This is characteristic of the fluctuating nature of chronic pain intensity (Dworkin & Whitney 1992). Neither a statistically, nor a clinically significant improvement in pain intensity can be reported.

On closer inspection of results it is noted that a high pain intensity report at the start of the pain management programme (see Graph 9 phase B) is not related to a fall in performance on measures of physical function (see Graphs 1–4). Nor is this increase in pain intensity associated with deterioration in self-reported disability level. It is also noted that, despite an obvious increase in pain intensity during phase A2, other measures taken at the same time do not appear to be greatly affected by this. Results suggest no relationship between self-reported pain intensity and self-report of mood, fear of movement, disability levels and physical function measures. This supports earlier studies suggesting that there is not a close correlation between the self-report of pain intensity and disability levels (Watson & Poulter 1997, Richards et al 1982).

It is important to comment on the study's external validity. This refers to the extent to which the results can be generalised. Generalisability is limited for this project. This is mainly due to the experimental design, single case study (n=1), which, by definition, provides poor external validity. Also, the subject included in this study was a patient referred to a specialised pain centre. Once referred, patients are assessed and selected for inclusion on a pain management programme. Following this selection process they are then asked to 'opt-into' the pain management programme. This referral system and filtering process further reduces generalisability of results. It could be argued that the study subject represented a highly motivated individual, more likely to do well with a self-management approach. She agreed to participate in this study and she also attended and completed all components of the pain management programme and follow-up assessments.

Within single case studies, all conditions apart from the treatment under investigation should remain constant so there can be no doubt that the differences observed result from true treatment effects. In practice this is not always possible. The study subject attended the pain management programme for a 3-week period, so it was not possible to control for external factors, perhaps in the home environment, which may have affected results e.g. influences of others, significant life events. It is also not possible to say which aspects of the pain management programme led to the observed improvement, as the treatment approach is multidisciplinary, including a number of interventions.

Despite these limitations, the investigation supports the multidimensional treatment of fibromyalgia and recommendations for a cognitive-behavioural approach (Rossy et al 1999, White & Neilson 1995). It is clear from the results outlined, that an improvement in measures of physical function, self-reported disability, fear of movement and depressive symptomatology can be seen. An effect on pain intensity levels is not observed. Pain self-report was extremely variable; this is characteristic of fibromyalgia and other chronic pain conditions (Dworkin & Whitney 1992).

Since the aims of a pain management programme are to reduce the disability and distress caused by chronic pain rather than affect the pain per se (Pain Society 1997), the results of this investigation are consistent with these aims.

Conclusion

This small single case study supports the multidimensional treatment of fibromyalgia and recommendations for a cognitive-behavioural approach.

A primary problem in pain research in evaluating treatment efficacy is the definition of outcome criteria. Variation in the length of follow-up, outcome measurements, programme delivery and programme content between different pain management programmes, confirm that there is no clear agreement on when patients should be followed up and how they ought to be evaluated. Future multi-patient research might address such issues making comparisons between different pain management programmes possible.

ACKNOWLEDGEMENTS

This single case study was carried out as part of the modular MSc (physiotherapy) degree at Manchester School of Physiotherapy, UK. I would like to thank Paul Watson for his supervision and helpful comments and Steve Goldingay for his assistance with data collection.

REFERENCES

Bailey A, Starr L, Alderson M, Moreland J 1999 A comparative evaluation of a fibromyalgia rehabilitation programme. Arthritis Care and Research 12(5):336–340

Barlow D, Hersen M 1988 Single Case Experimental Designs 2nd edition. Pergamon Press, London

Bennett R M 1996 Multidisciplinary group programs to treat fibromyalgia patients. Rheumatic Disease Clinics of North America 22(2):351–367

Boissevain MD, McCain GA 1991 Toward an integrated understanding of fibromyalgia syndrome I. Medical and pathphysiological aspects. Pain 45:227–238

Burckhardt CS, Mannerkorpi K, Hedenbers L, Bjelle A 1994 A randomised, controlled trial of education and physical training for women with fibromyalgia. Journal of Rheumatology 21:714–720

Carette S, Bell MJ, Reynolds WJ et al 1994 Comparison of amitriptyline, cyclobenzapine and placebo in the treatment of fibromyalgia. Arthritis and Rheumatism 37:32–40

Chaitow L 2000 The history and definition of fibromyalgia. In: Chaitow L (ed) Fibromyalgia Syndrome: a practitioners guide to treatment. Churchill Livingstone, Edinburgh

Consensus report on fibromyalgia 1996 The fibromyalgia syndrome: A consensus report on fibromyalgia and disability. The Journal of Rheumatology; 23(3):534–537

Consensus document on fibromyalgia: The Copenhagen declaration 1992 Lancet 340 (September 12)

Croft P, Rigby AS, Boswell R, Schollum J, Silman A 1993 The prevalence of chronic widespread pain in the general population. The Journal of Rheumatology 20(4):710–713

Dworkin SF, Whitney CW 1992 Relying on objective and subjective measures of chronic pain: Guidelines for use and interpretation. In: Turk DC, Melzack R (eds) Handbook of Pain Assessment. The Guildford Press, London

Harding V 1998 Application of the cognitive-behavioural approach. In: Pitt-Brooke, Reid H, Lockwood J, Kerr K (eds) Rehabilitation of Movement. W B Saunders, London

Harding V, Williams ACdeC 1995 Extending physiotherapy skills using a psychological approach: Cognitive-behavioural management of chronic pain. Physiotherapy 81(11):681–688

Harding V, Williams ACdeC, Richardson PH, Nicholas MK, Jackson JL, Richardson I, Pither CE 1994 The development of a battery of measures for assessing physical functioning of chronic pain patients. Pain 58:367–375

Henriksson KG 1994 Chronic muscular pain: Aetiology and pathogenesis. In: Masi AT (ed) Ballieres Clinical Rheumatology. Balliere Tindall, London

Henriksson KG, Mense S 1994 Pain and nociception in fibromyalgia: Clinical and neurobiological considerations on aetiology and pathogenesis. Pain Reviews 1:245–260

Hicks CM 1999 Research methods for clinical therapists 3rd edn. Churchill Livingstone, Edinburgh

Hunt IM, Silman AJ, Benjamin S, McBeth J, Macfarlane GJ 1999 The prevalence and associated features of chronic widespread pain in the community using the 'Manchester' definition of chronic widespread pain. Rheumatology 38:275–279

Kazdin A 1982 Single Case Research Designs. Oxford University Press, Oxford

Kirwan JR, Reeback JS 1986 Stanford health assessment questionnaire modified to assess disability in British patients with rheumatoid arthritis. British Journal of Rheumatology 25:206–209

Kori SH, Miller RP, Todd DD 1990 Kinisophobia: A new view of chronic pain behaviour. Pain Management Jan/Feb 35–43

Ledingham J, Doherty S, Doherty M 1993 Primary fibromyalgia syndrome—an outcome study. British Journal of Rheumatology 32:139–142

Mason LW, Goolkasian P, McCain G A 1998 Evaluation of a multimodal treatment program for fibromyalgia. Journal of Behavioral Medicine 21(2):163–178

MacFarlane GJ, Croft PR, Schollum J, Silman A J 1996 Widespread pain: Is an improved classification possible? Journal of Rheumatology 23:1628–1632

McDermid AJ, Rollman GB, McCain GA 1996 Generalized hypervigilance in fibromyalgia: evidence of perceptual amplification. Pain 66:133–144

Main CJ 1984 Psychological factors in chronic low back pain. Doctoral thesis, University of Glasgow, UK

Melzack RA 1987 The short form McGill questionnaire: Major properties and scoring methods. Pain 1:277–299

Melzack RA, Wall PD 1996 The Challenge of Pain. Penguin Books, London

Morley S, Eccleston C, Williams A 1999 Systematic review and meta-analysis of randomized controlled trials of cognitive-behaviour therapy and behaviour therapy for chronic pain in adults, excluding headache. Pain 80:1–13

Pain Society (1997) Report of a working party of the Pain Society of Great Britain and Ireland: Desirable criteria for pain management programmes. Pain Society London

Peat GM (1998) Functional limitation in chronic low back pain. Doctoral thesis, University of Manchester, UK

Peat GM, Moores LL, Goldingay S, Hunter M 2001 Pain management programme follow-ups: A national survey of current practice in the United Kingdom. Journal of Pain and Symptom Management, 21(3):218–226

Pellegrino M 2000 Physical medicine and a rehabilitation approach to treating fibromyalgia. In: Chaitow L (ed) Fibromyalgia Syndrome: a practitioners guide to treatment. Churchill Livingstone, Edinburgh

Richards J S, Nepomuceno C, Riles M, Suer Z 1982 Assessing pain behaviour: The UAB pain behaviour scale. Pain 31:65–75

Rosen 1994 Physical medicine and rehabilitation approaches to the management of myofascial pain and fibromyalgia syndromes. In: Masi AT (ed) Ballieres Clinical Rheumatology. Balliere Tindall, London

Rossy LA, Buckelew SP, Dorr N, Hagglund L et al 1999 A meta-analysis of fibromyalgia treatment interventions. Annals of Behavioral Medicine 21(2):180–191

Sandstrom MJ, Keefe FJ 1998 Self-management of fibromyalgia: The role of formal coping skills training and physical exercise training programs. Arthritis Care and Research 11(6):432–447

Spanswick CC, Peat GM 2000 Audit of pain management programmes. In: Lack JA, White LA, Thomas GM, Rollin AM (eds) Raising the Standard: A compendium of audit recipes for continuous quality improvement in anaesthesia. Royal College of Anaesthetists, London

Sweet CA 1995 Presentation to Rheumatology Forum, University of Manchester

Vlaeyen JWS, Teeken-Gruben NJG et al 1996 Cognitive-educational treatment of fibromyalgia: A randomised clinical trial, I. Clinical effects. Journal of Rheumatology 23(7):1237–1245

Watson PJ, Poulter ME 1997 The development of a functional task orientated measure of pain behaviour in chronic low back pain patients. Journal of Back and Musculoskeletal Rehabilitation 9:57–59

White KP, Harth M 1996 An analytical review of 24 controlled trials for fibromyalgia syndrome (FMS). Pain 64:211–219

White KP, Nielson WR 1995 Cognitive-behavioural treatment of fibromyalgia syndrome: A follow-up assessment. Journal of Rheumatology 22:717–721

Wigers SH, Stiles TC, Vogel PA 1996 Effects of aerobic exercise versus stress management treatment in fibromyalgia. Scandinavian Journal of Rheumatology 25:77–86

Wolfe F, Ross K, Anderson J, Russell IJ 1995 Aspects of fibromyalgia in the general population: Sex pain threshold and fibromyalgia symptoms. Journal of Rheumatology 22:151–156

Wolfe F, Smythe HA, Yunus MB et al 1990 The American College of Rheumatology criteria for the classification of fibromyalgia. Report of the multi-centre criteria committee. Arthritis and Rheumatism, 33(2):160–172

Yunus MB 1992 Towards a model of pathophysiology of fibromyalgia: Aberrant central pain mechanisms with peripheral modulation. Journal of Rheumatology 19:846–850

Appendix

Order and details of the physical function tests used in the investigation

5 minute walking distance

The number of 20 metre laps covered in a 5 minute time period (Harding et al 1994).

The subject was instructed to walk as many laps of a 20 metre corridor as she could in 5 minutes. They were told that it was up to them to determine their own walking pace. The subject was informed they could rest at any time during the test if they wanted to. A chair was in place at either end of the corridor. The use of walking aids was not permitted but the subject was allowed to use the wall for support. The observer did not converse with the patient during the test except to tell them when 2 minutes had elapsed and when 1 minute of the test remained. The completion of 1 lap was counted when the subject touched the line at each end of the corridor. If the subject had covered half or more of one length of the corridor the score was rounded up. If less than half a lap was completed the score was rounded down.

Step-up test

The number of completed step-ups achieved in a 30 second time period using a 20cm step-up block (adapted from Harding et al 1994).

The step-up test was carried out using a 20cm reinforced polystyrene block. The subject stood directly in front of the block and was instructed to step onto it with both feet. The use of walking aids was not allowed.

The subject was told that it did not matter which leg they led with and they were allowed to hold onto the wall or a set of nearby wall bars for light support only. The subject was instructed to perform as many step-ups as they could in 30-seconds.

The observer did not converse with the subject during the test only to tell them when 15-seconds had elapsed. The number of completed step-ups was recorded.

Psychophysical lifting test

The maximum load lifted and transferred from a plinth onto a chair and back up onto the plinth (Sweet 1995).

During this test a wide selection of sandbag weights up to the total value of 51.75Kg was positioned at waist height for the subject on an adjustable height plinth. A strong plastic basket was placed next to the weights.

A wooden stool approximately 10cm lower than the plinth was placed, slightly to the left and in front of the plinth. The subject was instructed to place as many of the sandbags as they felt they could lift into the basket. They were then asked to move the basket with both hands down onto the stool and then lift it back up onto the plinth. The subject was explicitly told to 'test out' the weight they had selected, by lifting the basket a little before carrying out the full test, so that they were comfortable with the weight selected. The subject and observer were unaware exactly what weight was lifted at the time as the sandbags were coded. At the end of the assessment the observer recorded the actual weight lifted by consulting a list of codes with corresponding weights in kg for each bag.

Timed 20 metre speed walk

The time taken to walk 20 metres measured in seconds (Harding et al 1994).

The subject was instructed to walk, as quickly as possible, a distance of 20 metres. The subject began the test behind a line at one end of the corridor when the observer gave the instruction 'Ready, set, go'. The use of walking aids was not permitted but the use of the walls for support was allowed.

The time was recorded when the subject crossed the line at the opposite end of the corridor.

Results as Tables and Graphs

Table 1 20 metre fast walk (time taken in seconds)

Phase A1		Phase B	Phase A2	6-month follow-up
15.4		16.2	10.0	9.9
14.9		16.1	13.1	
16.6		12.1	—	
15.9		11.0	11.6	
16.1		12.1	11.7	
16.8		9.7	10.6	
Mean =	2 SD =		Mean =	
15.95	1.43527		11.4	

Graph 1 20 metre fast walk

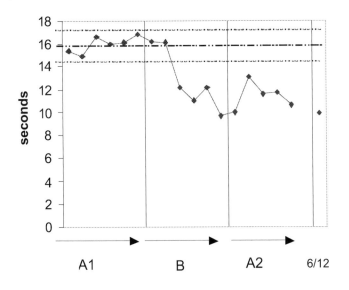

Graph 1 represents data for the 20 metre speed walk. Measurements taken during phase A1 reveal a stable baseline. It can be seen that during phase B the time taken to walk 20 metres reduces steadily. The last 4 measurements during phase B fall outside the 2 standard deviation band, as do all measures during phase A2 and 6-month follow-up. This indicates a statistically significant increase in walking speed has occurred during phase B that is maintained during phase A2 and at the 6-month follow-up stage.

Table 2 5 minute walk (number of 20-metre laps comleted)

Phase A1		Phase B	Phase A2	6-month follow-up
11		13	17	18
14		13	15	
13		14	—	
12		17	15	
11		15	15	
12		17	16	
Mean =	2 SD =		Mean =	
12.16	2.33		15.6	

Graph 2 5 minute walk

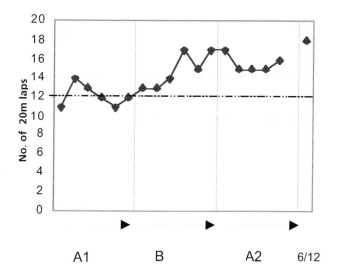

Graph 2 presents data for the 5 minute walking test. The baseline phase A1 is stable as all measures during this phase fall within 2 standard deviations of the mean. During phase B the number of 20 metre laps walked in 5 minutes steadily increases to above the 2 standard deviation band for the last 3 consecutive observations taken during this phase. This statistically significant improvement is maintained for all measurements taken throughout phase A2 and at the 6-month follow-up phase.

Table 3 Psychophysical lift (weight lifted in kg)

Phase A1	Phase B	Phase A2	6-month follow-up
8.75	9.0	12.5	15.75
13.25	10.0	9.5	
10.5	11.0	—	
8.5	12.5	9.0	
9.25	12.0	14.75	
9.25	13.5	15.0	
Mean = 2 SD =		Mean =	
9.9 3.54		12.15	

Graph 3 Psychophysical lift

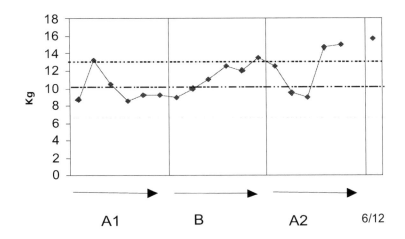

Graph 3 represents data collected for the psychophysical lifting test. Phase A1 indicates a fairly stable baseline as with the exception of one measurement during week 1 of the investigation all measures fall within 2 standard deviations. Measurements taken during phase B reveal a steady increase in weight lifted; however, only 1 measurement (the last) during phase B falls outside the 2 standard deviation band. During phase A2 the last 2 measurements taken fall outside the 2 standard deviation band and this is maintained at the 6-month follow-up assessment.

Table 4 Number of step-ups in 30 seconds

Phase A1		Phase B	Phase A2	6-month follow-up
14		13	13	14
11		9	9	
13		10	—	
9		10	9	
9		10	12	
9		12	12	
Mean =	2 SD =		Mean =	
10.83	4.45		11	

Graph 4 Number of step-ups in 30 seconds

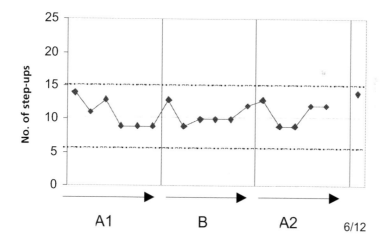

Graph 4 represents the data collected for the number of step-ups achieved in 30 seconds. A deteriorating baseline is noted initially, which then becomes stable for the last 3 recorded measurements. During phase B there is an initial increase followed by a decline in the number of step-ups performed in 30 seconds. At no point during the investigation do 2 successive data points fall outside the 2 standard deviation band. Therefore, results indicate that there was no significant change identifiable with this measure.

Table 5 Disability score (measured using the Kirwan and Reeback questionnaire)

Phase A1		Phase B	Phase A2	6-month follow-up
4.875		3.625	3.0	2.75
3.75		3.25	3.375	
3.875		3.25	—	
4.25		3.25	3.25	
3.875		3.25	3.125	
4.5		2.875	2.875	
Mean = 4.1875	2 SD = 0.877	3.25		

Graph 5 Disability score

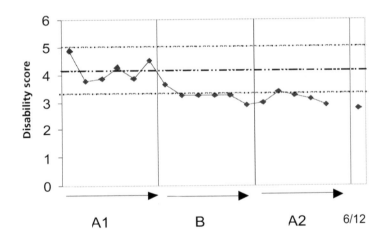

Graph 5 presents data for the level of disability. After a stable baseline, phase B disability scores gradually decrease, so that all but the first data point fall outside the 2 standard deviation band during phase B. This is maintained for all but the 2nd measurement taken during phase A2. The single data point at 6-months reveals that this change is maintained. This indicates that a statistically significant change occurred during the intervention phase, which was maintained during the follow-up phase A2.

234

Table 6 TSK (fear of movement and re-injury)

Phase A1		Phase B	Phase A2	6-month follow-up
31			24	26
27			25	
33			—	
33			24	
31			26	
34		20	24	
Mean = 31.5	2 SD = 5.01			

Graph 6 TSK

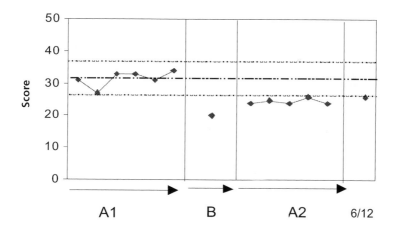

Graph 6 represents the data collected to assess fear of movement and re-injury. A stable baseline is noted. It can then be seen clearly that the measurement taken during phase B at the post programme assessment indicates a considerable reduction in the fear score falling outside the 2 standard deviation band. This significant change is maintained for all measurements taken during phase A2 and is also evident at the 6-month assessment stage.

Table 7 Modified Zung (depressive symptomatology)

Phase A1	Phase B	Phase A2	6-month follow-up
44		25	25
41		30	
42		—	
47		32	
48		33	
49	22	26	
Mean = 45.17	2 SD = 6.62		

Graph 7 Modified Zung

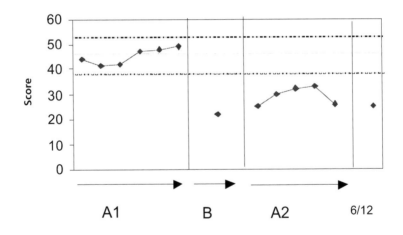

In Graph 7 phase A1 indicates a stable baseline for the results of the Modified Zung questionnaire. A marked reduction in the depression score is clearly seen at the post programme assessment stage during phase B. This score falls well outside the 2 standard deviation band. This change is maintained for all scores during phase A2 and at the 6-month follow up stage.

236

Table 8 MSPQ (somatic symptoms)

Phase A1		Phase B	Phase A2	6-month follow-up
27			8	10
18			12	
17			—	
16			12	
14			9	
23		10	9	
Mean = 19.167	2 SD = 9.75			

Graph 8 MSPQ

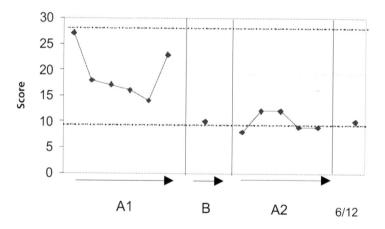

Graph 8 represents data for the Modified Somatic Perception Questionnaire. During phase A1 all measures fall within 2 standard deviations of the mean. However, measurements during phase A1 fluctuate. Initially an improvement is noted, however, an increase in somatic symptoms is seen just prior to the start of the pain management programme. The single measurement taken during phase B falls marginally inside the 2 standard deviation band. The first measurement during phase A2 falls outside the 2 standard deviation band, following which somatic awareness increases and scores fall inside the 2 standard deviation band. The final 2 successive measurements taken during phase A2 fall marginally outside the 2 standard deviation band. At 6-month follow-up the MSPQ score does not fall outside the band.

Table 9 Pain intensity (Visual Analogue Scale)

Phase A1		Phase B	Phase A2	6-month follow-up
24		93	22	12
51		61	84	
43		53	—	
64		25	64	
71		47	50	
80		61	39	
Mean = 55.5	2 SD = 40.81			

Graph 9 Pain intensity

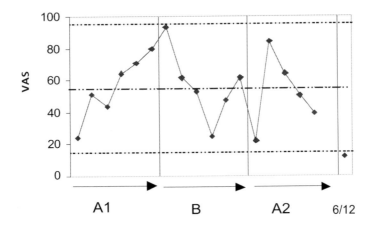

Graph 9 indicates that during phase A1 there is a steep increase in self-reported pain intensity measured on a visual analogue scale. The first 4 measures taken in phase B show a sharp decrease in intensity before a steep increase again with the last 2 measures in Phase B. A similar fluctuating pattern can be seen in phase A2. At no point during the A1, B, A2 phases do 2 successive measurements fall outside the 2 standard deviation band. At 6-month follow up the pain intensity score falls marginally outside the 2 standard deviation band. These results show that there was no significant change in self-reported pain intensity.

Table 10 Pain intensity (sensory component)

Phase A1		Phase B	Phase A2	6-month follow-up
2		5	0	0
3		0	3	
1		2	—	
4		1	2	
4		1	2	
10		2	2	
Mean = 4	2 SD = 6.3			

Graph 10 Pain intensity

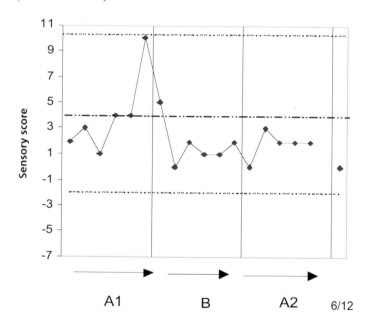

Graph 10 demonstrates that there is considerable variability in the sensory pain scores of the McGill pain questionnaire. A peak is noted just prior to the start of the pain management programme. A significant change cannot be detected.

Table 11 Pain intensity (Affective component)

Phase A1		Phase B	Phase A2	6-month follow-up
6		25	5	5
17		14	21	
14		12	—	
17		7	15	
23		9	9	
29		17	8	
Mean =	2 SD =			
55.5	40.8			

Graph 11 Pain intensity

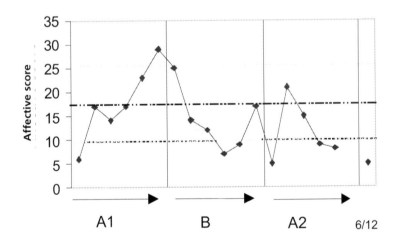

Graph 11 shows there is considerable fluctuation in the affective component of the McGill pain questionnaire. A peak in intensity can be seen just before the start of the pain management programme. The last two consecutive measures taken in phase A2 fall outside the 2 standard deviation band. Given the variability of these scores, it is not possible to say that a significant reduction in the affective score of pain intensity has occurred.

13

The epidemiology of chronic musculoskeletal pain

ANN C PAPAGEORGIOU

The role of epidemiology

Epidemiology involves the study of the distribution of disease in the population. The Arthritis Research Campaign's (ARC) Unit in Manchester specifically focuses on the distribution of musculoskeletal disorders. This chapter will address some of the problems encountered when studying such disorders in the community, especially those of case definition, and describe a study of low back pain undertaken in south Manchester. The relevance of these results, and issues they raise, will be discussed.

Epidemiology has three main concerns:

- to describe and measure the distribution of disease in the population
- to investigate the causes and influences on its occurrence
- to evaluate the impact of any interventions.

This chapter will address for first two of these in relation to musculoskeletal pain. There are three levels at which musculoskeletal pain can be studied:

- in the population
- in primary care
- in the hospital or specialist setting.

Data from each source will provide a different picture of the nature and distribution of musculoskeletal pain. Each year, of every seven people with back pain only one will consult their general practitioner, and only a minority of these are referred to a specialist clinic, or are treated by a physiotherapist or other health professional—the vast majority remain 'out there' in the community. Population surveys are one way to obtain a handle on the distribution of this hidden pain.

Why should we be interested? Is it important? Musculoskeletal pain is the second most common symptom presented to the general practitioner (McCormick et al 1995), the diagnosis of fibromyalgia is increasingly common (Croft et al 1994), and there has been an exponential rise in sickness absence due to back pain in the past ten years (CSAG 1994). Musculoskeletal pain is not usually life-threatening—the endpoint is rarely death—but it is responsible for a huge amount of disability and suffering and, as such, constitutes a major economic and health problem for society as well as for individuals and their families.

Is this increase 'real'? And why has it occurred? The pain is very 'real' to those experiencing it, but its increased prevalence could reflect either social changes in people's attitude towards pain (maybe a belief that pain can be cured has lead to an increasing propensity to seek treatment), or changes in how information about musculoskeletal pain is collected. Of course, the increase could also be 'real'—some change in society or our life-style could be making us more vulnerable to chronic musculoskeletal pain. One way to examine if the increase is 'real' is to look at trends in the reporting of pain in the population over time using an *identical definition* of pain at each time-point. Only then can one start investigating why such change in the apparent prevalence of pain has occurred.

Defining pain for population surveys

Pain can be many different things, as illustrated in the following quote:

> What kind of pain are you interested in? Are you interested in the pain that is racking my body right now and from which I will never recover? Are you asking about the pain of my life when I lost my daughter? Are you talking about the pain of my loneliness because I have no one who cares? (Autton 1986).

The detail and focus of questions asked about pain will vary depending on the purpose for which that information is to be used. For example, when making a diagnosis the physician requires a detailed description of the symptom, such as the character, severity, site, duration, frequency and special times of occurrence, and factors that aggravate and relieve the pain (Ryle 1948).

For clinical trails and in-depth qualitative studies the researcher may ask about pain intensity, whether it lead to a consultation or time off work, and its impact on a person's life and activities.

However, in defining pain for prevalence studies the emphasis has to be on clarity and consistency. The primary concern is to identify cases from non-cases based on whether certain defining criteria are reported. In such studies it is not feasible to explore the subtle association between the sensory and affective elements of pain.

In population surveys there are three important parameters when defining cases of musculoskeletal pain from non-cases: the anatomical site, the duration of pain, and the time period in which the pain occurred.

Information on the *anatomical site* may be elicited in a variety of ways.

a) **A direct question** 'Have you had any pain in your (shoulder) during the past month?' This leaves the spatial definition of 'shoulder' and the duration of pain unspecified. This form of question is commonly used in general health surveys.

b) **With reference to a diagram** with the anatomical site shaded, a question asking about any pain in the shaded area during the past month. This focuses attending on a defined area, but still leaves the duration unspecified.

c) **A general question** asking 'During the past month have you experienced any ache or pain which has lasted for one day or longer?' If answering 'Yes', the subject is asked to shade in the site of any ache or pain on a blank manikin. This is then coded by the researcher using a perspex template on which the defined area of interest is marked.

In studies using more than one definition, we have found the lowest prevalence is recorded with the direct question, although this will clearly depend on how the broadly anatomical area is defined on the manikin for the particular study.

The use of the blank manikin has several advantages. First, it permits pain reported in a particular part of the body to be understood in the context of other pains the person may experience. Second, the anatomical site can be redefined if necessary after the data collection is completed; this can be particularly useful when relating the area of pain to disability or outcome. Third, it avoids directing a person towards a particular site of pain.

Having established the anatomical site, the *duration of pain* is considered. Is the study concerned with any pain, pain lasting one day or more, or chronic pain defined as persisting for three months or longer? So as to discount trivial pain we have usually opted for a duration of 'one day or longer'. However this is not without its problems. When a sample of survey responders were subsequently interviewed it was clear that 'one day or longer' was often interpreted as having pain for *at least part of the time* on more than one day. For example, back pain each morning, or shoulder pain experienced each time a young child was lifted would be included under the duration criteria of pain lasting 'one day or longer' in the past month. Providing we know what respondents include within a given definition, subjects giving similar responses can be grouped together, and the results interpreted. However, we do not know how *consistently* our criteria are thus interpreted, and more work is needed to clarify this.

The third aspect to defining pain is the *recall period*. To ask about pain 'today' or 'now' will provide a point-prevalence—a snap-shot of pain in the population at that point in time. However, this is likely to over-estimate those with constant problems, and under-estimate the number with episodic pain, which may be absent on the day in question. More commonly a one-month or one-year prevalence is obtained by wording such as 'Thinking back over the past month (or year) have you experienced pain lasting for one day or longer?' Alternatively, lifetime prevalence can be obtained by asking 'Have you ever experienced pain lasting...?' The longer the time period, the less reliable the person's recall is likely to be. Using identical definitions of low back pain, there was no difference between the one month prevalence of low back pain (39%) in the south Manchester study (Papageorgiou et al 1995) and the one-year prevalence reported by Walsh et al (36%) (1992) and by Mason (37%) (1994).

The *incidence* of pain relates to 'new' cases. For disorders that are clearly defined and require medical attention, such as cancer or hip fracture, monitoring the number of new 'incident' cases during a set period of time (conventionally a year) is relatively unproblematic. However, such definitions are not so easy with musculoskeletal pain, such as back pain, which is likely to follow a different course with each individual. It might be a single acute episode or, more frequently, repeated episodes over a period of time. These might be exacerbations overlying a chronic aching of the back, and, occasionally, the pain might be both chronic and severe. Croft (1996) suggests that the course of low back pain is best considered as individual histories, no two being identical (Croft 1996, Croft et al 1997). In this case 'incidence' is usually taken to refer to the first new episode of back pain during the year in someone who has been pain free for a given period, conventionally one or three months. Even this can be problematic when 'pain free' can be interpreted as a residual 'ache', but the absence of acute pain. A new episode, however defined, is rarely the first ever episode of back pain the person has experienced and is more correctly referred to as the 'one year cumulative incidence'.

The three essential aspects for defining pain in population surveys, outlined above, are the site, duration of pain and period of recall. In studies of chronic pain there is also the continuance of pain to be considered. As both the American College of Rheumatology (ACR) (Woolfe et al 1990) definition for fibromyalgia, and earlier studies of back pain refer to chronic pain as that lasting for three months or longer, we have adopted the same time-period in our studies.

Intervention or follow-up studies often include questions about the severity of pain and related disability. Raspe and Kohlmann (1994) recommend using an eleven-point numerical rating scale (from 0=no pain to 10=intolerable pain) for assessing pain severity. There are several well-validated measures of disability both for general health problems and for specific musculoskeletal disorders. The inclusion of such additional information enables degrees of pain severity and its disabling affects to be monitored and can be particularly useful when assessing interventions which may lead to a reduction in pain or disability, but not its eradication.

I will illustrate the type of epidemiological survey of musculoskeletal pain we have undertaken with reference to a large population study of low back pain, and then compare the results with those of similar studies of chronic widespread pain.

South Manchester back pain study

The aims of this study were to identify:

- risk factors for the development of a new episode of low back pain
- factors which predict the chronicity of such symptoms.

The first step was to collect information on potential risk factors in subjects identified as free of back pain. We did this by means of a survey questionnaire.

The study populations comprised all 7669 adults, aged between 18 and 75 years, registered with two general practices in south Manchester. These were sent an initial survey questionnaire, which asked if pain lasting for one day or longer had been experienced during the past month. Those responding positively were asked to shade the site of such pain on a blank manikin. Additional questions asked about a past history of back pain and neck pain. As well as sociodemographic data, information was also obtained on potential risk factors for back pain including physical activity at work and leisure, psychosocial factors (such as satisfaction with work and income), and psychological status. Psychological distress was assessed using the 12-item General Health Questionnaire (GHQ), a well–validated instrument for identifying symptoms of anxiety and depression of recent onset in the general population (Goldberg & Williams 1988). Social class was obtained from the present or last job title using the OPCS (now renamed as the Office for National Statistics—ONS) Standard Occupational Classification (1991).

After two reminders, the recruitment questionnaire was returned by 4501 subjects—a response rate of 59%. The 2715 respondents with no pain in the past month, or pain shaded on the manikin outside the areas defined as the low back (that is, not between the 12th rib and the gluteal folds) were deemed to be free of low back pain. These formed the back-pain free cohort for the follow-up study.

The second step was to identify all new episodes of back pain in this cohort. As most people with low back pain do not consult their general practitioner, two approaches were required. First, both general practices routinely recorded the reason for each consultation on their computer records. At the end of each week these were checked to identify subjects who had consulted because of low back pain. Those who had previously returned the recruitment survey were asked to agree to a home visit by a research nurse. Information about low back pain in people who did *not* consult their general practitioner was obtained by means of a second survey questionnaire sent out twelve months after the initial recruitment survey. This asked about the presence, duration and consequences of any low back pain during the previous year, and was returned by 1638 subjects (64%) after two reminders.

The second aim of this study was to identify predictors of chronicity by following the progress of back pain and disability in those who developed a new episode. For practical reasons, this could only be carried out in those presenting to primary care and, again, two approaches were involved. First,

245

a research nurse visited subjects within two weeks of their having consulted the general practitioner, and again three and twelve months later. At the initial interview information was obtained about both the present episode of back pain, and any past history of the symptom. The follow-up visits allowed the course of the back pain to be monitored. At each visit pain severity was recorded on a numerical rating scale, associated disability was measured using the Hanover Back Pain Daily Activity Schedule (Kohlmann & Raspe 1996), and an assessment of spinal mobility was carried out.

Second, the case records of all subjects consulting the general practitioner because of low back pain were reviewed and information obtained on the number of consultations for back pain that had taken place in the three months following the initial visit. Those with no record of consultations beyond three months were deemed to have recovered from the back pain for which they had initially sought treatment.

Results

Of the 4501 adults returning the initial survey questionnaire, 39% reported low back symptoms in the previous month. Even after adjusting for potential non-response bias, the prevalence of low back pain (as defined above) was still between 35% and 37%. The life-time prevalence of low back pain was 59% (Papageorgiou et al 1995).

During the follow-up year 490 people consulted their general practitioner at least once because of low back pain, making a cumulative consultation

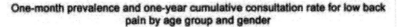

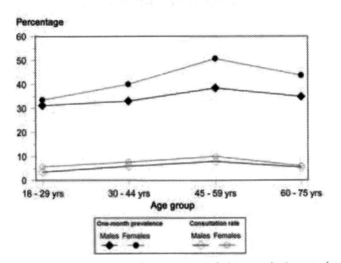

Fig 13.1 One month prevalence and one year cumulative consultation rate for low back pain by age group and gender.

rate of 6.4% (men 5.6%, women 7.1%). This is almost identical to that reported in government statistics (McCormick et al 1995). However, of the 4501 responders to the recruitment survey, only 109 (2.4%) had recorded no current back pain and were, therefore, consulting with a new episode. Of those initially free of back pain, 31% reported a new episode for which they did not consult.

Both the prevalence and incidence followed the same pattern as recorded in previous population studies of back pain, with the rates for women being higher than those for men, and rates for both genders increasing up to the 45–59 year age-group and then decreasing in the elderly (see Fig. 13.1). The possible reasons for this decrease are discussed later. However, these differences were not great with just over a 50% increase between the lowest prevalence of low back pain (31% in males aged 18–29 years) to the highest (49% in women aged between 45 and 59 years).

As stated earlier, one aim of this study was to identify risk factors for developing a new episode of low back pain. To do so we first identified a group of people free of current back pain and collected information on potential risk factors for this symptom, and then identified those who developed a new back pain episode. This enabled us to examine which factors were reported significantly more frequently at recruitment by those who developed back pain compared to those who did not. In Table 13.1 these are presented as odds ratios. These differences are generally considered 'significant' when the 95% confidence interval (CI) does not cross 1.

Table 13.1 Risk for a new episode of low back pain during the follow-up year

Risk	Consulting OR (95% CI)	Non-consulting OR (95% CI)
Psychological distress (GHQ)		
lowest v highest tertile	2.0 (1.2-3.2)	1.8 (1.4-2.4)
Previous history LBP		
males	1.9 (0.9-3.8)	4.8 (3.3-7.1)
females	2.9 (1.7-5.1)	2.2 (1.6-3.0)
Current 'other' musculoskeletal pain		
males	2.7 (1.3-5.8)	1.4 (0.9-2.1)
females	1.8 (1.0-3.4)	1.9 (1.3-2.7)
Work related (psychosocial)		
dissatisfaction	0.8 (0.2-2.7)	2.0 (1.2-3.3)
inadequate income	3.6 (1.8-7.2)	1.3 (0.8-2.1)
social class IV or V	4.8 (2.0-11.5)	0.8 (0.5-1.3)
Work related (physical)		
regular lifting > 11kg		
males	1.2 (0.5-3.0)	1.1 (0.7-1.7)
females	2.3 (1.1-5.0)	2.5 (1.5-4.1)
standing/walking > 2 hrs		
males	2.1 (0.7-6.4)	0.9 (0.6-1.5)
females	3.5 (1.4-8.8)	1.8 (1.1-2.8)

Table 13.1 shows that, in people free of current back pain:

- **Psychological distress** doubled the risk of developing a subsequent new back pain episode (that is, those in the highest third of GHQ scores at baseline were twice as likely to develop back pain in the follow-up year compared to those with the lowest third of GHQ scores) (Croft et al 1995).
- A **previous history** of back pain was an even stronger risk. These risks were expected as they have been reported in previous studies. However, the use of a shaded manikin to record all aches and pain lasting for at least 24 hours during the previous month provided us with information about pain in **other sites** of the body. This showed that people reporting pain in sites other than the low back at baseline were again more likely to develop back pain in the following year (Papageorgiou et al 1996).
- Several **work-place** based studies have reported that employee dissatisfied with their work are more prone to develop back pain. We found similar results in that *dissatisfaction* was a risk for workers to report a new back pain episode, but *not for consulting* with this symptom. Conversely, workers who reported their *income* as inadequate for their needs, and those in *social class IV or V* were, independently, at greater risk only *for consulting* the general practitioner because of back problems in the follow-up year. The reporting of back pain for which no consultation was sought was similar across all social classes and perceptions of income.

As our study was population based, information on the degree of satisfaction with non-employed status, social class and perception of income were also available for those not currently in employment. Surprisingly this showed an identical pattern of risks for back pain as found in persons currently employed (Papageorgiou 1998). This raises questions about attributing 'dissatisfaction' solely to work-related back pain.

Turning to **physical activity** at work:

- Table 13.1 shows these risks to be more pronounced in women than in men.
- In this study, *sitting* for more than two hours continuously was found to lessen the risk of developing back pain; this could be because those whose work involved long periods seated were less likely to be exposed to lifting, or prolonged standing/walking (Macfarlane et al 1997).

The second aim of the south Manchester back pain study was to identify predictors for the outcome of back pain once a new episode had developed. We were able to compare two different sources of outcome data at three months: that collected from the general practice records on the number of repeat consultations, and that from the nurse's home visits on degree of pain and disability. Unresolved back pain was defined, respectively, as back pain consultations which continued beyond three months, and back pain (recorded on a numerical scale) or back-related disability which persisted beyond a minimal level.

Overall 60% of subjects consulted only once for the back pain episode (80% of those under 30 years, compared to half of subjects aged 30 or over), a third had repeated consultations within three months, and only 9% had evidence in their medical records of consultations extending beyond that period. These results could be interpreted as 90% of back pain having resolved within three months.

However, the information collected at the home visit showed a very different three-month outcome with *75% of those followed up still reporting some degree pain and/or disability related to their back*. This figure was little changed at the one-year follow-up visit (Croft et al 1998).

Finally we looked at predictors of outcome using data collected both at the recruitment survey (prior to the onset of back pain) and at the first nurse-administered interview and examination. This identified the strongest independent *pre-morbid* risks of poor outcome (defined as continued pain and disability at three and twelve months) to be:

- female gender
- a previous history of low back pain
- dissatisfaction.
  Predictors of poor outcome identified at the *first* home visit were:
- pain in other areas of the body
- two or more spinal restrictions (both of which tripled the risk of a poor outcome)
- and, to a lesser extent, radiating leg pain.

Only 6% of subjects with two or less of these risk factors developed persistent disabling back pain, compared to 70% of those with five or all six factors present (Thomas et al 1999).

Chronic widespread pain

Similar survey methods have been used to monitor the prevalence and course of chronic widespread pain in the adult populations registered with two general practices in Cheshire (Croft et al 1993, Macfarlane et al 1996). Again, asking that the site of pain lasting for one day or longer in the past month be shaded on a blank manikin, we were able to identify subjects whose pain was 'widespread'. As recommended by the ACR criteria for fibromyalgia (Wolfe et al 1990), this was defined as pain affecting the axial skeleton and at least two contralateral quadrants of the body. A further question asked if the pain had persisted for three months or more. A sample of respondents were visited by a research nurse who obtained additional information on symptoms and carried out an examination of tender points. Subjects with widespread pain lasting for longer than three months, and with eleven or more tender points (out of 18 sites examined) met the ACR criteria for fibromyalgia. On the initial postal survey 13% of respondents had chronic widespread pain (men 9.4%, women 15.6%). When this was adjusted for the age and gender distribution of England and Wales, the estimated prevalence of chronic widespread pain in the population was 11.2%. However, only 40% of those with chronic widespread pain met the ACR criteria for fibromyalgia (with eleven or more tender points) resulting in an estimated prevalence of fibromyalgia of 4.8% in the population as a whole.

The research nurse revisited all subjects three years later and similar information was collected.

- Only about a third of subjects with chronic widespread pain initially still met these criteria on the second visit.
- However, one in five of subjects with regional pain (defined as pain not satisfying the criteria for chronic widespread pain) on the original survey had developed pain which was both chronic and widespread at the three-year follow-up.

Factors that predicted either the persistence or development of chronic widespread pain at follow-up were:

- older age
- female gender
- fewer educational qualifications
- longer reported duration of aches and pain
- higher levels of psychological distress
- fatigue
- sleep problems
- abdominal pain and headaches.

A further population-based prospective study looked at predictors for developing chronic widespread pain in two groups of subjects, one pain-free and a second with regional pain. Again, similar results were obtained, with subjects who reported psychological distress, somatic symptoms, fatigue or disability on the initial survey at least *twice as likely* to report chronic widespread pain one year later compared to those not reporting these problems. These results were not explained by the subjects' age, gender or initial pain category (McBeth et al 2001).

Discussion

This chapter has addressed some of the methodological issues met when studying musculoskeletal pain in the population. In epidemiology, in order to count 'cases' these must be clearly identified from 'non-cases'. For subjective symptoms, such as pain, fatigue and stiffness, this is problematic. What is pain to one person might be considered a minor ache by another. The best a researcher can achieve in large population surveys is to put limits to what is, and is not, classified as a 'case'. This may be achieved by a single question ('Within the last month have you suffered from any problems with headaches?') or a series of questions corresponding to criteria. Only subjects providing a positive response to each question would meet the study's definition of pain, and therefore be counted as a 'case'.

The back pain study also illustrates how the source of data, and the definition used, may lead to quite different conclusions. Based on the general practice records it could be concluded that 90% of low back pain had resolved within three months of the subjects having first consulted their general practitioner. This figure is often quoted in relation to the one-month resolution of back pain and can be traced back to a 1972 meeting when general practitioner from London, Dr Fry, reported that 86% of patients attending his practice with acute back pain were better within four weeks. However, when back pain is defined as continued pain (on a numerical rating scale) or back-related disability then, *after three months, only 25% of subjects no longer had back problems.* Similarly, while around 15% of the population will report having consulted their general practitioner because of back pain in the past year, less than half this number (around 6% of the population) will have evidence of such a consultation in their practice records. (CSAG 1994, Walsh et al 1992).

Pain is a subjective sensation, and the epidemiology of pain is not the same as the epidemiology of impairment. For example, using MRI *75% of people complaining of low back pain have a disc abnormality,* which might suggest a reasonable association between back pain and impairment. However, *a quarter will show no disc abnormality* and, when the same technique was used on *subjects with no back pain, 70% showed the same abnormalities.* Similarly, only half of subjects showing changes on their hip X-rays consistent with hip osteoarthritis will have complained of hip pain (Croft 1996).

Epidemiologists are generally wary of committing themselves to the term 'causal' because of potential confounding factors, and two related terms are usually preferred: risk factors and temporal relationships. As well as monitoring the outcome of any intervention, prospective (or follow-up) studies, such as those described earlier in this chapter, are used to identify risk factors. Cross-sectional studies are able to identify associations, such as between pain and psychological distress, but are unable to show the direction of any temporal relationship. It is equally feasible to conclude that people with pain are more likely to become distressed, as to argue that someone who is psychologically distressed is more likely to develop pain. In prospective studies potential risk factors can be identified in subjects free of pain and these subjects are then observed to see which factors predict the subsequent development of pain. Similarly, a cross-sectional study of back pain might show that lifting at work is associated with a reduction in back pain symptoms (as shown for men in Table 13.1). However, only a longer term prospective study will show if this is due to the so-called 'healthy worker' effect—those with back pain will tend to undertake work which does not include lifting weights, leaving this type of work to a 'healthy back' group. We found that men with back pain had worked for fewer years in jobs involving repeated lifting compared to those free of pain. This suggests that either a 'healthy worker' effect was indeed present, or that a 'training' effect had occurred, in that good lifting techniques had been learned with experience, and strong back muscles had developed (Macfarlane et al 1997).

Another consideration when studying pain and its chronicity is the fluctuating nature of this symptom. Population surveys provide 'snap-shots' of the current situation, and even repeated surveys cannot provide reliable information about what is experienced between times. Because a person is free of pain at three time points throughout a year, it cannot be assumed that she has been free of pain throughout the whole year.

In studies using population surveys to ascertain the prevalence of any disease or symptom, a high response rate is important. People with a disease or symptom are more likely to respond to survey questionnaires than those without symptoms. Falsely high prevalence estimates can be reported if this potential 'non-response' bias is not considered. Although the response rate in the back pain study, described previously, was only 60%, we had information (from the general practice registers) on the non-responders, and so were able to adjust the prevalence for age and gender to take account of non-responders. However, the principal way to minimise any non-response bias is to ensure a high response rate, preferably over 80%.

Both the prevalence of back pain at the initial survey, and the incidence throughout the following year, showed the highest rates to be in the 45–59 age group, with a small but consistent drop in the elderly. There are four possible explanations for this.

- It could be a cohort effect—there was something in the lives of those born before 1930 which protected them from developing back pain (possible reasons might be more exercise as children, no heavy school bags to carry, dietary factors).
- It could be a physiological effect—the older spine is less flexible and therefore less prone to injury, or the elderly are less likely to undertake activities that might injure their spine.
- It could be perception of pain—either older people have so many other aches and pain, that a bit of back pain is disregarded, or they have a different attitude towards pain; they may, for example, be reluctant to admit to pain (this might also be a 'cohort' effect).
- Although unlikely, this could be a 'healthy survivor' effect—those with back pain having died, leaving a healthy back-pain-free group to complete survey questionnaires.

This gives some idea of how data from epidemiological studies can be interpreted and form the basis of hypothesis for future studies using similar or alternative research methods.

Conclusions

Ideally, an internationally agreed definition (or criteria) should be applied when studying pain, as is the case for rheumatoid arthritis and many other diseases. In the absence of this, epidemiological studies of pain should clearly state how pain has been defined for the study, and any follow-up or comparisons should utilise identical definitions.

This chapter describes just some of the studies of musculoskeletal pain undertaken at the ARC Unit in Manchester, from which three consistent factors are emerging:

1. Whatever the site of pain being studied (lower back, shoulder, hip, or widespread pain) similar risk factors are identified—and these are predominantly psychosocial factors (psychological distress, dissatisfaction, social status). The risks associated with physical factors that put stress on a particular joint or muscles, while still important, are less marked. These results would reaffirm the approach to the research of musculoskeletal pain that adopts the biopsychosocial model which encompasses the biological, psychological and social aspects of pain (Waddell 1992).

2. Our studies show that pain is rarely experienced in isolation from other somatic symptoms. If pain is reported in one site (especially chronic pain), that individual is likely to have, or develop, musculoskeletal pain in other sites of their body. This may be due to a heightened awareness of pain, or to some changes in the chemical or neurological physiology of the body as a consequence of the continual pain, which heightens pain perception.

3. Previous pain experience has been shown to be a strong predictor of future pain, and already by 15 years of age, about one in every five school children report having experienced low back pain in the previous year (Burton et al 1996). It is difficult to know the hereditary role for this, or how parental attitudes towards pain and illness influence the reporting of symptoms by children. However, it could equally well be due to physical factors affecting young people today (such as heavy school bags, less walking and sports, etc), and we are currently undertaking a study of a thousand school-children to investigate this hypothesis.

Over the past years there has been a noticeable move in musculoskeletal epidemiology research towards more common problems, such as back and other joint pains. At the same time there has been increasing realisation that the key to chronic musculoskeletal pain lies not solely in the test-tube, but also in the person and the social environment in which they live. These various perspectives are encompassed in the biopsychosocial model. Linked to this—and the reverse side of the coin—is the notion that pain, although initially restricted to one anatomical region, can, if persistent, become the precursor of other less-well-defined pains and somatic symptoms, where 'the notion of episode has been lost and it is seen as a long-term problem, regardless of current severity' (Croft et al 1997 p. 8). There is an accepted body of evidence that psychological distress and other psychosocial factors influence the occurrence and outcome of non-acute musculoskeletal pain, but what interventions can be used, the role of other factors (such as altered biochemistry, family and childhood influences, social attitudes) and the interplay between these remains an important challenge for future research.

Meanwhile—the person, their pain and their cries for help must remain centre stage.

253

ACKNOWLEDGEMENT

While I take full responsibility for the views expressed in this chapter, the research reported therein was very much a team effort by members of the ARC Research Unit, past and present. Nor can such research be undertaken without the co-operation of the doctors, staff, and patients at the medical centres in south Manchester and Cheshire (especially Brooklands, Bowland Road, Bollington, Wilmslow Road and Altrincham).

REFERENCES

Autton N 1986 Pain: an exploration. Darton, Longman & Todd, London

Burton AK, Clarke RD, McClune TD, Tillotson KM 1996 The natural history of low back pain in adolescents. Spine 21:2323–2328

Clinical Standards Advisory Group 1994. Epidemiology review: the epidemiology and cost of back pain. HMSO, London

Croft P 1996 The epidemiology of pain: The more you have, the more you get. Annals of the Rheumatic Diseases 55:859–860

Croft P, Rigby A, Boswell R, Schollum J, Silman A 1993 The prevalence of chronic widespread pain in the general population. Journal of Rheumatology 20(4):710–713

Croft P, Schollum J, Silman A 1994 Population study of tender point counts and pain as evidence of fibromyalgia. British Medical Journal 309:696–699

Croft PR, Papageorgiou AC, Ferry S, Jayson MIV, Silman AJ 1995 Psychological distress and low back pain: Evidence from a prospective study in the general population. Spine 20:2731–2737

Croft P, Papageorgiou A, McNally R 1997 Low back pain. Health care needs assessment. In: Stevens A, Raftery J (eds)The Epidemiologically Based Needs Assessment Reviews. Second series. Radcliffe Medical Press, Oxford

Croft PR, Macfarlane GJ, Papageorgiou AC, Thomas E, Silman AJ 1998 Outcome of low back pain in general practice: A prospective study. British Medical Journal 316:1356–1359

Goldberg D, Williams P 1988 A User's Guide to the General Health Questionnaire. NFER-Nelson, Windsor

Kohlmann T, Raspe H 1996 Der Funktionsbeeintrachtigung durch Ruckenschmerzen (FFbH-R). Rehabilitation 35:I–VIII

McBeth J, Macfarlane G J, Benjamin S, Silman A J 2001 Features of somatization predict the onset of chronic widespread pain: Results from a large population-based study. Arthritis and Rheumatism 44(4):940-946

McCormick A, Flemming D, Charlton J 1995 Morbidity statistics from general practice. Fourth national study 1991–1992. Office of Population Censuses and Surveys. HMSO (Series MB5 No 3), London

Macfarlane GJ, Thomas E, Papageorgiou AC, Schollum J, Croft PR, Silman A J 1996 The natural history of chronic pain in the community: a better prognosis than in the clinic Journal of Rheumatology 23(9):1617–1620

Macfarlane GJ, Thomas E, Papageorgiou AC, Croft PR, Jayson MIV, Silman AJ 1997 Employment and physical work activities as predictors of future low back pain. Spine 22:1143–1149

Mason V 1994 The prevalence of back pain in Great Britain. Office of Population Censuses and Surveys. Social Survey Division. HMSO, London

Papageorgiou AC, Croft PR, Ferry S, Jayson MIV, Silman AJ 1995 Estimating the prevalence of low back pain in the general population. Spine 20:1889–1894

Papageorgiou AC, Croft PR, Thomas E, Ferry S, Jayson MIV, Silman AJ 1996 Influence of previous pain experience on the episode incidence of low back pain: results from the south Manchester back pain study. Pain 66:181–185

Papageorgiou AC, Croft PR, Thomas E, Silman AJ, Macfarlane GJ 1998 Psychosocial risks for low back pain: Are these related to work? Annals of the Rheumatic Diseases 57:500–502

Raspe H, Kohlmann T 1994 Disorders characterised by pain: A methodological review of population surveys. Journal of Epidemiology and Community Health 48:531–537

Ryle JA 1948 The Natural History of Disease 2nd edn. Oxford University Press, London

Standard Occupation Classification 1991 Office of Population Censuses and Surveys. HMSO, London

Thomas E, Silman AJ, Croft PR, Papageorgiou AC, Jayson MIV, Macfarlane GJ 1999 Predicting who develops chronic low back pain in primary care: A prospective study. British Medical Journal 318:1662–1667

Waddell G 1992. Biopsychosocial analysis of low back pain. Bailliere's Clinics in Rheumatology 6:523–557

Walsh K, Cruddas M, Coggon D 1992 Low back pain in eight areas of Britain. Journal of Epidemiology and Community Health 46:227–230

Wolfe F, Smith HA, Yunus MB et al 1990 The American College of Rheumatology 1990 criteria for the classification of fibromyalgia. Report of the multicenter criteria committee. Arthritis and Rheumatism 33:160–172

Index

Now Available...

Editor: Louis Gifford

Topical Issues in Pain 1

Introductory Essay Integrating pain awareness into physiotherapy wise action for the future
David Butler

Part 1 **Whiplash: science and management**
Michael Thacker, Louis Gifford, Vicki Harding, Suzanne Shorland and Katharine Treves.

Part 2 **Fear avoidance beliefs and behaviour**
Patrick Hill, Dr Michael Rose, Vicki Harding and Max Zusman

Topical Issues in Pain 2

Introductory Essays The patient in front of us: from genes to environment *Louis Gifford*
Interpreting the results of treatment *George Peat*

The challenge of change in practice *Heather Muncey*

Exercise for low back pain: clinical outcomes, costs and preferences
Jennifer Klaber Moffett et al.

Part 1 **Biopsychosocial assessment and management**
Lisa Roberts, Paul Watson, Nicholas Kendall, Jennifer Klaber Moffett

Part 2 **Relationships and pain**
Hazel O'Dowd, Toby Newton-John, Suzanne Brook, Christina Papadopoulos and Vicki Harding

Topical Issues in Pain 3

Topical Issues in Pain 4

Review:Topical Issues in Pain 1: Whiplash Science and Management. Fear Avoidance Beliefs and Behaviour. Editor Louis Gifford

By Professor Patrick Wall, best known for the Gate control theory of pain and author of the best selling books 'The Challenge of Pain' (with Ronald Melzack),'Pain the Science of Suffering' and 'The Textbook of Pain' (with Ronald Melzack).

It is not an exaggeration to say that this book marks a milestone not only for an understanding of pain but also for the maturation of physiotherapy. For centuries physiotherapy has been placed in a minor subservient role among the medical arts. This low status encouraged a passive intuitive acceptance of therapy in a barren desert of intellectual questioning. The present rapid evolution of attitude no longer permits untested acceptance. The authors of this book and the organisers of the Physiotherapy Pain Association are clearly pioneers leading their profession out of the desert. They have been reading and experiencing and questioning everything to the conditions, which are treated rather than restricting themselves to the classical physiotherapy texts, which are often dull, repetitive and trivial. In addition to an open-minded education, they point to the almost unique opportunity characteristic of physiotherapy, which remains the close prolonged interaction with patients. Social pressure has removed this from almost every other branch of the medical arts.

The practical pragmatic obsession of old-school physiotherapy assigned questioning and investigation to a separate and distant other class who in practise in fact ignored the problems. Research was assigned to some non-existent class of intellectuals and thought to be beyond the scope of physiotherapists. A striking example is that to be found on page 94 where 20 therapies for whiplash are listed. Of these two are thought to be useless, two useful and the other 16 have not been adequately investigated. This vagueness is a threat to patients and to physiotherapists and to an understanding of pain. Research can not be the responsibility of others. It does not require huge high tech resources. The results are not to be feared. The discovery that a therapy depends on a placebo response should be welcomed with relief because it liberates the therapist into a positive area to explore the economics and the precise nature of the placebo component of the therapy.

Work over the past thirty years has rejected the model of a pain mechanism as caused by a fixed rigid modality-dedicated mechanism. The process, which produces pain, is plastic and changes sequentially with time. That essential mobility of mechanism exists in damaged tissue, in the peripheral nerves and spinal cord. This movement of pathology from periphery to centre proceeds with the triggering of reactive processes in the brain. It presents the therapist with a migrating distributed target. For that reason, I was particularly impressed by the chapter by Gifford on the "Mature Organism Model" which places pain in an integrated context without any permission to accept the old dualistic split that pain must be either in the body or in the mind.

I look forward to this series and to the activities of the Physiotherapy Pain Association because they promise to revolutionise the morale, dignity and way of thinking of physiotherapists and thereby to affect everyone concerned with pain.

Patrick Wall   26.11.98

(Reproduced with permission from : Physiotherapy, February 1999/vol 85/no 2 page 101-102).

Review: Topical Issues in Pain 2: Biopsychosocial assessment and management; Relationships and pain Editor: Louis Gifford

By Gordon Waddell, Consultant Orthopaedic Surgeon and author of 'The Back Pain Revolution'.

The first year book from the Physiotherapy Pain Association was a hard act to follow, but this second year book is even better.

This a diverse collection of essays on selected aspects of pain which is inevitably somewhat disjointed and variable in style and quality, but that lets it explore a number of rarely visited, fascinating topics. Although the authors come from a range of professional backgrounds, they all have considerable "hands on" clinical experience of physiotherapy for patients with pain. Indeed, one of the major achievements and attractions of this book is the highly successful blend of the latest concepts and research on pain with practical illustrations of how that can be applied in practice. That practice ranges all the way from routine out-patient physiotherapy to a tertiary pain management clinic, and the one general criticism is that sometimes the setting of a particular essay is not made clear. For example, lessons from the highly selected patients in a pain management programme are not always applied to more routine practice. However, once the reader realises that different authors may sometimes be talking about different patients, it is possible to draw these lessons from oneself.

Altogether, this is a rich kaleidoscope of the latest thinking and research, which includes some real gems. Each reader will find their own favourites, but a very personal selection that tickled my fancy included the chapters on interpreting the results of treatment, the challenge of change in practice, the impact of patient preferences on treatment outcome, applying yellow flags in clinical practice, pain perceptions and attitudes, and most of the section on "relationships" including in particular pain stories, pain couples and the INPUT Patient Handout on Chronic Pain and Pregnancy. These include some original, highly pertinent and stimulating perspectives. The major achievement and value throughout the book are the many examples of how biopsychosocial principles can be applied in clinical practice.

This is a delightful little book for all physiotherapists and indeed all other health professionals who actually treat patients with pain, not only for those working in pain clinics. The Physiotherapy Pain Association and the editor, Louis Gifford, are once again to be congratulated on producing such a marvellous collection of essays.

Gordon Waddell DSc MD FRCS
(Reproduced with permission Physiotherapy Dec 2000 vol 86(12):665)

Topical Issues in Pain 1

Reader's comments:

'one of the best and most useful Physiotherapy books I've read'

'clinically relevant and up to date stuff'

'keep this sort of material coming!'

Topical Issues in Pain 2

Reader's comments:

'Excellent, another useful and extremely usable book'

'We have found the case history in chapter 4 invaluable in our in-service training of the biopsychosocial model and assessment'

'Should be a standard text in all Physiotherapy undergraduate and post graduate education programmes'

'Easy to read, easy to understand and I've read it from cover to cover (I don't normally get passed chapter 1!!)'.

Topical Issues in Pain 3

Reader's comments:

> *'congratulations on Topical Issues in Pain 3,*
> *a tremendous piece of work.'*

> *'a vital resource'*

> *'I learnt some more very interesting things about the*
> *sympathetic nervous system, a really comprehensive guide.'*

> *'the usual high standard and easy to read'*

The Physiotherapy Pain Association - PPA

Formed in 1994 as a Special Interest Group of the Chartered Society of Physiotherapy

Membership is open to CSP members. Associate membership is available for physiotherapists who are not members of the CSP and includes other professions.

Website: www.ppaonline.co.uk

Publications: PPA News twice yearly
                        Topical Issues in Pain book series

Regional Network: PPA North

For further information contact:

                        The Chartered Society Of Physiotherapy,
                        14 Bedford Row,
                        London
                        WC1R 4ED.

                        www.csp.org.uk